MINIMAL ACCESS SURGERY IN ONCOLOGY

MINIMAL ACCESS SURGERY IN ONCOLOGY

Edited by
James G. Geraghty
Howard L. Young
Jonathan M. Sackier

Associate Editors
H. Stephan Stoldt
Riccardo A. Audisio

© 1998

GREENWICH MEDICAL MEDIA LTD
219 The Linen Hall
162-168 Regent Street
London
W1R 5TB

ISBN 1 900151 022

First Published 1998

Apart from any fair dealing for the purposes of research or private study, or criticism or review, as permitted under the UK Copyright Designs and Patents Act, 1988, this publication may not be reproduced, stored, or transmitted, in any form or by any means, without the prior permission in writing of the publishers, or in the case of reprographic reproduction only in accordance with the terms of the licences issued by the Copyright Licensing Agency in the UK, or in accordance with the terms of the licences issued by the appropriate Reproduction Rights Organization outside the UK. Enquiries concerning reproduction outside the terms stated here should be sent to the publishers at the London address printed above.

The right of J.G. Geraghty, J.M. Sackier and H.L. Young to be identified as editors of this work has been asserted by them in accordance with the Copyright, Designs and Patents Acts 1988.

The publisher makes no representation, express or implied, with regard to the accuracy of the information contained in this book and cannot accept any legal responsibility or liability for any errors or omissions that may be made.

British Library Cataloguing in Publication Data
A catalogue record for this book is available from the British Library.

Distributed worldwide by
Oxford University Press

Project Manager
Gavin Smith

Designed and Produced by
Derek Virtue, DataNet

Printed in Hong Kong by Dah Hua

Contents

Contributors vii

Foreword ix

Introduction xi

CHAPTER 1

Minimal access surgery and the biology of cancer 1
Richard L. Whelan, John D. Allendorf and Marc Bessler

CHAPTER 2

Oncologic principles and minimal access surgery 17
Frederick L. Greene

CHAPTER 3

Role of laparoscopic diagnosis and staging of intra-abdominal malignancy 23
Timothy G. John, K.K. Madhaven an O. James Garden

CHAPTER 4

Endoscopic management of gastrointestinal malignancies 45
Frederick L. Greene

CHAPTER 5

Laparoscopic cholecystectomy: lessons learned from gallbladder cancer 61
Frank H. Chae and Jonathan M. Sackier

CHAPTER 6

Laparoscopic colectomy: the concerns and the benefits 69
Steven D. Wexner and Eric G. Weiss

CHAPTER 7

Role of video-assisted thoracic surgery in the management of pulmonary cancer and tumors of the mediastinum 83
Joseph S. Friedberg and Larry R. Kaiser

CHAPTER 8

Minimally invasive techniques in the management of esophageal cancer 99
Cathal J. Kelly, David Galvin and Patrick J. Broe

CHAPTER 9

Laparoscopy and other minimally invasive techniques in patients with advanced intraperitoneal malignant disease 107
David M. Thompson, Cihat Tetik and Maurice E. Arregui

CHAPTER 10

Operative laparoscopy in gynecologic oncology 121
Joel M. Childers and Earl A. Surwit

CHAPTER 11

Application of minimal access surgery in the management of diverse malignancies 135
H. Stephan Stoldt, Riccardo A. Audisio, Amy L. Halverson and Jonathan M. Sackier

CHAPTER 12

Minimal access surgery in the evaluation of lymph nodes: lessons from breast cancer 145
Theodore N. Tsangaris

CHAPTER 13

Future of minimal access in surgical oncology 157
Amy L. Halverson and Jonathan M. Sackier

Index 163

Contributors

John D. Allendorf
MD
*Department of Surgery,
Columbia University College
of Physicians & Surgeons,
New York, USA*

Maurice E. Arregui
MD, FACS
DIRECTOR OF FELLOWSHIP
IN LAPAROSCOPY, ENDOSCOPY
AND ULTRASOUND
*St Vincent Hospital and
Health Center,
Indianapolis, Indiana, USA*

Riccardo A. Audisio
MD
DIRECTOR, GENERAL SURGERY
*MultiMedica
Milan, Italy*

Marc Bessler
MD
*Department of Surgery,
Columbia University College
of Physicians & Surgeons,
New York, USA*

Patrick J. Broe
FRCSI
CONSULTANT SURGEON
*Department of Surgery,
Royal College of Surgeons
in Ireland,
Beaumont Hospital,
Dublin, Ireland*

Frank H. Chae
MD, CM
*Department of Surgery,
The George Washington
University Medical Center,
Washington DC, USA*

Joel M. Childers
MD
*The University Physicians,
Gynecologic Oncology,
Tucson, Arizona, USA*

Joseph S. Friedberg
MD
ASSISTANT PROFESSOR OF SURGERY
*Department of Surgery,
University of Pennsylvania
Medical Center,
Philadelphia, USA*

David Galvin
MB
*Department of Surgery,
Royal College of Surgeons
in Ireland,
Beaumont Hospital,
Dublin, Ireland*

O. James Garden
BSc MBChB FRCS(Ed & Glas)
MD
PROFESSOR OF SURGERY
*Department of Surgery,
The University of Edinburgh,
Edinburgh, UK*

James G. Geraghty
PhD MCh FRCSI
CONSULTANT SURGEON
*Professorial Department of Surgery
Nottingham City Hospital
Nottingham, UK*

Frederick L. Greene
MD
PROFESSOR OF SURGERY
DIRECTOR OF SURGICAL
ONCOLOGY AND ENDOSCOPY
*Department of Surgery,
University of South Carolina,
South Carolina, USA*

Amy L. Halverson
MD
*Department of General Surgery,
The George Washington
University Medical Center,
Washington DC, USA*

Timothy G. John
MBChB FRCSEd(Gen)
SENIOR SURGICAL REGISTAR
*Department of Surgery,
The University of Edinburgh,
Edinburgh, UK*

Larry R. Kaiser
MD
ASSOCIATE PROFESSOR OF SURGERY
*Department of Surgery,
University of Pennsylvania
Medical Center,
Philadelphia, USA*

Cathal J. Kelly,
FRCSI
*Department of Surgery,
Royal College of Surgeons
in Ireland,
Beaumont Hospital,
Dublin, Ireland*

K. K. Madhaven
MBChB FRCSEd(Gen)
CONSULTANT SURGEON
*Department of Surgery,
The University of Edinburgh,
Edinburgh, UK*

Jonathan M. Sackier
MD FRCS FACS
PROFESSOR OF SURGERY
DIRECTOR, ENDO-SURGICAL
EDUCATION & RESEARCH CENTER
*The George Washington
University Medical Center,
Washington DC, USA*

H. Stephan Stoldt
MD
*Department of General
Surgical Oncology,
European Institute of Oncology,
Milan, Italy*

Earl A. Surwit
MD
*Hematology and Oncology
Physicians P.C.,
Tucson,
Arizona, USA*

Cihat Tetik
MD
FELLOW IN LAPAROSCOPY,
ENDOSCOPY AND ULTRASOUND
DIRECTOR OF FELLOWSHIP IN
LAPAROSCOPY, ENDOSCOPY AND
ULTRASOUND
*St Vincent Hospital and Health
Center,
Indianapolis,
Indiana, USA*

David M. Thompson
MD
FELLOW IN LAPAROSCOPY,
ENDOSCOPY AND ULTRASOUND
DIRECTOR OF FELLOWSHIP IN
LAPAROSCOPY, ENDOSCOPY AND
ULTRASOUND
*St Vincent Hospital and Health
Center,
Indianapolis,
Indiana, USA*

Theodore N. Tsangaris
MD FACS
ASSOCIATE PROFESSOR OF SURGERY
DIRECTOR
*Breast Surgical Service,
Georgetown University
Medical Center,
Washington DC, USA*

Eric G. Weiss
MD
*Department of Colorectal Surgery,
Cleveland Clinic Florida,
Fort Lauderdale,
Florida, USA*

Steven D. Wexner
MD
CHAIRMAN AND RESIDENCY
PROGRAM DIRECTOR
*Department of Colorectal Surgery,
Cleveland Clinic Florida,
Fort Lauderdale,
Florida, USA*

R. Larry Whelan
MD
ASSISTANT PROFESSOR OF SURGERY
*Department of Surgery,
Columbia University College
of Physicians & Surgeons,
New York, USA*

Howard L. Young
MBChB, ChM, MBA,
FRCS(Eng)
DEPUTY DIRECTOR OF
POSTGRADUATE STUDIES
*The School of Postgraduate
Medical and Dental Education,
University of Wales College of
Medicine,
Cardiff,
Wales, UK*

Foreword

This is a very exciting era in the field of surgical oncology. Advances in technology now give the option of performing surgical procedures previously carried out by using "open" surgery, with approaches which cause less surgical trauma to the patient. I remember well advocating this philosophy many years ago in my own special area of interest in breast cancer. It was not easy to convince people of the advantages of quadrantectomy over mastectomy, yet this more conservative approach is now an accepted way of treating breast cancer. The key issue in this minimalist era in cancer is not so much about technical competence, but more about the long term outcome of the patient undergoing such minimalist approaches.

This is the main reason why this book is so important. There is no technical burden, instead this text gives a scientific appraisal of the oncological acceptability of performing cancer surgery using a minimalist approach. Each author has clearly been instructed to provide a text based solely on existing evidence and as such, each chapter provides the information in a manner which will easily allow the reader to draw conclusions uninfluenced by the bias of the author. Its scientific content is also demonstrated by one chapter specifically dedicated to the impact of laparoscopy itself on biological and immune aspects of cancer.

The book is well written and is comprehensive in its coverage of a variety of tumor types. It is also striking that this book, both from an editorial and contributor standpoint, represents both sides of the Atlantic. This mix adds greatly to the book's value as a balanced statement of the current state of the art in minimally invasive surgery in oncology.

This book is essential reading for the individual whose task is to decide if a minimalist approach should be employed in oncology. Given the multidisciplinary nature of this specialty and its emphasis on oncological merit rather than technique, this book is also important reading for all those involved in the management of the cancer patient.

Umberto Veronesi,
1998

Introduction

Since the introduction of minimal access surgery (MAS), with its ability to access organs through small incisions, there is an ever-increasing number of applications being implemented using this new technology. For many surgeons, the term minimal access surgery is linked to the introduction of laparoscopic cholecystectomy. When Mouret reported the first laparoscopic cholecystectomy in 1987, it was met with mixed reactions. The protagonists firmly supported its more widespread use whilst others were very concerned about its introduction, particularly in view of the reported higher incidence of common bile duct injury. Reduced postoperative pain, length of hospital stay and early return to work were heralded as key advantages to its introduction. The term minimal access surgery now encompasses a variety of other techniques including fibreoptic endoscopy, transanal endoscopic microsurgery as well as the well-documented laparoscopic and thoracoscopic approaches for a variety of conditions. Advances in technology now mean that, in the majority of such cases, a minimalist approach is a feasible alternative to the more conventional option of open surgery.

Emphasis is now being firmly placed on the appropriateness of such a policy rather than technical feasability alone. Can the minimalist approach achieve as good a result as its "open" counterpart? Nowhere is this more relevant than in the field of oncology where adequacy of both resection and regional lymphadenectomy are key issues. This book is designed to address these vital questions and as such examines the current evidence-base for a minimalist approach in a variety of tumour types. This book therefore is not so much about the technical aspects of minimally invasive surgery – there is already extensive literature in this field. It accepts technical competence but questions whether oncological principles are upheld and results are acceptable in this era of minimally invasive surgery.

Addressing these issues is not so simple. Before one debates concerns such as adequacy of resection or completeness of lymphadenectomy, there is much to suggest that minimalist approaches such as laparoscopy in itself can have profound effects on areas such as immune function with consequent impact on host-tumour relationship. The initial section of this book concentrates on this key area as well as the ongoing related concern of port-site metastases. These factors are of great importance to the clinician as they will impact on disease-free interval and survival. These latter parameters are the standards against which the minimalist approach is judged in the remainder of the book. Whilst shortened recovery time and reduced hospital stay must be one of the main goals of minimally invasive surgery, it is unacceptable to achieve this goal at the expense of a compromise, or potential compromise, in survival. The problem remains that the evidence base in some instances is not sufficient to give formal guidelines to clinicians and varies greatly from one tumour to another. The reality is that many clinicians around the world are employing a minimalist approach, and that this number is increasing rapidly.

The time is therefore ripe to put the scientific evidence together so that some conclusions can be drawn and advice given to those performing these procedures. That is the purpose of this book. It is not designed to give biased viewpoints, but to put the relevant evidence in a succinct form to allow the reader to draw conclusions for him/herself. The length of the chapters is dependent on the evidence-base which remains small in certain tumour types. The number of publications will continue to increase in this field and it is hoped that this book will provide a solid platform against which to judge such literature.

We hope you will enjoy reading this book and that decision-making in the area of minimally invasive surgery in oncology will be enhanced as a result.

James G. Geraghty, Howard L. Young,
Jonathan M. Sackier

1

Minimal Access Surgery and the Biology of Cancer

R. Larry Whelan, John D. Allendorf and Marc Bessler

The use of laparoscopic techniques for the curative resection of malignancies is the most controversial issue surrounding minimally invasive surgery today. Critics question whether equivalent resections can be accomplished laparoscopically and are concerned that long-term survival may be adversely affected. Early publications reporting port-site tumor recurrences have raised the concern that there may be something inherently dangerous about minimal access surgery in the setting of malignancy. In general, this criticism has placed the supporters of the new methods on the defensive. In the absence of long-term outcome data, proponents are presently trying to prove that laparoscopic methods are as good as open methods via randomized prospective clinical trials.

Interestingly, in the face of these reasonable concerns, there is a growing body of animal data that suggests that minimally invasive techniques may offer those with cancer immuologic and oncologic advantages in the early postoperative period. These studies suggest that minimizing the trauma to the abdominal wall favorably influences the body's ability to limit the growth and spread of tumors after surgery.

The use of laparoscopic techniques raises complex issues. Are the fears mentioned above reasonable? What is the clinical data regarding adequacy of resection and long-term outcome? What is known about immune function and tumor growth after open and laparoscopic surgery? Are the benefits found in animal models likely also to be found in humans? What is the clinical and laboratory data regarding port-site tumors. This chapter addresses these questions and the issues surrounding them.

SURGICAL ISSUES

Resection results

Although this chapter is mainly concerned with the impact of surgical techniques on cancer biology, the surgical issues raised above are briefly addressed. The vast majority of data available regarding laparoscopic resection of cancers concerns colorectal malignancies. Published reports suggest that, when compared to the results of open resection, an equivalent colon resection in terms of lymph node harvest as well as bowel and mesenteric margins, can be accomplished laparoscopically.[1-11] Franklin et al.[9] in a prospective study of colon cancer patients comparing 191 laparoscopic and 224 open resection patients found that there were no significant differences in the resection parameters mentioned. Similarly, preliminary results from the NCI sponsored Clinical Outcomes of Surgery Trial (COST), a randomized and prospective trial, also demonstrate equivalence between the open and laparoscopic groups with regard to gross pathological parameters.[12]

It must be realized that laparoscopic colon resection is highly operator dependent. The surgeons who generated the data mentioned above are the most experienced laparoscopists. Laparoscopic-assisted colon resection (LACR) is a difficult procedure to master and has a lengthy learning curve. Most laparoscopic surgeons agree that curative cancer resections should not be attempted until the surgeon has gained considerable experience by performing at least 20 resections for benign pathology.

Long-term outcome

Because LACR is a relatively new procedure, 5-year results are not yet available. The longest follow-up data available are for the prospective study mentioned above.[9] The mean length of follow-up varied from 30 to 37 months for stage I, II and III patients. There were no significant differences in survival, local recurrence rates or rates of distant metastases when the open and laparoscopic groups were compared stage for stage. There was a trend in stage III patients toward improved survival in the laparoscopic group. In the next few years, 5-year results will become available for a number of prospective studies currently underway.

IMMUNE FUNCTION FOLLOWING SURGERY

Human data

Is immune function important in cancer patients? Numerous investigators believe that cell-mediated and natural immune systems are involved in limiting the spread of certain tumor cells.[13-18] Furthermore, preoperative anergy is associated with a significantly lower rate of resectability in cancer patients going to surgery.[19] Not surprisingly, the incidence of postoperative sepsis and infection has been shown to be significantly higher in anergic patients.[20] Lastly, immunosuppressed patient populations have a well-documented higher incidence of certain malignancies compared to the general population.[21]

Is immune function impaired after open surgery? It has been well documented that immune function is suppressed after major open surgical procedures. The degree of suppression roughly correlates with the magnitude of the surgical procedure. Almost all studies looking into postoperative immune function have dealt with cell-mediated immune activities. Impairment of the following cell-mediated functions has been found: lymphocyte and neutrophil chemotaxis; natural killer T-cell activity; lymphocyte and macrophage interactions; and delayed type hypersensitivity (DTH) responses.[22-26]

Do laparoscopically performed procedures suppress cell-mediated immune function to the same degree as open ones? By comparing preoperative and postoperative DTH responses, it is possible to assess the functional status of the cell-mediated immune system at various points in time. A series of intradermal challenges are carried out with an antigen to which the subject has been previously sensitized. The areas of induration of the postoperative challenges are compared to the preoperative wheal, which represents the baseline response. Significantly, diminished DTH responses have been documented after major open surgery in humans and have been shown to persist for 6-9 days.[27] Kloosterman et al.[28] demonstrated that the DTH responses in laparoscopic cholecystectomy patients were preserved after surgery compared to the open group which manifested significantly smaller DTH wheals. A similar DTH study concerning colectomy patients at Columbia University was begun in mid 1995. A preliminary analysis of the results to date indicate that there appears to be a significantly larger decrease in DTH response postoperatively in the open colectomy group compared to the minimally invasive group (Whelan et al., unpublished results). Other than these two DTH studies, postoperative immune function has not been directly studied in humans.

A number of investigators have determined the levels of several markers of stress after open and laparoscopic procedures. For example, interleukin 6 (IL-6) and C-reactive protein are both thought to be nonspecific indicators of surgical trauma and stress. The majority of studies comparing laparoscopic and open cholecystectomy report significantly lower IL-6 levels in the laparoscopic groups.[28-31] Similar studies comparing laparoscopic-assisted and open colectomy have not yielded consistent results. Harmon et al.[32] found significantly lower IL-6 levels in the laparoscopic group whereas Fukushima et al.[33] found the opposite to be true. Similarly, the results concerning C-reactive peptide are inconclusive.[28,33] Furthermore, most investigators have not been able to demonstrate differences in cortisol and catecholamine responses when comparing minimally invasive and open procedures.

Animal data

In addition to the limited human data mentioned above, there is a growing body of animal data regarding immune function after minimally invasive surgery.

Horgan et al.[34] compared lymphocyte proliferation rates of mice undergoing either laparoscopy, laparotomy or anesthesia alone. They found that the laparotomy group demonstrated significantly lower lymphocyte proliferation rates than the control group but there were no significant differences between the laparoscopy and control groups. The conclusion of this study was that less immunosuppression follows laparoscopy compared with laparotomy. A series of DTH studies in rodents were carried out at Columbia University to investigate the immunologic effects of laparoscopic techniques.

In the first study, abdominal exposure techniques alone were compared and no intra-abdominal procedure was carried out. The three study groups were: 1) sham full laparotomy; 2) CO_2 pneumoperitoneum; and 3) anesthesia control, and the procedure length was standardized to 30 min. The rats were challenged preoperatively, on the day of surgery and on the second postoperative day to Keyhole limpet hemocyanin (KLH) and phytohemagglutinin (PHA). The area of the wheal was measured 24 and 48 hours after each challenge. The laparotomy group demonstrated significantly smaller DTH responses than the pneumoperitoneum and control groups for both postoperative challenges (Fig. 1.1). Importantly, there were no significant differences between the insufflation and anesthesia contol groups at any of the time points. These results suggest that there was significant cell-mediated immunosuppression following laparotomy but not after insufflation alone.[35] It was hypothesized that the immunosuppression related to the sizeable open abdominal incision. A more recent animal study at Johns Hopkins reported similar DTH differences when sham laparotomy was compared to CO_2 pneumoperitoneum in a mouse model.[36]

The goal of the second study was to determine if the difference in DTH response persists when an actual intra-abdominal procedure, in this case a cecal resection, is carried out.[37] The rat cecum is several

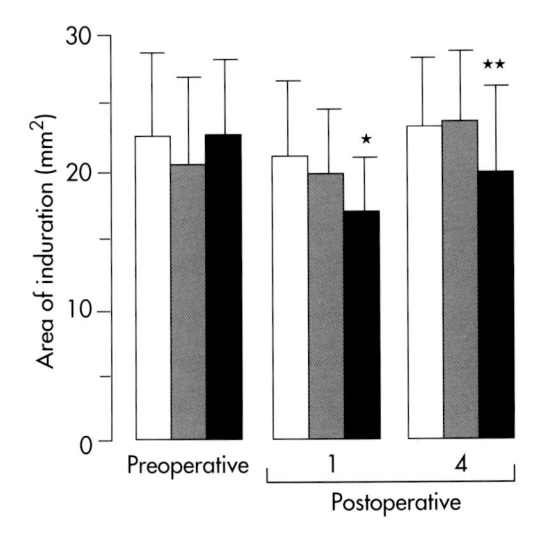

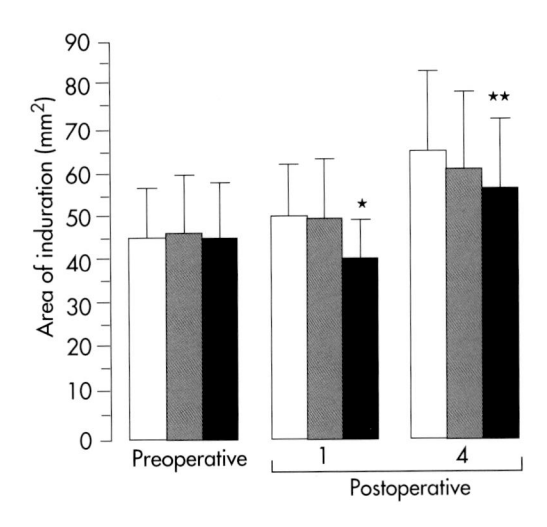

Figure 1.1 – Delayed type hypersensitivity response to phytohemagglutinin at 24 hours. Open bars = control group; shaded bars = insufflation group; solid bars = lapartomy group. ★ = p<0.05 versus insufflation and control; ★★ = p<0.01 versus insufflation and control. POD = postoperative day.

Figure 1.2 – Delayed type hypersensitivity response to phytomemagglutinin at 24 hours. Open bars = control group; shaded bars = laparoscopic resection group; solid bars = laparotomy group. ★ = p<0.01 versus control and laparoscopic resection on postoperative day (POD) 1; ★★ = p<0.05 versus control on POD 3.

centimeters long which permits a bowel resection without necessitating an anastomosis which would be technically demanding. Open resection via a full length incision was compared to both laparoscopic-assisted resection and anesthesia alone in over 120 rats. The animals were challenged with the same antigens and response measured 24 and 48 hours later as described for the above experiment. The open resection group responses were significantly smaller than the anesthesia control rats at all postoperative time points. Similarly, the open group responses were smaller than the laparoscopic-assisted group responses at all postprocedure time points (Fig. 1.2).[38] Therefore, the observed differences in DTH response after sham procedures persisted despite the additon of a bowel resection.

In the third study, the relationship of the length of the abdominal incision to postoperative immune function was investigated. Five groups were compared: 1) sham full laparotomy; 2) mini-laparotomy (half the xyphoid to pubis distance); 3) open cecal resection (via full laparotomy); 4) laparoscopic-assisted cecal resection; and 5) anesthesia control. Challenges with KLH and PHA were carried out in a similar fashion to the previous studies. Significantly smaller DTH responses were observed in the full laparotomy and open cecal resection when compared to the laparoscopic-assisted resection group and anesthesia controls. Of note, the mini-laparotomy group DTH responses were not significantly different from the minimally invasive groups or the controls.[39] These results support the hypothesis that immunosuppression relates to the overall length of the abdominal incision.

Watson et al.[40] examined monocyte function, a measure of the natural or native immune system, after sham laparotomy and pneumoperitoneum. They documented decreased peritoneal macrophage phagocytic function as well as increased macrophage production of tumor necrosis factor (TNF) and superoxide anion (inflammatory mediators) after laparotomy when compared to a CO_2 pneumoperitoneum. Interestingly, they do not believe that these differences in immune function relate to the size of the abdominal incision and instead believe that exposure of the peritoneal cavity to factors found in air results in translocation of endotoxin (lipopolysaccharide), generated by Gram negative bacteria in the gut, into and across the bowel wall. The endotoxin then interacts with macrophages, monocytes and neutrophils in the peritoneal cavity and the circulation, thus resulting in immunosuppression.[40]

In summary, laparoscopy and laparoscopic-assisted bowel resection in animals and humans appears to be associated with significantly less immunosuppression than a full laparotomy or open bowel resection carried out via a full laparotomy. The reason for these immune function differences is unclear; however, the authors believe that the length of the abdominal incision is one determining factor. Clearly, more detailed and specific human and animal studies looking at lymphocyte proliferation rates, lymphocyte subpopulations and parameters of natural immune function need to be carrried out to verify the results presented above and to determine the mechanism of the observed differences in immune function.

TUMOR GROWTH AFTER SURGERY

Does the method of access to the abdominal cavity influence the growth or spread of tumors after surgery? Several investigators have demonstrated that tumor growth in rats and mice is accelerated following laparotomy when compared to anesthesia controls.[41-43] In an effort to determine whether minimally invasive surgical methods have a similar effect on postoperative tumor growth, a series of tumor experiments have been carried out in mice and rats.

Allendorf et al.[44] performed two studies that utilized the mouse mammary carcinoma (MMC-2) cell line. MMC is an immunogeneic tumor line that is syngeneic to the C3H/He mouse strain. Characteristically, once established, MMC tumors increase in size for about 12 days and then begin spontaneously to regress. MMC tumor regression is thought to be immune mediated.[45] Tumor nodules that could be easily assessed were established by intradermally injecting the dorsal skin of the mice with tumor cells.

The purpose of the first experiment was to determine if the growth rates of tumors established at the time of surgery would differ when the two different abdominal exposure techniques were compared. Animals were injected with a high dose of tumor cells on the day of laparotomy, insufflation or anesthesia alone for 30 min and 12 days post procedure the mice were sacrificed and the tumors excised and weighed (Fig. 1.3). Tumor establishment was noted in practically all animals. The tumors of the laparotomy group were significantly larger than the lesions found in both the insufflation and control groups, an 80% ($p<0.013$) and almost 300% difference ($p<0.001$), respectively. It is important to note that the insufflation group tumors were significantly larger than the control group's ($p<0.037$).[44]

The purpose of the second experiment was to determine if the rate of tumor establishment from tumor cells implanted at the time of surgery was different following insufflation and laparotomy. A lower 'threshold' dose of cells was administered. At this dose, only a small percentage of controls animals were expected to develop tumors. The mice underwent anesthesia alone, insufflation or full sham laparotomy for 30 min and 30 days after the interventions, they were sacrificed and the dorsal skin reflected to confirm the presence or absence of tumor. Tumors had developed in 75% of the laparotomy group, 37% of the insufflation group and 25% of the control mice ($p<0.04$ open vs insufflation, $p<0.01$ open vs control) (Fig. 1.4). There was no significant difference between the insufflation and control groups.[45]

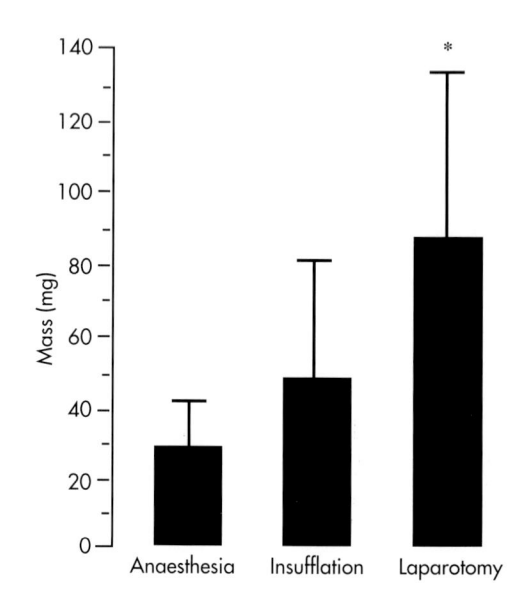

Figure 1.3 – Tumor mass for anesthesia (control), insufflation and laparotomy treatment groups. ★ = $p<0.01$ versus insufflation and $p<0.01$ versus insufflation and anesthesia.

Figure 1.4 – Incidence of tumor establishment by postoperative day 30 after intradermal injection of 10 000 tumor cells. ★ = $p<0.04$ versus insufflation and $p<0.01$ versus control.

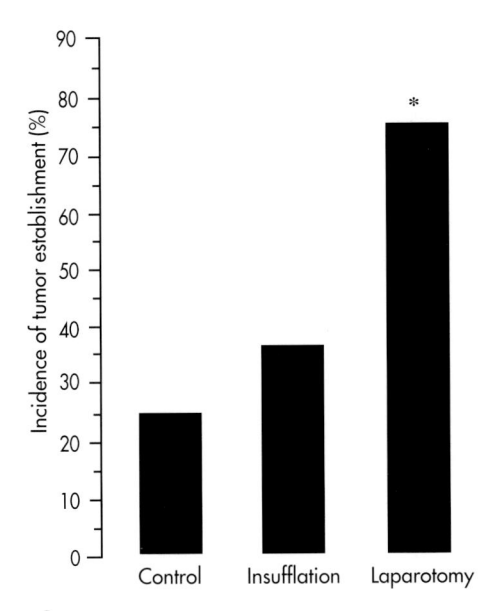

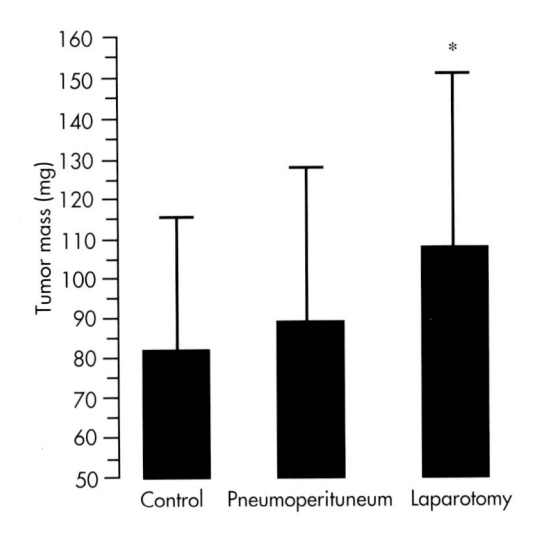

Figure 1.5 – Colon-26 tumor mass on postoperative day 12 after laparotomy versus pneumoperitoneum in mice. $p<0.05$ laparomtomy versus control; $p<0.05$ laparotomy versus pneumoperitoneum; $p<0.3$ control versus pneumoperitoneum.

These results are not specific to the MMC cell line and have also been demonstrated with the colon-26 and melanoma B-16 tumor cell lines which are not immunogenic (Fig. 1.5) (Southall *et al.*, unpublished results).

The results of these sham procedure studies suggest that following a full laparotomy tumors grow faster and are more easily established than after a pneumoperitoneum. Futhermore, these differences in tumor growth do not appear to be tumor-line dependent. This work led to the next group of studies which compared open and minimally invasive interventions that included an actual intra-abdominal procedure.

Allendorf *et al.*[46] utilized the MMC tumor line and the C3H/He mouse strain for two experiments comparing cecal resections carried out using either open (via full laparotomy) or laparoscopic-assisted technique. Similar to the rat, the mouse cecum is several centimeters long which lends itself to easy resection without the need for an anastomosis.[37]

The first study utilized a high-dose intradermal tumor injection on the day of the procedure to compare the early postoperative growth of tumors established at the time of bowel resection. Three groups were compared: 1) anesthesia control; 2) laparoscopic-assisted resection; and 3) open cecal resection. Twelve days post-procedure the mice were sacrificed and the tumors excised and weighed. Tumors were noted in practically all the animals. Similar to the results of the high-dose sham study, there was a stepwise increase in tumor size from the control to the laparoscopic to the open group (Fig. 1.6). The open resection group tumors were 150% larger than the laparoscopic-assisted group lesions ($p<0.01$) and 230% larger than the anesthesia control group tumors ($p<0.01$). Although smaller than the open group tumors, the laparoscopic group lesions were significantly larger than the anesthesia control group's ($p<0.02$).[46]

The purpose of the second study was to compare the rate of tumor establishment for the two different resection methods and controls after low-dose, day-of-surgery tumor injections. Thirty days following bowel resection the mice were sacrificed, the dorsal skin over the site of injection reflected, and the presence or absence of a tumor nodule confirmed for each animal. As for the sham study, tumors were established in far more of the open resection group

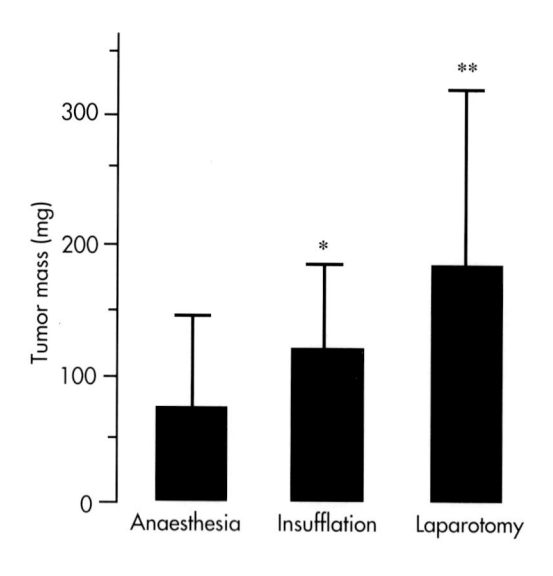

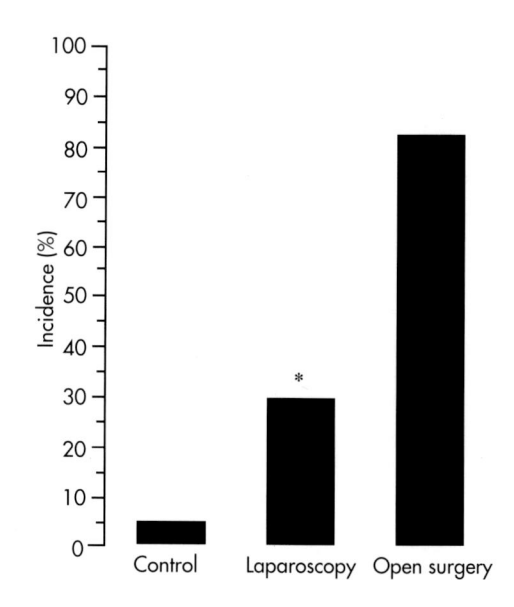

Figure 1.6 – Tumor mass on postoperative day 12 after open versus laparoscopic cecetomy. ★ = p<0.02 versus control; ★★ = p<0.01 versus control and laparoscopy.

Figure 1.7 – Incidence of tumor establishment by postoperative day 30 after open versus laparoscopic cececetomy. ★ = p<0.01 versus control and open surgery; ★★ = p<0.01 versus control and laparoscopy.

(83%) than either the laparoscopic-assisted (30%) or anesthesia control (5%) groups (Fig. 1.7). Significant differences were found for all comparisons between the three groups.[46]

Bouvey et al.,[47] using a rat small bowel resection model that involved a hand-sutured bowel anastomosis, demonstrated significantly slower tumor growth after laparoscopic resection than after open bowel resection. In this model a uniformly sized piece of colon tumor (CC531) was implanted beneath the renal capsule and 2 weeks later the tumors were excised and weighed. Therefore, despite the addition of an intra-abdominal procedure, tumors have been found to grow more quickly and to establish more easily after open versus laparoscopic surgery. Although differences in tumor growth were documented, the etiology of these differences remained obscure.

To determine if the observed differences in postoperative immune function are an important factor in determining tumor behavior following open and laparoscopic surgery, Allendorf et al.[48] (and unpublished results) utilized the MMC tumor cell line in two different strains of mice: athymic (nude, nu -/-) and immunocompetent mice (NCR nude (nu +/-) heterozygous mice), which differ in only one allele. The athymic mice serve as controls as they have no T-cells and therefore lack cell-mediated immune function, regardless of the operative method they are subjected to. Sham interventions for 20 min without actual intra-abdominal procedures were compared. At surgery, high-dose injections of tumor cells were used and tumor mass at 12 days was the endpoint. The immunocompetent mice demonstrated the familiar stepwise increase in tumor size from the anesthesia control to the pneumoperitoneum to the laparotomy group, but in the nude mice, there was no significant difference noted in tumor size between the laparotomy and pneumoperitoneum groups (Fig. 1.8). However, both the open and pneumoperitoneum groups' tumors were significantly larger than the anesthesia control group tumors. These results suggest that although cell-mediated immune function influences tumor behavior after surgery, other factors are also at work.

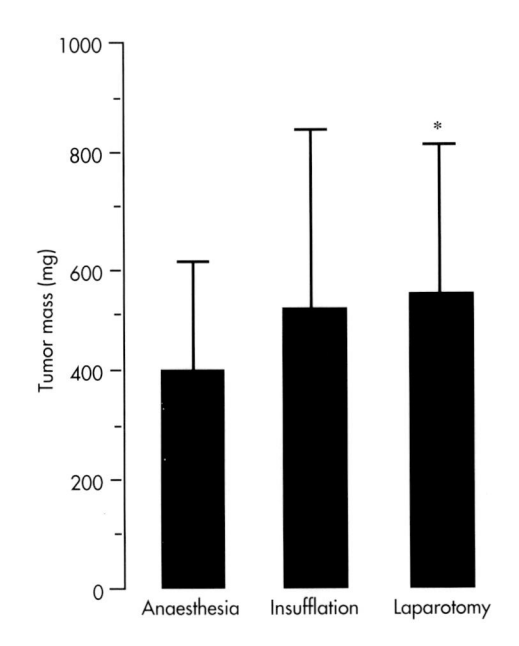

Figure 1.8 – Tumor mass on postoperative day 12 after pneumoperitoneum and laparotomy in NCR nude mice (nu -/-). * = p<0.02 versus pneumoperitoneum and laparotomy.

It is difficult to explain these findings on the basis of the observed differences in postoperative immune function. One would anticipate that the cell-mediated immune system interacts with immunogenic tumors by increasing tumor destruction and not by limiting proliferation. The explanation for these findings is, therefore, as yet unclear. It is possible that differences in the levels of one or several growth factors may contribute to the observed differences in cell proliferation. Nonetheless, this study has brought to light a previously undemonstrated benefit of laparoscopy in the setting of malignancy.

Does the type of gas used for insufflation influence perioperative tumor growth? In an effort to address this question, the Columbia University group carried out the following experiment. After a high-dose, day-of-surgery, intradermal MMC tumor injection, mice were subjected to sham laparotomy, CO_2 pneumoperitoneum or air pneumoperitoneum. Air was chosen as the alternative gas in order indirectly to test Watson *et al's* hypothesis (see p. 00) that factors in air are responsible for the immunosuppression that follows laparotomy.[40] The animals were sacrificed 12 days postoperatively and the tumors excised and weighed. The laparotomy group was found to have significantly larger tumors than the other two groups. There were no significant differences between the CO_2 and air pneumoperitoneum groups (Fig. 1.9) (Southall *et al.*, unpublished results). These results suggest that the particular type of gas used for insufflation does not significantly influence early postoperative tumor growth and do not support Watson *et al's* hypothesis.[40]

In contrast, Jacobi *et al.*[48] in a recent rat study that utilized a colon cancer cell line showed that postoperative tumor growth was significantly greater after CO_2 compared with helium pneumoperitoneum. Similarly, *in vitro* and *ex vivo* experiments comparing CO_2 and helium also demonstrated greater tumor growth in the CO_2 groups. It is possible that different tumor lines do not react in the same way to a CO_2 pneumoperitoneum. Interestingly, Jacobi *et al's* findings[48] are consistent with several of Allendorf *et al's* tumor studies which have shown significantly larger tumors in the CO_2 pneumoperitneum groups both with and without interventions and in immunocompetent and athymic mice.[44,46] A study comparing both helium and lifting techniques to CO_2 pneumoperitoneum is underway at Columbia University and will, hopefully, shed further light on this important area.

Allendorf *et al.*[46] assessed tumor cell proliferation rates after sham laparotomy, CO_2 pneumoperitoneum and anesthesia alone. A high-dose intradermal injection of MMC tumor cells was administered immediately prior to the surgical intervention which was 20 min long. A proliferation index for each study group was determined using the immunohistochemical assay for proliferating cell nuclear antigen (PCNA), an intranuclear polypeptide which is primarily synthesized during the S-phase of the cell cycle and is essential for DNA synthesis. This assay has been shown to provide an accurate assessment of tumor cell proliferation. The tumors were harvested either 6 or 12 days after the intervention. A stepwise increase in the proliferation index from the anesthesia control to the pneumoperitoneum to the laparotomy group was found at both time points. The proliferation index of the laparotomy group was significantly higher than both the pneumoperitoneum and anesthesia control groups 6 and 12 days after surgery. Similarly, the pneumoperitoneum group's proliferation rate, although less than that of the open group, was significantly higher than the anesthesia control group's on postoperative days 6 and 12.[46]

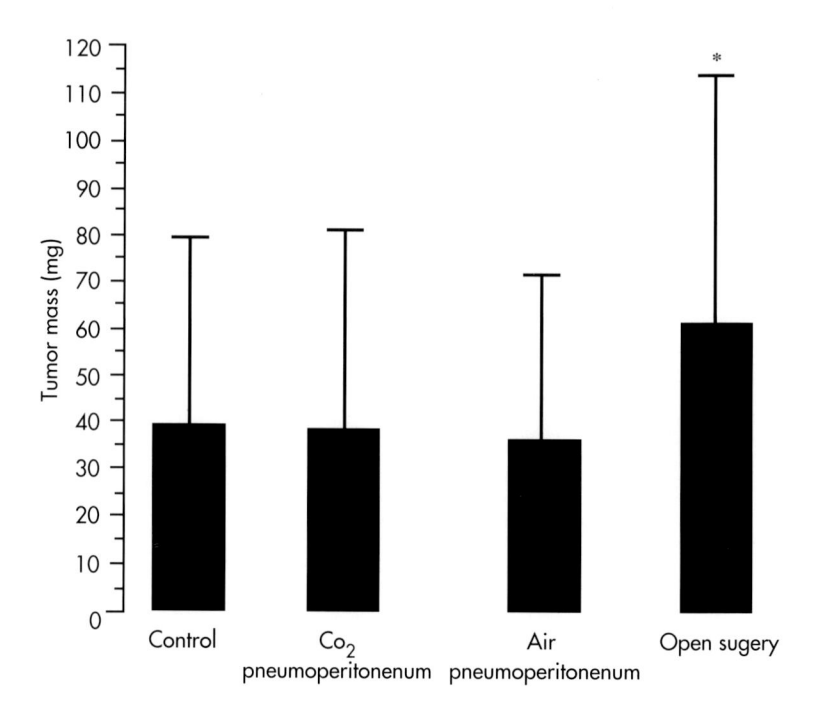

Figure 1.9 – Tumor mass on postoperative day 12 after CO_2 pneumoperitoneum, air pneumoperitoneum and laparotomy in mice. p<0.025 open versus control, CO_2 and air. P values were not significant for other comparisons.

In summary, it has been demonstrated, in four different tumor cell lines, that a full laparotomy is associated with faster tumor growth in the early postoperative period than pneumoperitoneum. The rate of tumor establishment and the proliferation rate of tumor cells are also significantly higher after laparotomy. Futhermore, the tumor growth and establishment differences persist despite the addition of a bowel resection. Differences in cell-mediated immune function after surgery account for at least part of the observed tumor growth differences. Despite the fact that tumor growth after CO_2 pneumo-peritoneum is slower than after a full laparotomy, CO_2 pneumoperitoneum appears to promote tumor growth compared to helium or anesthesia alone. Clearly, further studies are needed better to understand the oncologic effects of both open and minimally invasive surgical techniques.

PORT-SITE TUMORS

Any discussion of the impact of laparoscopic methods on tumor biology must include consideration of port-site tumor recurrences. Although port-site tumors have been reported after minimally invasive resection of gallbladder, ovarian, lung and other malignancies, the greatest number have been reported after colectomy. To date, over 35 port-site tumors have been reported following LACR for colonic malignancies[49-53] and these have raised serious concerns about the safety of LACR for colon cancer. The true incidence of port-site tumors is unknown; estimates range from 0 to 21%.[49] The most recent data from two large colectomy series with mean follow-up of over 2 years places the incidence between 0 and 1.2%.[9,12] Incisional recurrences occur after open surgery as well; two large series of open colectomy patients, each involving over 1000 cancer cases, have reported incisional tumor incidences of 0.6 and 0.68%.[54,55] What is the cause of port-site tumor recurrences? Thus far only a limited number of animal studies have addressed this question and the etiology remains obscure.

On anatomic grounds, it is unlikely that port-site tumors are the result of hematogenous or lymphatic spread. Direct implantation of tumor cells in the port site or wound is the most likely mechanism. Such seeding might occur at the time of specimen removal through the enlarged trocar site incision, especially if the tumor has invaded through the bowel wall and the wound is unprotected. This mechanism, however, would not explain the development of tumors at ports remote from the specimen extraction site. Logic dictates that two conditions must be met in order to seed these other port wounds: first, the presence of free and viable tumor cells in the peritoneal cavity and second, that the liberated cells must be transported to the port wound in some manner.

How do tumor cells become separated from the primary lesion? Patients with carcinomatosis demonstrate that, on rare occasions, tumors may spontaneously shed viable cells that can implant on peritoneal surfaces. However, this does not occur in the vast majority of patients. It is possible that a CO_2 pseudoperitoneum alone, in some way encourages cells to be shed. A more likely mechanism would be direct trauma to the tumor during the operation. Poor surgical technique, e.g. direct handling of the tumor during bowel mobilization and resection, may result in tumor cells being shed into the peritoneal cavity or onto the instruments themselves.

How are the liberated cells transported to the port wounds? The removal of a contaminated instrument through an intact port might carry the cells to the port. Removal of a contaminated port at the end of surgery might also result in wound seeding. The pneumoperitoneum via desufflation events, either inadvertent or intentional, may provide transportation for aerosolized cells or free cells in liquid suspension. Free intraperitoneal fluid that contains tumor cells may seed the wounds via position changes during or after surgery. It is also possible that the CO_2 pseudoperitoneum in some way creates conditions conducive to tumor establishment.

Most studies to investigate the etiology of port-site tumors have used liquid tumor cell suspensions. Hewitt et al.[56] injected a solution containing 10-15 million tumor cells into pigs. A CO_2 pneumoperitoneum was established and three ports placed. Fifty liters of CO_2 was allowed to escape through a filter attached to one of the ports. After changing the filter, a further 50 liters was allowed to escape while the bowel was manipulated with an endoscopic grasper through a second port, and finally 50 liters was allowed to escape while the bowel was manipulated through the port to which the filter was attached. The instruments, ports and filters were washed with saline, which was collected and sent for analysis. Tumor cells were found on the grasping instrument in 40% of animals and on the ports in 20%, but only on 1 of 30 (3.3%) port filters. This filter was from a port through which the bowel had been maniputated while the CO_2 was escaping. This study suggests that once tumor cells are liberated they are most likely transported via instruments and ports that have become contaminated during the procedure.

Whelan et al.[57] subjected liquid tumor cell suspensions in vitro to a variety of high pressure CO_2 environments but observed no tumor growth in any of the the test culture dishes following desufflation through sterile culture medium, or any non-viable cells in the CO_2. This and results from a similar in vivo rat model suggest that aerolization has not occurred. In a separate in vitro study it was demonstrated that droplets of fluid containing tumor cells could be transported via sudden desufflation but only after coating the entire inner surface of the study apparatus with the cell suspension.[57]

Allandyce et al.[58] performed a cell suspension study in a porcine model that determined tumor cell distribution following laparoscopic colectomy carried out via a CO_2 pneumoperitoneum or 'gasless' abdominal wall lifting. Tumor cells were found in all the locations sampled (port sites, diaphragm and peritoneum overlying the kidney) and on all instruments regardless of the method of laparoscopic exposure. There was a 2-8 fold higher number of cells recovered from the ports used by the operating surgeon compared to the number recovered from those used to retract the bowel. Presumably, there are more instrument exchanges and movements at the former ports. There was a trend towards higher cell counts in wounds where the port and stability thread (to prevent port dislodgement) were withdrawn before tissue samples were taken compared to those where samples were taken with the port and thread intact. It is important to note that avoidance of a CO_2 peritoneum by mechanically elevating the abdominal wall did not prevent tumor cell seeding of the abdominal wounds.

Jones et al.[59] sought to determine the impact of a CO_2 pneumoperitoneum on the incidence of abdominal wall tumors using a cell suspension study in a hamster model. All animals underwent a 1 cm midline incision and placement of four ports, followed by injection of the tumor cell suspension via the midline incision. After closing the midline incision, half the animals were subjected to a 10 min CO_2 pneumoperitoneum. Six weeks later the incidence of tumors at the port wounds and midline incision was found to be significantly greater in these animals than in the controls. With few exceptions, tumors only developed at sites of peritoneal or visceral injury and the study suggests that a CO_2 pneumoperitoneum, in the absence of instrumentation or performance of an intra-abdominal procedure, encourages development of port wound tumors. This speculation is supported by the findings of Jacobi et al.[48] that in a cell suspension study in a rat model, significantly more animals developed tumors at the abdominal wounds following a 30 min CO_2 pneumoperitoneum than animals either subjected to a 30 min helium pneumoperitoneum or anesthesia controls.

Bouvy et al.,[60] utilizing a rat model, compared CO_2 pneumoperitoneum, gasless laparotomy (abdominal wall lifting) and sham laparotomy after injection of tumor cells. The three groups demonstrated similar tumor growth after 4 weeks on the liver, kidney and retroperitoneum, but the volume of peritoneal tumor at the port sites and abdominal incision was significantly larger for the laparotomy group than the other two groups, and the volume for the CO_2 pneumoperitoneum group was significantly larger than for the gasless group. The authors attributed the difference between the laparoscopy groups to the turbulence caused by the CO_2 pneumoperitoneum. In an earlier cell suspension study in a rat model, these authors had shown that laparoscopic methods, when compared to open techniques, are associated with signficantly less tumor take at the abdominal wall.[61]

Sellers et al.[62] sought to determine the impact of sudden desufflation of a CO_2 pneumoperitoneum on the incidence of abdominal tumors in a cell suspension study in mice. The hypothesis was that sudden desufflation would provide an opportunity for free tumor cells to be transported to the port wounds by the rapidly moving CO_2. A trend was shown toward larger tumor volumes in mice groups that underwent multiple port dislodgements and reinsertions after desufflation compared to groups that had a single port insertion and removal. However, the largest tumors by far were seen in the laparotomy group. The authors hypothesized that the size of wound tumor was directly related to the amount of abdominal wall injury incurred and that multiple port insertions were likely to result in more peritoneal injury than a single insertion and removal. Obviously, the open group incurred the largest peritoneal injury. This observation may help to integrate the results of the studies described above, which at first glance appear to be contradictory.

Jones et al.[57] found that a CO_2 pneumoperitoneum is associated with a higher incidence of wound tumors, whereas most of the other studies, which looked at tumor volume, found the largest tumors in the open control groups. A close examination of these studies, however, reveals important differences in their design and this may explain the seemingly disparate results. It is probably unreasonable to compare abdominal wall tumor volumes unless the amount of trauma to the abdominal wall, in the form of trocar sites and incisions, is the same. Much more peritoneum is disrupted with a laparotomy incision than with 2-3 port wounds. The design of Jones et al's study[59] allows comparison since all animals had both an incision and ports placed, whereas the other studies[60-62] did not control for incision length and, not surprisingly, found the largest abdominal tumor volumes in the laparotomy groups. In the latter studies, the larger tumors in the open group may reflect differences in wound size and may not be related to pneumoperitoneum or minimally invasive techniques.

Hubens et al.[63] compared tumor growth following sham laparotomy, pneumoperitoneum and anesthesia alone and injection of a relatively small dose of tumor cells (10^4 cells compared with the 10^5 or greater doses employed in the other studies). Unlike the other studies, tumors did not grow in all animals and were only found in 50-60% of all animals in the three groups. A port-site tumor only grew in 1 of 10 animals in the pneumoperitoneum group and no abdominal tumors were noted in the open group at the incision site. The authors concluded that a pneumoperitoneum alone did not increase the implantation rate of free tumor cells.

Cell suspension experiments are easy to perform but the above studies point out the many problems associated with them. They are unrealistic because they involve a huge number of viable cells that uniformly result in tumor deposits at numerous parietal, peritoneal and visceral locations which is certainly not analogous to the human setting. In several studies where tumor growth was found at all abdominal wound sites, the investigators, by necessity, compared peritoneal tumor volume or masses instead of tumor incidence. The validity of this type of comparison is unclear. Futhermore, cell suspension studies assess only the manner in which free cells implant. Using this model, it is not possible to assess how often tumor cells become liberated or by what means they become free. Because of these reservations, the results of these studies have to be evaluated very carefully. It is not at all clear that it is reasonable to extrapolate to the human setting which, in almost every way, is different. Nonetheless, these studies have served to raise the suspicion that a CO_2

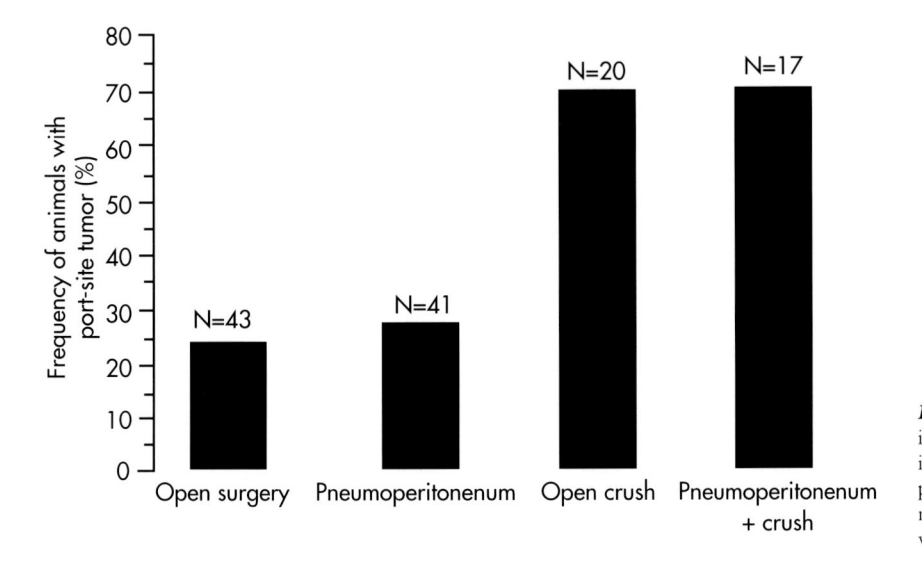

Figure 1.10 – Comparison by intervention of tumor implantation at trocar sites. p<0.7 open versus pneumoperitoneum; p<0.01 open versus open crush.

pneumoperitoneum may be deleterious with regards to wound tumors.

A second type of study utilizes solid tumor pieces which are introduced into the abdomen at the beginning of the study and then removed at the end of the intervention. Many of the objections voiced about cell suspension studies apply to this model as well. Bouvy et al.[60] inserted a lump of solid tumor into the abdomen of each animal via a port wound and after 20 min removed it via either the midline wound or the same port wound. After 6 weeks tumors were found in all abdominal wounds and at various other places in the abdomen and, not surprisingly, those that developed at the port used for insertion and removal of the tumor were significantly larger than the tumors at the other ports. There were no significant differences in tumor volumes when the CO_2 pneumoperitoneum and gassless groups were compared, which contrasts with the results of cell suspension studies from the same group.[60,61]

A third category of study better approximates the human situation. An isolated tumor that has been established in an intra-abdominal organ can be excised under a variety of conditions using a number of different techniques. Using this type of model it is possible to assess how tumor cells are shed in addition to determining what happens to the liberated cells. Unfortunately, this is the most difficult type of model to establish. Recently, a new rodent model has been developed that will, hopefully, allow more realistic port-site tumor studies. A splenic tumor(s) is established in mice by injecting tumor cells into the spleen after it has been exteriorized via a 1 cm subcostal incision at the initial procedure. Seven to 10 days later the mice are re-explored via the same subcostal incision and those that have developed isolated splenic tumors then undergo splenectomy under a variety of conditions (with and without a pneumoperitoneum). The animals are sacrificed 7-10 days later at which time the number of abdominal wound and visceral tumor metastases are noted.

A preliminary study using this model evaluated the influence of a CO_2 pneumoperitoneum and poor technique on the incidence of abdominal wall tumors. All animals had three ports placed well away from the subcostal incision before resection, and all underwent splenectomy via the left subcostal incision. However, the animals were divided into 4 study groups depending on the method of resection: 1) careful resection and anesthesia alone; 2) tumor crush, resection and anesthesia; 3) careful resection and 20-min CO_2 pneumoperitoneum; and 4) tumor crush, resection and 20-min CO_2 pneumoperitoneum. The presence of a CO_2 pneumoperitoneum did not significantly change the incidence of abdominal wall tumors but significantly more tumors were found in the two groups whose tumors had been crushed than in the groups for which careful resection had been carried out (Fig. 1.10).[68] One major shortcoming of this study is that no procedure or manipulation was carried out during the pneumoperitoneum.

Summary of port-site studies

Clinically, the true incidence of port-site tumors is unknown. Initial fears that the incidence would be very high appear to be unfounded. The etiology also remains unclear. Common sense dictates that poor surgical technique should greatly increase the chances of port site tumors developing. The instruments may carry the cells to the ports. The CO_2 pneumoperitoneum may also play a role, either through desufflation or via some, as yet unexplained, physiologic effect. Aerosolization of tumor cells seems an unlikely explanation. Much of the available animal data must be carefully scrutinized because the model used for the bulk of these is insensitive and, in many ways, unrealistic. Futhermore, the results of the cell suspension studies are contradictory in many regards. Newer, more realistic, animal models are being developed that will, hopefully, shed more light on the cause of port-site tumors. Animal and human studies looking into alternative laparoscopic exposure techniques need to be carried out. Both the efficacy and oncologic impact of these methods need to be determined. In the meantime, the following technique recommendations seem prudent: 1) routine use of specimen bags or wound protectors; 2) minimizing tumor manipulation; 3) avoidance of sudden desufflation and slow CO_2 leaks; 4) washing instruments and ports in the abdomen via irrigators before removal; and 5) careful and frequent suctioning of the abdomen. Finally, it is the authors' view that LACR for curative cancer resection should be limited to prospective and, preferably, randomized studies.

CONCLUSION

It appears that an equivalent cancer resection can be accomplished laparoscopically as can be carried out using open methods. The follow-up data available suggests the 3-year outcome is comparable in terms of survival and local recurrences. The final judgement regarding the utility of laparoscopic methods for curative cancer resections cannot be made until the port-site issue is settled and 5-year survival data is available. Recent human data suggests that the incidence of port-site tumors will be lower than initially feared. Randomized prospective trials will provide the best data. Surgical technique and the CO_2 pneumoperitoneum may be involved in port-site tumor formation. Prudence dictates that meticulous technique be used during laparoscopic cancer resections.

There is strong laboratory evidence suggesting that laparoscopic methods are associated with significantly better preserved postoperative immune function than open techniques. Similarly, the preliminary results of a human DTH study in colectomy patients noted more immunosuppression after open surgery. Furthermore, it appears that perioperative tumor growth in animals is significantly greater after open surgery than after minimally invasive surgery. It is unknown whether similar oncologic benefits will be found in humans. However, there exists the possibility that minimally invasive methods will be associated with improved long-term results when compared to open surgery. It goes without saying that further animal and human studies need to be carried out in this area.

REFERENCES

1. Saba AD, Kerlakian GM, Kasper GC et al. Laparoscopic-assisted colectomies versus open colectomy. *J Laparoendosc Surg* 1995;**5**:1-6.

2. Darzi A, Lewis C, Menzies-Gow N et al. Laparoscopic abdominoperineal excision of the rectum. *Surg Endosc* 1995;**9**:414-417.

3. Musser DJ, Boorse RD, Madera F et al. Laparoscopic colectomy: at what cost? *Surg Laparosc Endosc* 1994;**4**:1-5.

4. Tate JJT, Kwok S, Dawson JW et al. Prospective comparison of laparoscopic and conventional anterior resection. *Br J Surg* 1993;**80**:1396-1398.

5. Chindasub S, Charntaracharmnong C, Nimitvanit C et al. Laparoscopic abdominoperineal resection. *J Laparoendosc Surg* 1994;**4**:17-21.

6. Van Ye TM, Cattey RP, Henry LG. Laparoscopically assisted colon resections compare favorably with open technique. *Surg Laparosc Endosc* 1994;**4**:25-31

7. Ou H. Laparoscopic-assisted mini laparotomy with colectomy. *Dis Colon Rectum* 1995;**38**:324-326.

8. Hoffman GC, Baker JW, Fitchett CW et al. Laparoscopic-assisted cholectomy: initial experience. *Ann Surg* 1994;**21**:732-743.

9. Franklin ME, Rosenthal D, Abrego-Medina D et al. Prospective comparison of open versus laparoscopic colon surgery for carcinoma: Five year results. *Dis Colon Rectum* 1995;**39**(Suppl):s35-s46.

10. Baker R, Senagore AJ, Luchtefeld MA. Laparoscopic-assisted vs. open resection: rectopexy offers excellent results. *Dis Colon Rectum* 1995;**38**:199-201.

11. Gray D, Lee H, Schlinkert R et al. Adequacy of lymphadenectomy in laparoscopic-assisted colectomy for colorectal cancer: a preliminary report. *J Surg Oncol* 1994;**57**:8-10.

12. Fleshman JW, Nelson H, Peters WR et al. Early results of laparoscopic surgery of 372 patients treated by Clinical Outcomes of Surgical Therapy (COST) study group. *Dis Colon Rectum* 1996;**39**(Suppl):s53-s58.

13. Burnet FM. The concept of immunological surveillance. *Prog Exp Tumor Res* 1970;**13**:1-27.

14. Boon T. Toward a genetic analysis of human tumor rejection antigens. *Adv Cancer Res* 1992;**58**:177-210.

15. Herlyn M, Koprowski H. Melanoma antigens: immunological and biological characterization and clinical significance. *Ann Rev Immunol* 1988;**6**:283-308.

16. Prehn RT, Main MJ. Immunity to methylcholanthrene-induced sarcomas. *J Natl Cancer Inst* 1957;**18**:769-778.

17. Rosenberg SA, Lotze MT. Cancer immunotherapy using interleukin-2 and interleukin-2 activated lymphocytes. *Ann Rev Immunol* 1986;**4**:681-709.

18. Tonaka K, Yoshioka T, Bieberich C, Jay G. The role of the major histocompatibility complex class 1 antigens in tumor growth and metastasis. *Ann Rev Immunol* 1988;**6**:359-380.

19. Eilber FR, Morton DL. Impaired immunologic reactivity and recurrence follow cancer surgery. *Cancer* 1970;**25**:362-367.

20. Pietsch JB, Meakins JL, MacLean LD. The delayed hypersensitivity response: Application in clinical surgery. *Surgery* 1977;**82**:349-355.

21. Abbas AK, Lichtman AH, Pober JS. *Cellular and Molecular Immunology*. Philadelphia: WB Saunders, 1994, p.357.

22. Nielsen HJ, Pedersen BK, Moesgaard F. Effect of ranitidine on postoperative suppression of natural killer cell activity and delayed hypersenstivity. *Acta Chir Scand* 1989;**155**:377-382.

23. Christou NV, Superina R, Broadhead M et al. Postoperative depression of host resistance: Determinants and effect of peripheral protein-sparing therapy. *Surgery* 1982;**92**:786-792.

24. Lennard TWJ, Shenton BK, Borzotta A et al. The influence of surgical operations on components of the human immune system. *Br J Surg* 1985;**72**:771-776.

25. Nielsen HJ, Moesgaard F, Kehlet H. Ranitidine for prevention of postoperative suppression of delayed hypersenstivity. *Am J Surg* 1989;**157**:291-294.

26. Hjortso NC, Kehlet H. Influence of surgery, age and serum albumin on delayed hypersensitivity. *Acta Chir Scand* 1986;**152**:175-179.

27. Hammer JH, Nielsen HJ, Moesgaard F et al. Duration of postoperative immunosuppression assessed by repeated delayed type hypersensitivity skin tests. *Eur Surg Res* 1992;**24**:133-137.

28. Kloosterman T, von Bloomberg BE, Borgstein PJ et al. Unimpaired immune functions after laparoscopic cholecystectomy. *Surgery* 1994;**115**:424-428.

29. Jakeways MS, Mitchell V, Hashim IA et al. Metabolic and inflammatory responses after open and laparoscopic cholecystectomy. *Br J Surg* 1994;**81**:127-131.

30. Ueo H, Honda M, Adachi M et al. Minimal increase in serum interleukin-6 levels during laparoscopic cholecystectomy. *Am J Surg* 1994;**168**:358-360.

31. Goodale RL, Beebe DS, McNevin MP et al. Hemodynamic, respiratory and metabolic effects of laparoscopic cholecystectomy. *Am J Surg* 1993;**166**:533-537.

32. Harmon GD, Senagore AJ, Killbride MJ et al. Interleukin-6 response to laparoscopic and open colectomy. *Dis Colon Rectum* 1994;**37**:754-759.

33. Fukushima R, Kawamura YJ, Saito H et al. Interleukin-6 and stress hormone response after uncomplicated gasless laparoscopic-assisted and open sigmoid colectomy. *Dis Colon Rectum* 1996;**39**(Suppl):s29-s34.

34. Horgan PG, Fitzpatrick M, Couse NF et al. Laparoscopy is less immunotraumatic than laparotomy. *Minim Invasive Ther* 1992;**1**:241-244.

35. Trokel MJ, Bessler M, Treat MR, Whelan RL, Nowygrod R. Preservation of immune response after laparoscopy. *Surg Endosc* 1994;**8**:1385-1388.

36. Gitzelman CA, Mendoza-Sagaon M, Ahmad AS et al. Cell-mediated immune response: laparoscopy versus laparotomy. *Surg Forum* 1996;**XLVII**:148-150.

37. Allendorf JD, Bessler M, Whelan RL et al. A laparoscopic cecal resection model in mice. *Surg Endosc* (in press).

38. Allendorf JD, Bessler M, Whelan RL et al. Better preservation of immune function after laparoscopic-assisted vs. open bowel resection in a murine model. *Dis Colon Rectum* 1996;**10**(Suppl):s67-72.

39. Allendorf JD, Bessler M, Whelan RL et al. Postoperative immune function varies inversely with degree of sugical trauma. *Surg Endosc* (in press).

40. Watson RWG, Redmond HP, McCarthy J, Burke PE, Bouchier-Hayes D. Exposure of the peritoneal cavity to air regulates early inflammatory responses to surgery in a murine model. *Br J Surg* 1995;**82**:1060-1065.

41. Eggermont AM, Steller EP, Marquet RL et al. Local regional promotion of tumor growth after abdominal surgery is dominant over immunotherapy with interleukin-2 and lymphokine activated killer cells.

Cancer Detect Prevent 1988;**12**:421-429.
42. Goshima H, Saji S, Furata T *et al*. Experimental study on preventive effects of lung metastases using LAK cells induced from various lymphocytes - special reference to enhancement of lung metastasis after laparotomy stress. *J Jap Surg Soc* 1989;**90**:1245-1250.
43. Ratajczak HV, Lange RW, Sothern RB *et al*. Surgical influence on murine immunity and tumor growth: relationship of body temperature and hormones with splenocytes. *Proc Soc Exp Biol Med* 1992;**199**:432-440.
44. Allendorf JD, Bessler M, Kayton M, Whelan RL, Treat MR. Tumor growth after laparoscopy and laparotomy in a murine model. *Arch Surg* 1995;**130**:6 49-653.
45. Vaage J, Pepin K. Morphological observations during developing concomitant immunity against C3H/He mammary tumor. *Cancer Res* 1985;**45**:659-666.
46. Allendorf JD, Bessler M, Whelan RL *et al*. Differences in tumor growth after open versus laparoscopic surgery are lost in an athymic model and are associated with differences in tumor proliferative index. *Surg Forum* 1996;**XLVII**:150-152.
47. Bouvy ND, Marquet RL, Jeekel H *et al*. Gasles laparoscopy versus CO_2 pneumoperitoneum in relation to the development of adominal wall metastases. *Surg Endosc* 1996;**10**:186(Abstract).
48. Jacobi CA, Sabat R, Bohm B, Zieren HU, Volk HD, Muller JM. Pneumoperitoenum with carbon dioxide stimulates growth of malignant colonic cells. *Surgery* 1997;**121**:72-78.
49. Wexner SD, Cohen SM. Port site metastases after laparoscopic colorectal surgery for cure of malignancy. *Br J Surg* 1995;**82**:295-298.
50. Fusco MA, Paluzzi MW. Abdominal wall recurrence after laparoscopic-assisted colectomy for adenocarcinoma of the colon. *Dis Colon Rectum* 1993;**36**: 858-861.
51. Nduka CC, Monson JRT, Menzies-Gow N, Darzi A. Abdominal wall metastases following laparoscopy. *Br J Surg* 1994;**81**:648-652.
52. Berends FJ, Kazemier G, Bonjer HK, Lange JF. Subcutaneous metastases after laparoscopic colectomy. *Lancet* 1994;**344**:58(Letter).
53. Fingerhut A. Laparoscopic colectomy. The French experience. In: Jager R, Wexner SD (eds). *Laparoscopic Colorectal Surgery*. New York: Churchill Livingstone, 1995.
54. Hughes ESR, McDermott FT, Polglase AL *et al*. Tumor recurrence in the abdominal wall scar after large-bowel cancer surgery. *Dis Colon Rectum* 1983;**26**: 571-572.
55. Reilly WT, Nelson H, Schroeder G, Wieand HS *et al*. Wound recurrence following conventional treatment of colorectal cancer. *Dis Colon Rectum* 1996;**39**: 200-207.
56. Hewett PJ, Thomas WM, King G, Eaton M. Intraperitoneal cell movement during abdominal carbon dioxide insufflation and laparoscopy: An *in vivo* model. *Dis Colon Rectum* 1996;**39**:s62-s66.
57. Whelan RL, Sellers GJ, Allendorf JF *et al*. Trocar site recurrence is unlikely to result from aerolization of tumor cells. *Dis Colon Rectum* 1996;**39**(Suppl):s7-s13.
58. Allandyce R, Morreau P, Bagshaw P. Tumor cell distribution following laparoscopic colectomy in a porcine model. *Dis Colon Rectum* 1996;**39**(Suppl): s47-s52.
59. Jones DB, Guo L-W, Reinhard MK *et al*. Impact of pneumoperitoneum on trocar site implantation of colon cancer in hamster model. *Dis Colon Rectum* 1995;**38**:1182-1188.
60. Bouvy ND, Marquet RL, Jeekek H, Bonjer HJ. Impact of gas(less) laparoscocopy and laparotomy on peritoneal tumor growth and abdominal wall metastastases. *Ann Surg* 1996;**244**:694-701.
61. Bouvy ND, Marquet RL, Hamming JF, Jeekel J, Bonjer HJ. Laparoscopic surgery in the rat: beneficial effect on body weight and tumor take. *Surg Endosc* 1996;**10**:490-494
62. Sellers GJ, Van D, Whelan RL, Bessler M, Treat MR. A study of abdominal wall tumor implants in a murine model. *Dis Colon Rectum* 1996;**39**:A40(Abstract).
63. Jubens G, Pauwels M, Hubens A, Vermeulen P, Van Marck E, Eyskens E. The influence of a pneumoperitoneum on the peritoneal implantation of free intraperitoneal colon cancer cells. *Surg Endosc* 1996;**10**: 809-812.
64. Lee SW, Whelan RL, Southall BA, Bessler M. Pneumoperitoneum does not increase port site implantation rate of colon cancer in a murine model. (in press).

2

Oncologic Principles and Minimal Access Surgery

Frederick L. Greene

The principles governing the basic handling and dissection of solid tumors have evolved as surgeons have continued to play a major role in the diagnosis and management of cancer. Since the days of Hippocrates and Asklepois, the extirpation of cancer has been a major treatment modality and will no doubt continue to be important to future generations of surgeons. Surgical therapy has previously meant wide excision and radical dissection as illustrated by Halsted's original approach to breast cancer.[1] This has given way to a more conservative and less radical approach in the management of most cancers, although the importance of lymph node drainage and vascular supply to involved organs continues to be a principle that is considered sacrosanct.

Table 2.1 – Benefits of minimal access techniques in cancer management

Reduction of immune suppression compared to 'open' techniques[2]
Reduction in postoperative pain
Adjunct to preoperative staging[19]
Adequate nodal dissection and tumor margins[18]
Rapid return of gastrointestinal function
Lower postoperative analgesic needs
Application of chemotherapy and brachytherapy

BIOLOGICAL AND PHYSICAL EFFECTS

Many diagnostic and therapeutic maneuvers can now be approached using minimal access techniques. This may be of benefit when one considers that surgical manipulation and traumatic handling of tissue will adversely affect the patient's own immune mechanisms, allowing neoplastic cells to proliferate and eventually metastasize. The effect of minimal access techniques on the immune mechanism has been studied in both benign and malignant models in animals and in human patients.[2,3] Measurement of neutrophil function, cytokine levels, skin reactivity and other immunologic markers suggests that, at least transiently, minimal access procedures protect immune function.

However, associated maneuvers such as application of a pneumoperitoneum and use of general anesthesia may counteract this beneficial effect of less traumatic interventions (Tables 2.1 and 2.2). A CO_2 pneumoperitoneum has been shown to cause detrimental effects on cardiac and respiratory function.[4] Although little is known about the complete effect on the cancer patient, the creation of a pneumoperitoneum may be detrimental in some patients. It is well known that cancer patients are hypercoagulable, although the underlying mechanism is still debated. This hypercoagulability is manifested in the appearance of deep vein thrombophlebitis (DVT) and in the potential increase of lethal associated processes such as mesenteric venous thrombosis. Knowledge of these effects indicate that the addition of noxious stimuli, which might increase hypercoagulability, is to

Table 2.2 – Potential drawbacks of minimal access techniques in cancer management

Increased abdominal wound recurrence[15]
Increased coagulability secondary to vasopressin effect[6]
Increased potential of deep vein thrombosis secondary to pneumoperitoneum[5]
Reduced capability of intraoperative abdominal inspection[20]

be eschewed. It is known that creation of a pneumoperitoneum may increase the risk of a patient developing a DVT.[5] Virchow's triad defines venous stasis, hypercoagulability, and vascular trauma as predisposing factors for developing thromboembolism and a pneumoperitoneum induces the first two fo these. This hypercoagulability may be enhanced through the endogenous hypersecretion of arginine vasopressin (AVP),[6] which in turn may induce elevated levels of Factor VIII and von Willebrand's Factor. The endogenous production of AVP is directly attributed to the increase in abdominal pressure utilized during minimal access abdominal procedures. It is reasonable, therefore, either to perform these procedures under low levels of abdominal pressure or to abandon a pneumoperitoneum in favor of abdominal wall lift devices which may not induce increases in AVP.

TECHNICAL IMPLICATIONS

Although the metabolic consequences of minimal access techniques and the associated pneumoperitoneum are important, the oncologic principles of tissue handling and knowledge of regional node drainage of solid tumors are also highly influential in shaping the future role of both laparoscopy and thoracoscopy in the management of cancer patients. Gentle handling of neoplastic tissue was espoused by early surgeons in their effort to avoid dissemination of cancer cells and should be a principle that continues to direct oncologic surgical management. Since minimal access techniques may involve only small abdominal or chest incisions and small accessory instruments, it might be assumed that the potential for cellular dissemination is reduced. Unfortunately, the remote manipulation of instruments may result in inappropriate manipulation of solid tumors, both in diagnostic and therapeutic maneuvers. Anecdotal case reports[7] and registry data[8] both suggest that tumor embolization may be increased in the trocar sites created in the chest and abdominal walls. Reports have been documented for gallbladder,[9] pancreatic,[10] stomach,[11] colon,[12] and ovarian tumors[13] as well as manipulation of patients with lymphomas. Once again, the influence of the pneumoperitoneum in the dissemination of trocar or port-site metastases cannot be over-emphasized.

One important oncologic principle noted by previous generations of surgeons is the need to avoid placing a needle through skin into solid tumors if resection is likely to be the appropriate treatment. Today, especially with the use of diagnostic imaging, many tumors are biopsied with needles of various sizes for diagnostic confirmation prior to definitive oncologic resection. The risk of pleural or peritoneal seeding may well be forgotten in the fervor to obtain needle diagnoses for treatment planning. Similarly, diagnostic maneuvers through a thoracoscope or laparoscope with needle biopsy, wedge excision, or removal of tumor by forceps may enhance the spread of cancer cells to body cavities or the abdominal or chest wall.[14]

The true incidence of port-site metastases following laparoscopic intervention is not known. A retrospective analysis of registry data which followed up 280 patients found an incidence of 1.44%.[8] Unfortunately, port-site recurrence is not limited to patients with advanced tumors and is also seen in patients with early stage tumors, especially of colonic origin. These trocar problems may result not only from tumor manipulation in the abdominal cavity, but also from extraction techniques once cancers have been dissected within the chest or abdomen. During 'open' cancer procedures, surgeons have for many years advocated wound protection in order to reduce the possibility not only of infection but also the inoculation of the incision site by cancer cells. These principles must be adhered to especially when small trocar sites are utilized. If hemostasis is not carefully achieved in a trocar site, cancer cells may become entrapped in hematoma and will continue to flourish in this environment. The principles of wound care using appropriate suture and closure techniques as well as close attention to hemostasis must be followed.

Mechanisms of tumor metastases have been extensively studied for a variety of solid tumors. In terms of colorectal cancer, five mechanisms have been proposed: 1) hematogenous; 2) lymphatic spread of circulating tumor cells; 3) exfoliated (intramural) cells in the intestinal lumen; 4) free tumor cells in the peritoneal cavity; and 5) direct extension. It is established that tumor cells are released continuously into the vascular bed; however, no prognostic indicators are as yet known that link this intravascular dissemination to reduced survival. Studies of intracardiac injection of tumor cells have shown these cells to implant in laparotomy wounds.[15] It is interesting that wound recurrence, however, as shown by the classic paper of Hughes et al.[16] is actually quite low and generally is considered to occur in <1% of all laparotomy procedures involving colon resection for cancer. Data regarding implantation in the small wounds created for thoracoscopy and laparoscopy need to be collected and the potential for new mechanisms for dissemination remains great. The frequency of recurrence in trocar sites should be recorded carefully, especially in controlled trials dealing with the management of colon and lung cancer. The potential for further metastases may actually be enhanced when secondary tumor sites propagate since these 'remote' sites may serve as better foci than the original tumor for further metastases.

PRINCIPLES OF STAGING

An important principle in cancer management is the correct staging of solid tumors using the worldwide

TNM system supported by the Union International Centre Cancer (UICC) and the American Joint Committee on Cancer (AJCC) (see Table 5.2).[17] The staging of gastrointestinal cancer involves both clinical and pathological estimates of the depth of tumor penetration into the layers of the intestinal wall. The letter 'T' represents Tumor Extent and is assigned a number from 1 to 4 depending on the depth of tumor penetration. The designation T1 indicates tumor involvement of the mucosa and muscularis mucosae, while T3 denotes a malignancy that has penetrated the muscularis propria and serosa. This system is used throughout the gastrointestinal tract and differs from the 'T' designation in breast cancer, for example, which is based on the diameter of the primary cancer. Tumor depth may be judged by sophisticated endoscopic ultrasound probes that can visualize tumor margins in terms of mural depth of involvement. The 'gold standard' in the accurate delineation of tumor penetration, however, continues to be histologic examination by the pathologist after surgical extirpation. The 'T' stage is important in predicting patterns of recurrence and overall survival after treatment of most gastrointestinal tract malignancies.

The second staging indicator of the TNM system is the 'N' or nodal assessment. Traditional 'open' extirpation of a gastrointestinal malignancy has allowed careful anatomical dissection of lymphatic regions which drain both the upper and lower intestinal areas. The total number of nodes containing tumor emboli and the region of positive nodes in the mediastinal or mesenteric regions both have critical prognostic importance. Although preoperative imaging studies and endoscopic ultrasound may give valuable information as to the likelihood of nodal involvement, pathological evaluation remains the 'gold standard' in assigning the 'N' designation. Treatment options, especially the use of adjuvant radiation or chemotherapy, may depend on the accurate collection and pathological assessment of draining lymph nodes.

Both laparoscopic and thoracoscopic techniques must be able to identify appropriate nodal beds in the gastrointestinal tract and offer the same potential for nodal extirpation as formal celiotomy and thoracotomy. Recent descriptions of nodal retrieval during laparoscopic colectomy indicate that adequate mesenteric resection can be achieved when compared with traditional open techniques.[18] Laparoscopic staging has a potentially greater use in preoperative evaluation of patients with pancreatic cancer.[19]

Dissection of peripancreatic lymph nodes as well as evaluation of the direct extension of the cancer may reveal a subset of patients who will not benefit from formal celiotomy and attempts at pancreaticoduodenectomy. These patients may be candidates for bypass or stent placement of the biliary system which are also facilitated by minimal access techniques.

The third criterion of the TNM system is the 'M' or metastatic status of the primary tumor. For decades surgeons have been taught to assess patients preoperatively for obvious patterns of tumor metastasis using indirect indicators of liver function, protein tumor markers, nuclear medicine or radiologic studies, and careful concurrent examination of the entire abdominal cavity. Planned operative strategies are often changed after careful abdominal exploration. Biopsies of liver or other solid organs can be obtained to confirm the histology of the presumed metastatic implant. Once metastases are clinically or histologically proven, a designation of M1 is given which places any solid tumor in a category classified as Stage IV.

One potential drawback of minimal access techniques in the management of abdominal tumors is the difficulty of performing an initial examination of the entire peritoneal cavity.[20] Small metastases may be missed and as a result the abdominal malignancy may be understaged. The potential for inaccurate abdominal evaluation necessitates more aggressive use of preoperative imaging techniques such as computed tomography, magnetic resonance imaging or positron emission tomography. These studies guide the oncologic surgeon when laparoscopic cancer resection or staging is being performed. If implants are found, the laparoscope and thoracoscope are helpful in accurately performing needle or wedge biopsy of suspected metastatic implants.

PATIENT MANAGEMENT

Aside from the intraoperative use of minimal access techniques in cancer management, an important consideration is the effect of these techniques on the patient's quality of life. Patients with cancer should only undergo operative procedures which assure timely hospital discharge and a return to preoperative levels of activity. The use of laparoscopy and thoracoscopy for cancer management certainly enhances 'quality of life' issues and allows for earlier discharge of patients. When 'open' and minimal access techniques are compared, however, it is possible to overestimate the advantage of the minimal access technique in terms of the reduction of length of stay and return of function, e.g. gastrointestinal motility. Many patients who undergo traditional celiotomy may show a quicker return of gastrointestinal function and may even be managed without nasogastric intubation. An additional important consideration is the requirement for pain control in the postoperative cancer patient. Following minimal access approaches to the chest and abdomen, less narcotic is needed which may result in quicker restoration of gastrointestinal motility and a return of well being indicated by greater ambulation and activity.

THE FUTURE

The modern view of oncologic management is the 'team' approach, drawing on surgical, chemotherapeutic and irradiation expertise. Minimal access techniques may actually enhance the surgeon's role in helping to develop maneuvers which can more effectively deliver drugs and ionizing radiation to tumor areas and allow laparoscopic placement of after-loading catheters which can direct high energy radiation into the tumor bed. Although it is expected that surgeons will have less opportunity in the future for major extirpation or en bloc resection of cancer, the traditional picture of the surgeon as the leader in the management of cancer may be enhanced by minimal access techniques.

REFERENCES

1. Halsted WS. The results of operations for the care of cancer of the breast performed at the Johns Hopkins Hospital from June 1889 to January 1894. *Johns Hopkins Hosp Bull* 1894;**4**:297.
2. Borgstein RJ, Meijer S, Cuesta MA. Immunological alterations. In: Cohen RV (ed) *Metabolic and Systemic Responses Following Interventional Laparoscopy*. RG Landes Co Pub, 1994, pp. 55-66.
3. Kloosterman T, Blomberg B, Borgstein P et al. Unimpaired immune functions after laparoscopic cholecystectomy. *Surgery* 1994;**115**:424-428.
4. Liu SY, Leighton T, Davis I et al. Prospective analysis of cardiopulmonary responses to laparoscopic cholecystectomy. *J Laparoendosc Surg* 1991;**1**:241-246.
5. Caprini JA, Arcelus JI, Laubach M et al. Postoperative hypercoagulability and deep-vein thrombosis after laparoscopic cholecystectomy. *Surg Endosc* 1995;**9**:304-309.
6. Nussey SS, Bevan DH, Ang VT, Jenkins JS. Effects of arginine vasopressin (AVP) infusions on circulating concentrations of platelet AVP, Factor VIII: C and von Willebrand factor. *Thromb Haemostat* 1986;**55**:34-36.
7. Keate RF, Shaffer R. Seeding of hepatocellular carcinoma to peritoneoscopy insertion site. *Gastrointest Endosc* 1992;**38**:202-204.
8. Ramos JM, Gupta S, Anthone GJ et al. Laparoscopic bowel surgery registry. *Dis Colon Rectum* 1995;**38**:1110-1114.
9. Kim HJ, Roy T. Unexpected gallbladder cancer with cutaneous seeding after laparoscopic cholecystectomy. *South Med J* 1994;**87**:817-820.
10. Siriwardena A, Samarji WM. Cutaneous tumor seeding from a previous undiagnosed pancreatic carcinoma after laparoscopic cholecystectomy. *Ann R Coll Surg Engl* 1993;**75**:199-200.
11. Cava A, Roman J, Quintela AG et al. Subcutaneous metastasis following laparoscopy in gastric carcinoma. *Eur J Surg Oncol* 1990;**16**:63-67.
12. Berends FJ, Kazemier G, Bonjer HJ. Subcutaneous metastases after laparoscopic colectomy. *Lancet* 1994;**344**:58.
13. Hsin J, Given FT, Kemp GM. Tumor implantation after diagnostic laparoscopic biopsy of serous ovarian tumors of low malignant potential. *Obstet Gynecol* 1986;**68**:905-935.
14. Greene FL. Principles of cancer biology in relation to miminal access surgical techniques. *Sem Lap Surg* 1995;**2**:155-157.
15. Savalgi RS. Mechanism of abdominal wall recurrence after laparoscopic resection of colonic cancers. *Sem Lap Surg* 1995;**2**:158-162.
16. Hughes ESR, McDermott FT, Polglase AL. Tumor recurrence in the abdominal wall scar tissue after large-bowel cancer surgery. *Dis Colon Rectum* 1983;**9**:571-572.
17. Hutter RP. At last - worldwide agreement on the staging of cancer. *Arch Surg* 1987;**122**:1235-1239.
18. Hoffman GC, Baker JW, Doxey JB et al. Minimally invasive surgery for colorectal cancer: Initial follow-up. *Ann Surg* 1996;**223**:790-798.
19. John TG, Greig JD, Carter DC. Carcinoma of the pancreatic head and periampullary region. Tumor staging with laparoscopy and laparoscopic ultrasonography. *Ann Surg* 1995;**221**:156-164.
20. Slim K, Pezet D, Clark E et al. Malignant tumors missed at laparoscopic cholecystectomy. *Am J Surg* 1996;**171**:364-365.

3

Role of Laparoscopic Diagnosis and Staging of Intra-abdominal Malignancy

Timothy G. John, K.K. Madhaven and O. James Garden

The role of laparoscopy in the diagnosis and staging of intraabdominal malignancy has long been recognized, inspiring many of the breakthroughs in the evolution of the technique. Kelling first demonstrated the concept of 'coelioskopie' in 1901 by inspecting the abdominal cavities of dogs using air insufflation and a cystoscope.[1] At about the same time, the first laparoscopy in a human subject was performed by Ott, a Russian gynecologist.[2,3] Soon afterwards in Stockholm, Jacobeus developed his technique of 'laparoskopie', and showed its clinical use in establishing the diagnoses of liver cirrhosis, liver metastases, ascites and tuberculous peritonitis.[4] In 1911, Bernheim reported the first "organoscopy" in America, in a patient of Halsted's with pancreatic cancer.[5] A half-inch bore proctoscope was introduced through a small epigastric incision and was illuminated with an electric headlight. Prophetically, he speculated that the technique "...may reveal general metastases or a secondary nodule in the liver, thus rendering further procedures unnecessary and saving the patient a rather prolonged convalescence".[5] In the 1930's, Ruddock and Benedict extended the indications for diagnostic 'peritoneoscopy' and developed its clinical role in the evaluation of liver disease, ascites, and gastric, colorectal and gynecological malignancies.[6,7]

The concept of diagnostic laparoscopy was thus established and its continued evolution has been facilitated by technical advances such as improved instrumentation and the use of a second access port,[8] the use of CO_2 or O_2 instead of room air for the creation of a pneumoperitoneum,[9] and the development of the spring-loaded insufflation needle by Veress in 1938.[10] The development of forward-viewing optics, the Hopkins rod-lens optical system and the fiberoptic bundle to achieve enhanced light transmission[11,12] has lead to the development of contemporary videolaparoscopy systems providing high resolution laparoscopic images to multiple observers and enabling the findings to be recorded.[13]

GENERAL CONSIDERATIONS AND INDICATIONS

Until recently, diagnostic laparoscopy was used primarily by gynecologists and hepatologists, while its role in the evaluation of intra-abdominal malignancy was neglected by the majority of surgeons. However, the explosion of interest in minimal access surgery during the last decade, plus increasing recognition that laparoscopic inspection of the abdominal cavity provides an unrivalled opportunity to evaluate abdominal disease processes without resort to laparotomy, has renewed interest in diagnostic laparoscopy. Modern laparoscopic optics and light sources provide a magnified, high-resolution view of the peritoneal cavity which readily demonstrates intraperitoneal tumors, small quantities of malignant ascites and tiny metastatic lesions involving the peritoneum, omentum and liver. The clinical information yielded by laparoscopy is often able to address the limitations inherent in modern radiologic imaging techniques such as ultrasonography (US), computed tomography (CT), magnetic resonance imaging (MRI) and angiography, especially in the detection of disseminated 'minimal volume disease' within the abdominal cavity. Furthermore, the role of diagnostic laparoscopy in surgical oncology is enhanced by the opportunity for precise tissue sampling, improved imaging by laparoscopic ultrasonography (LapUS) and palliative laparoscopic bypass procedures. Thus, laparoscopy has become established firmly in the armamentarium of the general surgeon wishing to evaluate patients with suspected or established intra-abdominal malignancies.[14-16]

In this context, the indications for laparoscopy may be divided broadly between *diagnostic* and *staging* laparoscopy, although this distinction is often blurred in clinical practice. Diagnostic laparoscopy is usually performed to confirm or refute suspected intra-abdominal malignancy because of pain, a palpable mass, ascites or equivocal radiologic imaging signs. Staging laparoscopy is reserved for patients with an established diagnosis of malignancy in whom accurate tumor staging is important to define resectability and the appropriateness of adjuvant therapies.

Several studies testify to the contribution of laparoscopy in the management of patients with a variety of intra-abdominal malignancies encountered in general surgical practice. In Udwadia's series[17] of more than 2500 diagnostic laparoscopies, malignancy was confirmed in 215 of 507 patients (42%) with ascites, and in 177 of 181 patients (94%) with hepatomegaly. In Nagy and James' series,[18] abdominal malignancy was the indication for laparoscopy in 21 of 77 patients, of whom 14 (67%) were accurately assessed, thus averting laparotomy in 8 cases (38%). A recent audit by Cuschieri's team[15] revealed a "diagnostic yield" of 90%, "management benefit" of 30% and "management disadvantage" (i.e. understaging) in 4% of patients. This supported their earlier observation in 25 patients with suspected intra-abdominal malignant neoplasms where laparoscopy had confirmed the diagnosis in two-thirds of patients, with no known false negatives in the remainder.[19] Similarly, Schrenk et al.[20] performed laparoscopy in 33 patients presenting with suspected intra-abdominal malignancy and equivocal test results. They reported a diagnostic accuracy of 91%, and resorted to laparotomy in only 18% of cases. Hemming et al.[21] performed staging laparoscopy for a wide variety of intra-abdominal malignancies in 162 patients, obtaining information which prevented unnecessary laparotomy in 36% of cases and which was deemed to have been helpful in planning resection in another 30%.

The exact role of laparoscopy (and LapUS) in the evaluation of specific intra-abdominal malignancies continues to be evaluated. Its clinical impact is dependent upon the philosophy of the surgical team as regards the definition of resectability or operability, and also upon the availability of and expertise with other imaging modalities prevalent at individual institutions. Most work to date has focused on the preoperative evaluation of carcinoma of the pancreas and periampullary region, gastroesophageal carcinoma and primary and secondary liver malignancies.

PANCREATIC CANCER

The accurate diagnosis and staging of patients with suspected malignancy of the pancreas and periampullary region has long presented a clinical challenge because of its retroperitoneal location, its complex relationships with the peripancreatic blood vessels and viscera which are liable to local tumor invasion and the propensity of such lesions to have established occult intra-abdominal metastases at the time of presentation.[22] The dilemma is therefore to select reliably those patients for whom attempts at curative pancreatic resection are appropriate, while identifying those with factors which contraindicate surgery. The fallibility of modern radiologic imaging techniques in the assessment of pancreatic malignancy is well recognized, and reflected by reported non-therapeutic laparotomy rates of 12-39%.[23-26] The associated physical and psychological morbidity, and the cost-inefficiency of this strategy has led to increasing recognition that 'laparotomy and biopsy' is an unacceptable primary method of assessing such patients.[14] Furthermore, comparative studies have provided no evidence that surgical biliary bypass (with or without gastric drainage) should necessarily take precedence over biliary stent insertion in the palliation of malignant obstructive jaundice, which supports the rationale for nonoperative management in at least some patients with pancreatic malignancy.[25, 27-31]

Detection of metastatic disease

Laparoscopy has established an unique role in the preoperative assessment of patients with potentially resectable pancreatic cancers, mainly because of its sensitivity in detecting intra-abdominal metastases which are so prevalent in such cases (Figs 3.1 and 3.2, and Table 3.1).[32-41] Continuing on Bernheim's original theme (see above),[5] the utility of laparoscopy in this role has been supported by reports of the high prevalence of laparoscopically detected metastases in patients with pancreatic cancer.[32-34] In Cuschieri's experience, as well as the discovery of omental, serosal or liver metastases in 75% of patients, direct tumor invasion of adjacent organs (colon, mesocolon, duodenum and/or stomach) was detected in 21% of patients, and an overall histologic/cytologic diagnosis of pancreatic malignancy was achieved in 61 of 65 patients (92%).[32, 34] However, many of these patients had advanced tumors or pancreatic body cancers, and the relative absence of prior patient selection using less invasive imaging techniques diminishes the clinical impact of these findings. Subsequent work by Warshaw et al.[35, 36] suggested that truly unsuspected metastases had been apparent during laparoscopy in up to 41% of patients considered to be candidates for pancreatic resection on the basis of prior US and/or CT. Stepwise discriminant analysis confirmed the unique role played by staging laparoscopy in this context.[36] More recent experience with staging laparoscopy in Edinburgh[40, 42] and New York[41] has reproduced similar findings in 29-35% of patients who were otherwise thought to have 'curable' lesions (see Table 3.1).

Nevertheless, the concept of mandatory preoperative staging laparoscopy has failed to achieve widespread popularity in the management of patients with pancreatic cancer. A recent survey of national patterns of care for pancreatic cancer at 978 American institutions conducted by The Commission on Cancer of the American College of Surgeons reported that laparoscopy had been performed in only 6% of cases, a figure which had remained static between the

Table 3.1 – Staging laparoscopy and laparoscopic ultrasonography in the evaluation of pancreatic and periampullary cancer

Reference and year	Study details	Incidence of dissemination at laparoscopy (%)	Sensitivity for metastases (%)	Laparotomy avoided (%)
Cuschieri et al. [32,34] 1978-1988	n = 73 Lap only	75%	98%	30%
Ishida[33] 1983	n = 71 Lap only	43%	—	—
Warshaw et al.[35-37] 1988-1993	n = 86 Lap only	41%	96%	41%
John et al.[40] 1995	n = 40 Lap/LapUS vs US/CT	35%	83%	45%*
Bemelman et al.[38] 1995	n = 73 Lap vs US	23%	76%	17%*
Fernández-del Castillo et al.[39] 1995	n = 114 Lap vs CT/SVA	24%	93%	24%
Conlon et al.[41] 1996	n = 115 Lap vs US/CT	29%	75%**	36%
John et al (unpublished data)	n = 50 Lap/LapUS vs US/CT/SVA	30%	94%	38%*

Lap = laparoscopy; LapUS = laparoscopic ultrasonography; US = ultrasonography; CT = abdominal computerized tomography; SVA = selective visceral angiography; * includes LapUS findings; ** liver metastases only.

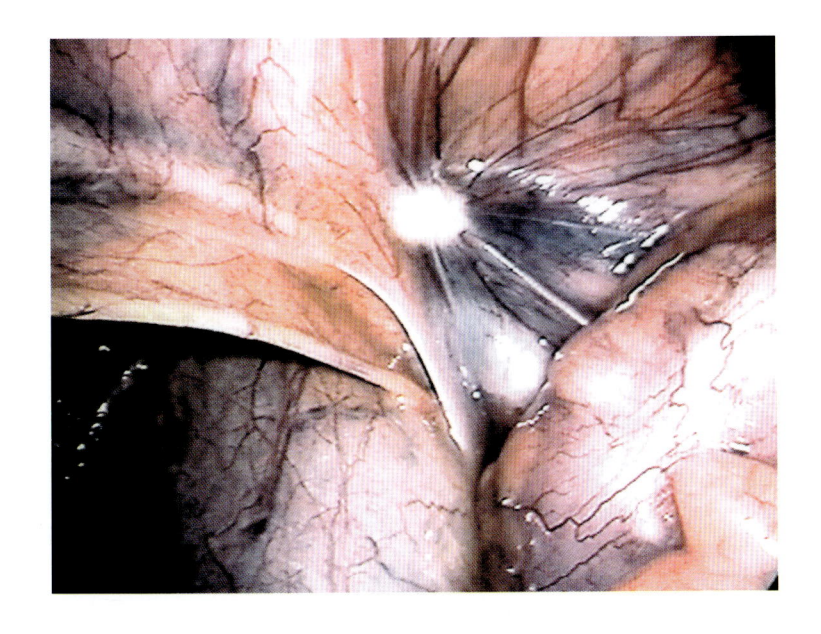

Figure 3.1 – Malignant peritoneal seedlings discovered during laparoscopy over the parietal peritoneum of the left inguinal region. Radiologic investigations had diagnosed a potentially resectable tumor of the periampullary region.

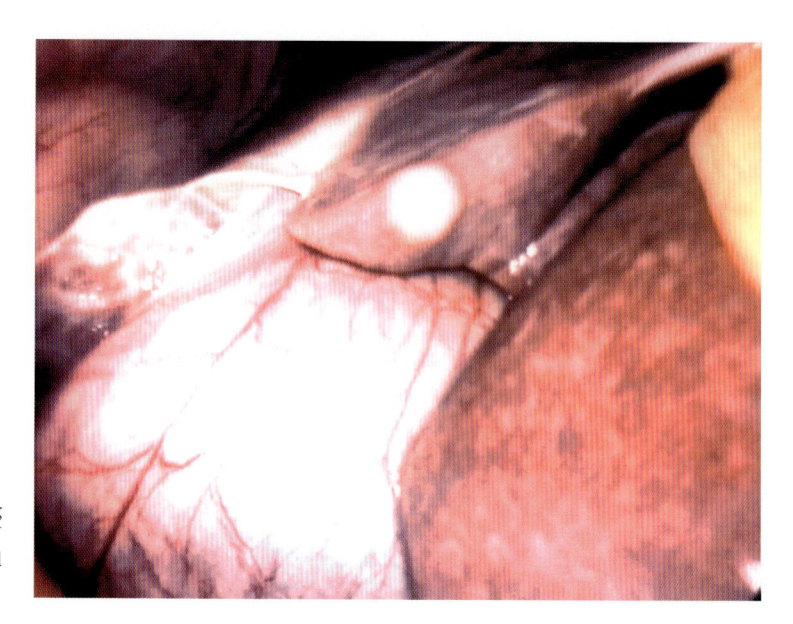

Figure 3.2 – Small liver metastasis arising from the capsule of hepatic segment IV within the umbilical fissure and discovered unexpectedly during staging laparoscopy.

1983-1985 period and 1990.[43] However, it seems unlikely that newer imaging modalities adopted in the assessment of pancreatic cancer such as endoscopic ultrasonography (EUS) and spiral CT scanning will address this apparent deficiency in preoperative staging. This has already been illustrated by Gmenwiesser et al.,[44] who documented the insensitivity of new generation helical CT technology in the detection of liver metastases in such patients.

Laparoscopic evaluation of locoregional disease

The retrogastric location of the pancreas, especially the pancreatic head, makes its examination difficult laparoscopically. The diagnosis of pancreatic malignancy during laparoscopy is therefore usually inferred by the presence of a retrogastric mass, and secondary signs such as the features of obstructive jaundice, ascites or metastases, and portal hypertension or splenomegaly due to underlying portal or splenic vein invasion (Fig. 3.3). Nevertheless, the feasibility of direct laparoscopic inspection of the pancreas by the techniques of 'supragastric pancreoscopy' (i.e. the pancreas is inspected through the intact gastrohepatic omentum[45]), 'supragastric bursoscopy' (i.e. the lesser sac is examined from within having incised the gastrohepatic omentum[46-48]) and 'infragastric bursoscopy' (i.e. the lesser sac is explored following incision of the gastrocolic omentum or mesocolon[32,49]) have all been reported. These techniques could also be used to facilitate laparoscopic biopsy of pancreatic masses under direct vision. Indeed, using the supragastric approach, Ishida[33] succesfully visualized tumors of the pancreatic body in 85% of cases, and established a laparoscopic-guided biopsy and/or cytologic diagnosis of pancreatic malignancy in 74% of pancreatic head tumors and 87.5% of body and tail tumors.

However, the success of supragastric pancreoscopy is dependent upon the quantity of fat in the lesser omentum, Meyer-Berg et al.[50] reported a success rate of only 60% using this approach. Furthermore, obliteration of the lesser sac with adhesions, inadequate access to the pancreatic head, and little available information regarding local tumor invasion of retroperitoneal structures were probable reasons for the failure of this approach to attain widespread acceptance as a viable method of evaluating pancreatic disease at a time when newer radiologic imaging techniques were gaining in popularity. Similarly, attempts to improve the diagnostic yield of laparoscopy in patients with suspected obstructive jaundice by laparoscopic cholecystcholangiography, where contrast radiography was performed following transhepatic needle puncture of the gallbladder, were rapidly superceded by techniques such as

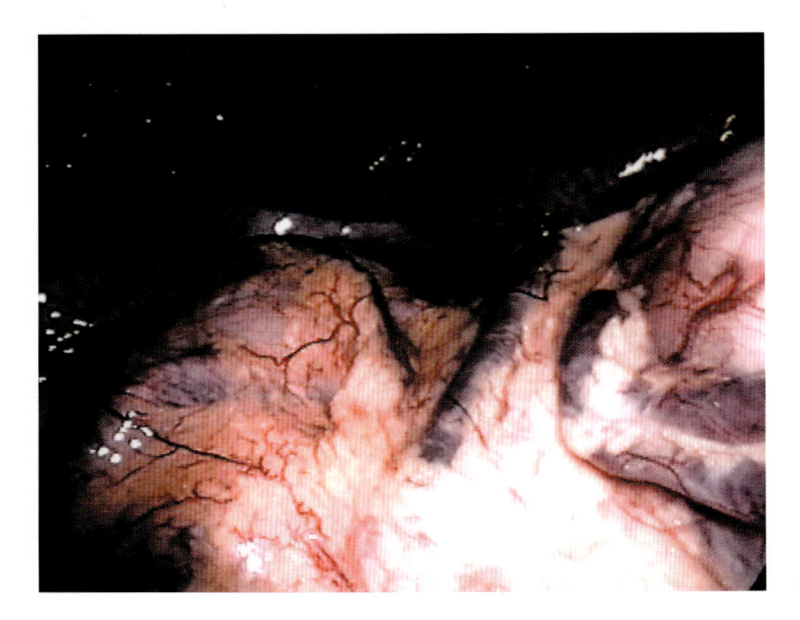

Figure 3.3 – Distended gastroepiploic veins and ascitic fluid in the region of the porta hepatis providing indirect evidence of portal vein invasion by carcinoma of the pancreatic head during staging laparoscopy.

percutaneous transhepatic and endoscopic retrograde cholangiography.[51,52] The limitations of laparoscopy in the evaluation of pancreatic lesions have been demonstrated by several studies where laparoscopy failed both to achieve a primary tumor diagnosis, and also to demonstrate local tumor invasion of structures such as the portal and superior mesenteric veins.[32,34-37,40,42] The role of laparoscopy alone in the staging of potentially resectable lesions in the head of the pancreas therefore appears limited.

Nevertheless, an endosurgical approach to the locoregional staging of potentially resectable peripancreatic malignancy, aiming to mimic open surgical exploration and trial dissection of tumor has been adopted by Conlon et al.[41] Using a four-port technique, maneuvres such as periportal lymph node biopsy, inspection of the mesenteric root and ligament of Treitz, and inspection of the lesser sac contents (caudate lobe, inferior vena cava and celiac axis) via the supragastric approach with biopsy of perigastric, portal and celiac nodes were performed following standard laparoscopic examination of the general peritoneal cavity. In addition to demonstrating extrapancreatic tumor spread in 29% of patients (Table 3.1), laparoscopic evidence of vascular invasion was obtained in 16 patients (15%). Ultimately, pancreatic resection was performed in 61 of the 67 patients considered potentially resectable following laparoscopic staging (i.e. a negative predictive value of 91%).[41] However, it remains to be seen whether such an invasive and time-consuming approach will be adopted widely as a prelude to exploratory laparotomy, especially following the development of relatively less intrusive techniques such as LapUS (see below).

Laparoscopic peritoneal cytology

Suggestions that cytological analysis of ascitic fluid or peritoneal washings might play an important role in the preoperative assessment of patients with pancreatic (and gastric) cancer,[53,54] both as a index of tumor resectability and as a determinant of prognosis, has stimulated interest in its role during laparoscopy. Furthermore, an association between positive peritoneal cytology and preceding operative tumor manipulation[53] or needle biopsy[54] has been hypothesized, implicating these maneuvres in the dissemination of malignant cells. However, the initially high reported incidence of positive peritoneal cytology of 25-30%[53, 54] has not been reproduced in several studies evaluating this technique during both laparotomy and laparoscopy where positive cytology rates of 7-17% have been reported (see Table 3.2).[39,55-58]

Table 3.2 – Summary of studies of peritoneal cytology in assessment of patients with pancreatic or periampullary carcinoma

Reference and year	Incidence of positive cytology (mode of retrieval)	Diagnostic accuracy in predicting unresectability
Martin et al.[53] 1986	5/20 = 25% (laparotomy)	Sensitivity = 28% Specificity = 100% PPV = 100% NPV = 13%
Warshaw[54] 1991	12/40 = 30% (laparoscopy 27) (laparotomy 13)	Sensitivity = 43% Specificity = 93% PPV = 90% NPV = 52%
Lei et al.[55] 1994	3/36 = 8% (laparotomy)	Sensitivity = 18% Specificity = 100% PPV = 100% NPV = 48%
Zerbi et al.[56] 1994	2/15 = 13% (laparotomy)	N/A
Fernández-del Castillo et al.[39] 1995	16/94 = 17% (laparoscopy)	N/A
Leach et al.[57] 1995	4/60 = 7% (laparoscopy 29) (laparotomy 31)	Sensitivity = 22% Specificity = 100% PPV = 100% NPV = 75%
John et al.[58] 1995	7/46 = 15% (laparoscopy)	Sensitivity = 21% Specificity = 100% PPV = 100% NPV = 33%

NPV = negative predictive value; PPV = positive predictive value; N/A = information not available.

Our experience in Edinburgh[58] with laparoscopic peritoneal cytology in the staging of patients with pancreatic and periampullary cancer is similar to that reported elsewhere.[55,57] Laparoscopic peritoneal cytology was insensitive in identifying patients with unresectable tumors (18-22%). Furthermore, this technique provided little information over that obtained by laparoscopic inspection of the peritoneal cavity, as all patients with positive cytology in our study also exhibited obvious signs of extrapancreatic tumor dissemination. It should be emphasized that none of the 49 patients with malignant peritoneal cytology reported in 7 studies (Table 3.2) had undergone curative pancreatic resection,[39,53-58] and such patients were found to have a significantly shortened survival.

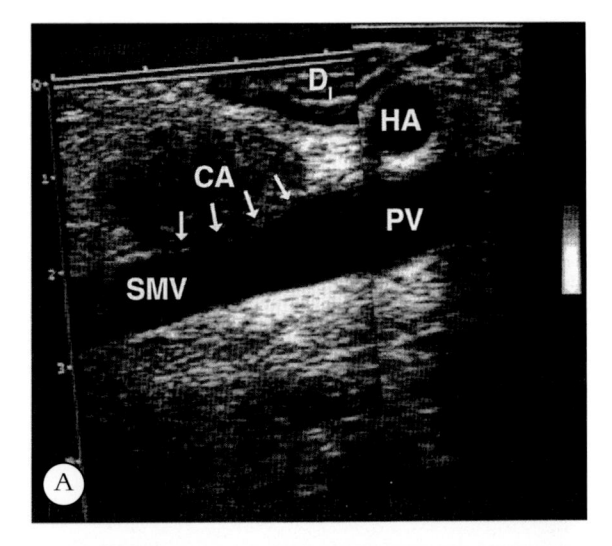

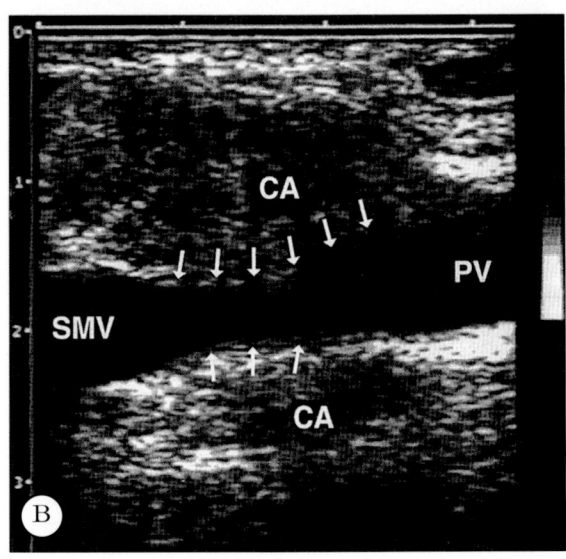

Figure 3.4 – Laparoscopic ultrasonography in the local staging of unresectable pancreatic cancer.
(A) Laparoscopic sonogram obtained in a parasagittal plane with the probe inserted via the umbilical port and transducer placed upon the pancreatic head. An hypoechoic carcinoma (CA) is shown extending into the pancreatic neck anterior to the superior mesenteric vein (SMV) and portal vein (PV). Loss of the hyperechoic interface between tumor and vein indicate local tumor infiltration (arrows). The tumor is clear of the common hepatic artery (HA) and first part of duodenum (D_1) at the superior pancreatic border. (B) Slight rotation of the probe shows the 'horseshoe' encroachment of the cancer posterior to the SMV.

Laparoscopic ultrasonography

Laparoscopic intraoperative ultrasonography (LapUS) utilizes the same principles as intraoperative ultrasonography (IOUS) and EUS during the laparoscopic examination. The fundamental advantage of LapUS compared with conventional transabdominal US derives from the placement of the ultrasound transducer in direct apposition with the intra-abdominal tissues. This maneuver permits the use of relatively high frequency transducers (7.5-10 MHz) which achieve correspondingly high image resolution, while minimizing the image degradation (or 'acoustic attenuation') experienced when scanning from outside the body wall due to the interposed body wall tissues, overlying viscera and bowel gas.

Early studies of LapUS used rather primitive 'A-mode' systems where the image consisted of a series of unidimensional spikes and which never found popularity in clinical practice. The forerunners of contemporary LapUS instruments were known as 'echolaparoscopes', incorporating B-mode scanners at the end of the laparoscopic telescope. In 1984 Okita et al.[59] in Japan reported their experience with prototype LapUS instruments which used an articulating 3.5-5 MHz linear array transducer at the flattened end of a 13 mm diameter laparoscope. They described the first successful application of LapUS imaging of a pancreatic carcinoma in a patient in whom CT, angiography and laparoscopy alone had been equivocal. Currently, LapUS is facilitated by the commercial availability of ultracompact, sterilizable probes with similar imaging specifications to contemporary high resolution IOUS systems, and which may be introduced through standard 10/11 mm diameter laparoscopic ports. Easily interpreted cross-sectional 'B-mode' images of the underlying tissues are generated in real-time and in fine detail.

In the evaluation of pancreatic malignancy, Lap US may be used to address some of the limitations of laparoscopy, such as detection of deep-seated intrahepatic metastases and regional lymph nodes, and demonstration of the primary tumor mass and its relationships with the peripancreatic vascular and ductal structures without resort to additional laparoscopic dissection (Figs 3.4 and 3.5). In this context, the impact of LapUS over laparoscopy was shown in a study of 38 patients considered to have potentially resectable tumors on the basis of US and/or CT.[40] Additional staging information (vascular invasion, regional lymphadenopathy, etc)

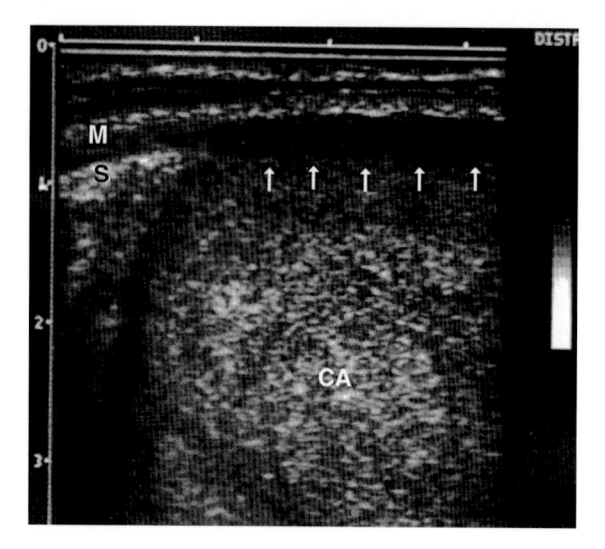

Figure 3.5 – Laparoscopic ultrasonography in the local staging of unresectable pancreatic cancer. A large isoechoic cancer of the pancreatic body (CA) is shown. The five echo layers of the posterior gastric wall lie anterior to the tumor. Local tumor invasion into the hypoechoic muscle layer (M) with loss of the hyperechoic plane defining the gastric serosa (S) is seen (arrows).

was obtained by LapUS in 20 patients (53%), whereas the clinical decision regarding tumor resectability was altered (i.e. upstaged) in 10 patients (25%). Laparoscopy combined with LapUS was more sensitive and accurate than laparoscopy alone in identifying tumor unresectability (88% and 89% versus 50% and 65%, respectively).[40]

Bemelman et al[38] also reported the efficacy of staging laparoscopy with LapUS in 70 patients with pancreatic cancer who had been considered to have potentially curable stage I disease following pre-operative endoscopic cholangiopancreatography (ERCP) and Doppler US. Laparotomy was avoided in 19% of patients due to the detection of liver, peritoneal and lymph node metastases, and the diagnosis of liver metastases was solely attributed to LapUS in 6 of 16 proven cases (38%). The preoperative stage was changed in 41% of patients examined, the therapeutic strategy was modified in 18 cases (25%) and the diagnostic accuracy of LapUS in predicting local tumor ingrowth was validated by surgical exploration. Vascular invasion was identified accurately by LapUS, with one false positive demonstrated following portal vein resection in a patient with local fibrosis due to previous irradiation (96% specificity; 93% positive predictive value).[38] However, histopathologic validation of resection margins revealed that despite the adoption of staging LapUS, underestimation of local tumor stage still occurred as reflected by a 59% sensitivity and 74% negative predictive value.

Similarly, stringent surgical and histopathologic validation of the TNM staging of pancreatic and periampullary cancer by laparoscopy with LapUS was performed in 50 patients in a recent study in Edinburgh, and the results compared with US, dynamic CT and angiography (unpublished data). Again, laparoscopic staging was significantly superior to the other three investigations in detecting intra-abdominal metastases (94% versus 29%, 33% and 0%, respectively). However, unlike the experience of Bemelman et al.,[38] the contribution of LapUS in detecting liver metastases which had not been seen during laparoscopy was marginal. Although exploration of the lesser sac was not attempted, and the laparoscopic diagnosis of pancreatic tumor never established, LapUS was at least as sensitive (96%) in imaging the primary lesion compared with the other modalities (82% US; 93% CT; 66% angiography).

Laparoscopic ultrasonography was at least as sensitive as Doppler US, CT and angiography in identifying locoregional invasion, although underestimation of T stage was encountered with all modalities (sensitivities of 68% versus 60%, 71% and 67%, respectively). Importantly, however, LapUS did not overstage local tumor invasion in the same way as the other modalities, as reflected by its specificity and positive predictive value of 100%. Unfortunately, in common with all other radiologic techniques, there are no reliable LapUS criteria for the diagnosis of regional malignant lymphadenopathy, and based upon node size alone N staging was found to be innacurate.

It may be concluded that sufficient evidence exists to justify routine preoperative laparoscopy in patients with suspected resectable peripancreatic malignancy based on its unique role in identifying occult intra-abdominal metastases. Laparoscopic ultrasonography may improve the locoregional evaluation of the primary tumor, although it is still fallible in defining soft tissue invasion and node staging. The morbidity of the technique is very low and consists of the occasional concealed port-site hemorrhage, minor wound infection and anecdotal reports of malignant port-site seeding (2 cases of which have been witnessed by the authors in patients with advanced peritoneal carcinomatosis).[60-63] A rationalized investigative algorithm based upon LapUS is

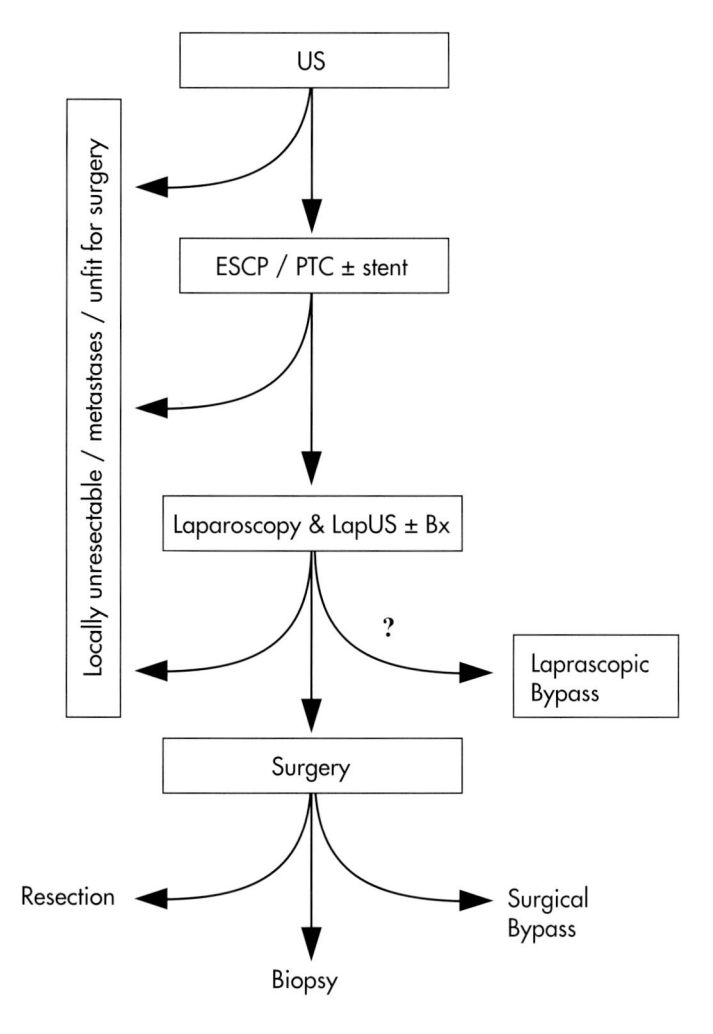

Figure 3.6 – Proposed algorithm for the investigation of patients with malignant obstructive jaundice utilizing laparoscopy with laparoscopic ultrasonography. USS = transabdominal ultrasonography; ERCP = endoscopic retrograde cholangiopancreatography; PTC = percutaneous transhepatic cholangiography; LapUS = laparoscopic ultrasonography; Bx = laparoscopic/LapUS-guided biopsy.

proposed for surgical laparoscopists who are enthusiastic about acquiring the appropriate skills (Fig. 3.6). Having established the likely diagnosis of distal bile duct obstruction or a pancreatic head mass with transabdominal US and/or ERCP, definitive tumor staging is performed with laparoscopy and LapUS, which may also provide the opportunity to obtain a tissue diagnosis and perform palliative laparoscopic biliary and/or duodenal bypass surgery.

GASTROESOPHAGEAL CANCER

Reference to the use of laparoscopy in the preoperative assessment of patients with esophageal cancer first appeared in the 1970's Russian literature.[64] The rationale for staging laparoscopy in gastroesophageal malignancy derives from its high sensitivity in detecting small metastases to the liver and serosal

Table 3.3 – Staging laparoscopy in the evaluation of gastroesophageal cancer

Reference and year	Study details	Incidence of dissemination at laparoscopy (%)	Sensitivity for metastases (%)	Laparotomy avoided (%)
Gross et al.[69] 1984	GC n = 46 Lap only	48†	100	52
Shandall and Johnson[70] 1985	GC & OC n = 37 Lap vs US/RIS	27* 14** 32***	96	54
Dagnini et al.[71] 1986	OC n = 369 Lap only	10* 7**	97	45
Possik et al.[72] 1986	GC n = 360 Lap vs US/RIS	16* 31** 45***	87* 83** 53***	34
Kriplani and Kapur[73] 1991	GC n = 40 Lap only	40	92	40
Bemelman et al.[74] 1995	OC n = 56 Lap/LapUS	9	83	5
Molloy et al.[75] 1995 see also[76]	OC n = 244 Lap vs US/CT	38†	96	42
Anderson et al.[77] 1996	OC & GC n = 44 LapUS vs US/CT	14†	83	16
Lowy et al.[78] 1996	GC n = 71 Lap vs CT	23 4* 25**	84 33* 94**	25
Finch et al.[79] 1997	OC & GC n = 26 Lap / LapUS vs CT	12	75	19

Lap = laparoscopy; LapUS = laparoscopic ultrasonography; US = ultrasonography; RIS = radioisotope scintigraphy; GC = gastric cancer; OC = cancer of the esophagus and gastric cardia; * liver metastases; ** peritoneal metastases; *** nodal metastases; † includes patients with locally advanced tumor.

surfaces, and its utility in demonstrating tumor invasion of adjacent organs and regional lymphadenopathy. The shortcomings of conventional radiologic techniques in this regard (particularly abdominal CT scanning) are well recognized.[65-67] The delayed discovery of disseminated tumor at exploratory laparotomy may preclude even palliative gastroesophageal resections, and avoidance of the implicit morbidity of unnecessary surgery remains an important goal in the management of such patients. Indeed, the incidence of laparotomy alone (with no resection or palliation) was 16.5% in a recent survey of 10 999 gastric cancer patients by the American College of Surgeons.[68] Although EUS has shown promise in refining the locoregional staging of gastroesphageal cancer, this technique has contributed little to the detection of distant abdominal metastases and has yet to achieve a significant impact on unnecessary laparotomy rates.

Studies which have investigated staging laparoscopy in the evaluation of carcinoma of the stomach, gastric cardia and/or esophagus are summarized in Table 3.3.[69-79] All testify to the sensitivity of laparoscopy in the detection and biopsy of intrabdominal metastases. Furthermore, Shandall and Johnson[70] and Possik et al.[72] reported the utility of laparoscopy in identifying malignant regional lymphadenopathy in 32-45% of patients. The lower yield of metastatic disease at laparoscopy (9-14%) reported in more recent studies[74,77,79] may reflect improved radiologic staging and patient selection prior to laparoscopy. Technical pitfalls such as failure to identify metastases concealed by adhesions or situated within the lesser sac also contribute to the false negative rate in most studies of laparoscopic staging. Nevertheless, unnecessary laparotomy was averted on the basis of laparoscopic findings in 16-54% of patients,[69-73,75-79] although the experience of Bemelman et al.[74] differed from this consensus. They ascribed little value to laparoscopic staging in patients with carcinoma of the middle and lower esophagus (albeit not neccessarily in those with tumors of the gastric cardia), although problems with obtaining representative laparoscopic tissue samples may have contributed to the diminished yield in their study.[74]

The role of laparoscopy in the locoregional staging of gastroesophageal cancer is less well defined. Tumor extension through the serosa of the anterior stomach wall and gross malignant invasion of adjacent structures such as the liver, colon, diaphragm and abdominal wall may be apparent during laparoscopic inspection.[69,72,74,75,77] However, demonstration of more subtle features of tumor advancement such as posterior invasion of the pancreas, 'lateral' intramural tumor spread and paraaortic lymphadenopathy may require a more invasive laparoscopic approach including exploration of the lesser sac. The advent of LapUS provides a less intrusive means of addressing the limitations of laparoscopy in the imaging of such concealed areas.[80]

The high resolution sonographic appearance of the wall of the gastrointestinal tract defines five distinct echo layers: 1) serosa-transducer interface (hyperechoic); 2) muscularis (hypoechoic); 3) submucosa (hyperechoic); 4) lamina propria (hypoechoic); and 5) mucosa (hyperechoic). Tumors appear as hypoechoic masses which disrupt this normal echo structure, and the T stage may by estimated by observing the extent to which the tumor invades these echo layers.[80] An assessment of the integrity of the hyperechoic plane separating the stomach and pancreas is of particular importance during staging LapUS as its obliteration by tumor ingrowth may indicate an unresectable T4 tumor (see also Fig. 3.5). However, cases of both overstaging and understaging of gastric and pancreatic cancers have been observed during LapUS and EUS,[79,81] and further experience is required before patients are denied operative assessment on the basis of this feature alone. An evaluation of intramural tumor extension may also be achieved during LapUS, paying particular attention to the gastroesophageal junction and its involvement with the tumor.[79] Such an approach may facilitate planning of the extent of resectional surgery.

Preliminary experience with staging LapUS in Edinburgh has shown it to be significantly more accurate in the overall TNM staging of gastroesophageal cancer compared with laparoscopy alone or abdominal CT.[79] More specifically, the impact of LapUS on staging laparoscopy was to reduce the false negative rate for T staging from 42% to 8%. These data reproduce those of Anderson et al.[77] who reported LapUS to be significantly more accurate than both abdominal CT and US in the T staging of upper gastrointestinal malignancies. Bartlett et al.[81] reported the utility of LapUS in defining accurately the T stage of gastric cancer where preceding investigations (CT and EUS) had overstaged local tumor spread with respect to invasion of the pancreas. This tendency for local tumor overstaging by CT is a cause for concern, and the role of LapUS in confirming or refuting such results was highlighted in a comparative study of CT and LapUS performed in Edinburgh.[79]

Laparoscopic ultrasonography facilitates the laparoscopic assessment of regional lymph node stage by demonstrating the size, site, shape and echogenicity of nodes in relatively inaccessible sites. Although lymph node staging with EUS and LapUS continues to evolve, and biopsy confirmation is still recommended in equivocal cases, sonographic features of malignant lymphadenopathy have been documented. In general, nodes which are more than 10 mm in diameter, spherical (rather than ovoid), hypoechoic and well-circumscribed (rather than hyperechoic and 'fuzzy') tend to characterize metastatic involvement.[82] Using these criteria, Finch et al.[79] reported LapUS to have improved the diagnostic accuracy of N staging compared with laparoscopy alone and CT (92% versus 84% versus 70%), whereas Anderson et al.[77] reported similar findings for laparoscopy/LapUS compared with CT (91% versus 62%). Nevertheless, the fallibility of all imaging modalities in identifying node metastases must be emphasized, and this highlights the desirability for the incorporation of guided fine-needle biopsy systems during LapUS (and EUS).

CHOLANGIOCARCINOMA AND GALLBLADDER CANCER

The pitfalls of evaluating malignancies of the biliary tree are well recognized as gallbladder carcinoma and proximal bile duct carcinomas may be very difficult to distinguish, locoregional staging without resort to laparotomy may be equivocal or misleading and a definitive tissue diagnosis may prove elusive. Although a combination of US and abdominal CT may demonstrate diffuse thickening of the wall or a mass in half of all patients,[83] both techniques have poor sensitivity in defining a gallbladder mass, as reflected by its frequent discovery during or after cholecystectomy for presumed benign disease. While angiography and cholangiography have become fundamental to the staging of biliary malignancies, the role of laparoscopy remains less certain, perhaps reflecting the apparent predilection of gallbladder carcinoma for port-site seeding.[62,84]

Nevertheless, the sensitivity of laparoscopy in establishing a diagnosis and demonstrating the intra-abdominal metastases of gallbladder carcinoma has been established by Daginini et al.[85] Kriplani et al.[86] provided further justification for this role in their study comparing laparoscopy with transabdominal US in 53 patients with suspected tumor cancer. The diagnostic sensitivity of laparoscopy was superior to that of US (96% versus 63%), and the specificity of laparoscopy was illustrated by its exclusion of gallbladder malignancy in 5 patients in whom equivocal findings had previously been observed. The unique role of staging laparoscopy was again highlighted by its superior sensitivity (95% versus 51%) in demonstrating intra-abdominal metastases which had been present in 41 patients (77%). The combination of US and laparoscopy resulted in 40 patients avoiding unnecessary laparotomy (75%), while 5 of 6 patients were correctly identified as being suitable for resectional surgery.[86] This investigative approach was therefore recommended for the evaluation of suspected gallbladder cancer, although no comparison with CT has been performed.

In the evaluation of biliary malignancy, LapUS seems well suited to the demonstration of small tumor masses, intrahepatic tumor invasion, regional lymphadenopathy and invasion of the hepatic arteries, portal veins and secondary biliary radicles. However, the inevitable presence of biliary stents, pneumobilia or gross intrahepatic biliary dilatation may diminish its impact. While the results of our prospective evaluation of biliary malignancy with laparoscopy and LapUS are awaited, the initial clinical impression is that the yield of LapUS in the locoregional staging of such tumors is not as beneficial as in patients with distal bile duct tumors and pancreatic malignancies. Although it is an attractive concept, speculation that the routine adoption of LapUS during laparoscopic cholecystectomy might identify early gallbladder carcinomas and so prevent inappropriate intervention (with the possible sequelae of distant dissemination) currently lacks any supporting evidence.

PRIMARY AND SECONDARY LIVER TUMORS

The utility of laparoscopy in the diagnosis of liver malignancy is well established. Although dependent on the absence of adhesions, most of the liver surface can be inspected laparoscopically. Recognition of liver tumors during laparoscopy requires that the tumor encroaches upon the liver surface or that its contour is distorted by the intrahepatic lesion. At least two-thirds of intrahepatic tumors may be detected laparoscopically and are amenable to laparoscopically directed needle biopsy. However, the fallibility of laparoscopy in detecting some deep-seated intrahepatic lesions was illustrated by Bleiberg et al.[87] who reported that 36% of negative laparoscopies performed in the staging of cancer patients had failed to demonstrate hepatic involvement subsequently confirmed at autopsy. In a series of 50 consecutive laparoscopic examinations in patients with suspected primary and secondary hepatic malignancies, direct visualization of the reference liver tumor was achieved in 34 patients (68%).[88]

The sensitivity of modern laparoscopic instruments in detecting tiny superficial and capsular liver lesions representing metastatic tumor deposits from distant primary sites, and beyond the threshold of detection by alternative modalities, has already been emphasized in the context of pancreatic, gastroesophageal and gallbladder malignancy. This principle is further illustrated by a series of diverse reports documenting the utility of diagnostic and staging laparoscopy in the assessment of patients with bronchogenic carcinoma,[89] ovarian tumors,[90] breast carcinoma,[91] malignant melanoma,[92] and lymphoma,[93, 94] without resort to laparotomy. The limitations of radiologic imaging techniques in demonstrating the subtle changes associated with diffuse liver abnormalities such as cirrhosis, fibrosis and steatosis are well recognized, although the fundamental contribution of diagnostic laparoscopy in this role has long been recognized by hepatologists.

Paradoxically, the deployment of laparoscopy as a preoperative staging tool in the selection of patients with known hepatic malignancy for liver resection has failed to find popularity. Most liver surgeons would regard as unresectable patients with primary or secondary liver tumors with evidence of extrahepatic or bilobar spread, or involvement of the major vascular trunks. There is no evidence that palliative surgery has anything to offer such patients, and avoidance of unnecessary laparotomy should be central to their management. This was highlighted by Lefor et al.[95] who reported the unexpected discovery of extrahepatic tumor spread at laparotomy in 28 of 107 patients (26%) considered to have potentially resectable colorectal liver metastases following abdominal CT scanning.

However, there is good evidence supporting preoperative staging laparoscopy in patients with liver tumors. Lightdale[96] performed laparoscopy in 16 patients with potentially resectable hepatocellular carcinoma, and discovered factors contraindicating surgery in 13 (80%) due to multifocal intrahepatic tumor spread, malignant peritoneal dissemination and/or coexisting severe cirrhosis. Similarly, Jeffers et al.[97] excluded from exploratory laparotomy a consecutive series of 27 patients with hepatocellular carcinoma following the laparoscopic discovery of similar findings. Brady et al.[98] performed diagnostic laparoscopy in 25 patients with suspected liver disease and negative CT scans and reported hepatic and/or peritoneal malignancy in 12 patients, as well as previously unsuspected cirrhosis in three. Babineau et al.[99] used staging laparoscopy to demonstrate factors contraindicating attempts at liver resection in 14 of 29 such patients (48%). Our experience in Edinburgh comprises a series of 50 patients with a variety of suspected liver tumors (colorectal liver metastases in 28 cases) otherwise considered potential candidates for liver resection. Laparoscopy revealed previously unsuspected factors contraindicating further operative intervention (extrahepatic dissemination (18 patients) and/or bilobar disease (11 patients)) in 23 patients (46%).[88]

Laparoscopic ultrasonography

As discussed above, laparoscopy alone fails to detect liver tumors in the remaining one-third of patients who have intrahepatic lesions situated away from the visible organ surface, and in those in whom the liver is partially obscured by adhesions. Also, the relative absence of anatomical markings on the liver surface hinders the laparoscopist's ability to determine the precise relationships between liver tumors and intrahepatic vascular structures. Intraoperative US has been an integral part of the development of liver surgery in recent years, facilitating the documentation of the site, size and number of liver tumors, and their pattern of involvement with respect to the segmental hepatic anatomy. Laparoscopic US can now exploit these principles during diagnostic and staging laparoscopy.

The first large series of LapUS examinations of the liver was reported by Furukawa et al.[100] who used a 360° sector scanning probe inserted through a separate port from the camera. They attributed 'diagnostic value' to 36 of 42 patients (86%) with a variety of liver tumors (and also described its use in localizing liver cysts). However, the limitations of radial scanning LapUS transducer designs in the laparoscopic evaluation of the liver was later highlighted by Fornari et al.[101] who reported their experience with a prototype 180° sector scanning LapUS probe. Problems were encountered in the detection of lesions in the posterolateral hepatic sector, in achieving adequate tissue penetration and in the ease of orientating the image with respect to the intrahepatic vasculature. Using a more sophisticated linear array probe design Okita et al.[59] described the utility of LapUS in imaging focal hepatocellular carcinoma within cirrhotic liver and venous invasion by tumor thrombus. The technique was later used to facilitate guided needle biopsy of laparoscopically invisible intrahepatic lesions.[102,103] In Edinburgh in 1991, an improvised LapUS system was devised for examination of the liver utilising a 16 mm diameter linear array endorectal ultrasound probe, and its clinical value in the assessment of hepatic malignancy reported.[104] Additional diagnostic information was obtained in 7 patients with liver tumors who had previously undergone CT scans, US and/or angiography, and LapUS was solely responsible for showing bilobar spread and/or portal vein invasion in 4 patients.

LapUS in a cohort of 43 patients undergoing preoperative staging laparoscopy yielded additional staging information in 18 of 43 patients examined (42%) (bilobar or multifocal liver tumor, hilar lymphadenopathy and main portal or hepatic venous invasion).[88] When compared with historical control patients at our hospital in whom no attempt at laparoscopic staging had been made, a significant increase in tumor resectability (58% versus 93%) was observed for the latter group of patients who had been evaluated using laparoscopy with LapUS.[88]

Further evidence supporting the unique role of staging laparoscopy in this context was recently provided by direct comparison with CT arterioportography (CTAP) in 37 patients with colorectal liver metastases.[105] Laparoscopy detected extrahepatic and bilobar tumor spread in 10 patients (27%), although the actual benefit attributable to LapUS was more marginal inasmuch as upstaging of disease occurred in just 3 of 37 patients (8%). However, it should be emphasized that false positive CTAP findings ('bilobar lesions and portal vein invasion') occurred in 6 of 37 patients (16%), all of which were refuted by laparoscopy with LapUS.

A further indication for LapUS which may find popularity is in the detection of occult hepatic metastases during laparoscopic resections of bowel malignancies. Accurate tumor staging at the time of the primary tumor resection has profound implications for the prognosis and continuing management of the patient with large bowel cancer. The early detection of occult liver metastases is important if informed decisions are to be made regarding the appropriateness of additional regional or systemic therapies, and such variables may affect the outcome of clinical trials evaluating both novel surgical procedures and regimens of adjuvant therapy. The rationale for the deployment of LapUS in this role is reflected by the utility of IOUS combined with operative palpation of the liver as the most sensitive staging procedure in the detection of occult hepatic metastases during laparotomy. This strategy seems destined to supplant the surgeon's palpating hand as a method of assessing the abdominal organs during minimal access colorectal cancer operations, and studies of the use of LapUS in this context are awaited.

Laparoscopic liver biopsy

Laparoscopic liver biopsy is indicated to resolve instances of diagnostic doubt, during staging laparoscopy when clinical management may be affected by the result and in the presence of diffuse parenchymal liver diseases such as steatosis, hepatitis and cirrhosis (especially when this may affect the resectability of hepatocellular carcinoma).

However, restraint should be exercised when contemplating biopsy of focal liver lesions. Biopsy of potentially resectable liver tumors is contraindicated because of the risk of malignant seeding into the peritoneal cavity, to the port site or to the needle track. This well described complication should be regarded as an avoidable catastrophe.[47,62,106-109] When focal liver tumors have been shown to occupy an anatomically resectable location, exploratory laparotomy is warranted with a view to liver resection, and histologic proof of malignancy is rarely, if ever, required. The biochemical, radiologic and/or laparoscopic findings and the clinical context of the case are usually sufficient under such circumstances.

The benefits of laparoscopic liver biopsy over blind percutaneous biopsy in patients with hepatic malignancy are well established, the positive yield of a single random percutaneous liver biopsy being less than 50%. More recently, the evolution of radiologic imaging techniques has challenged the role of laparoscopy as a means of obtaining guided-biopsy specimens,[110] and studies have failed to show a significant advantage for laparoscopy compared with scan-guided biopsy in diagnosing focal hepatic lesions. Fornari et al.[111] compared US-guided fine-needle aspiration cytology with laparoscopic-guided biopsy using core-cutting needles in 63 patients, and found no significant differences with respect to sensitivity and accuracy (76% versus 74%, and 84% versus 83%, respectively). Nevertheless, these results do not detract from the role of laparoscopy in providing additional information which may alter the surgical decision-making process.

TECHNICAL CONSIDERATIONS

Some surgeons recommend performing laparoscopy under local anesthesia as a day case, or as a prelude to a planned exploratory laparotomy under the same general anesthetic. However, it is the authors' preference to perform diagnostic and staging laparoscopy with LapUS as a separate operative procedure under general anesthesia, and we believe that the increased yield of diagnostic and staging information, and health economic factors, justify this approach. A second 10/11 mm diameter port is inserted, usually in the right flank, allowing the laparoscope and LapUS probe to be alternated.

A meticulous and systematic inspection of the peritoneal cavity is performed, utilizing the table tilt mechanism and probe to displace the omentum and bowel loops, ensuring that areas such as the pelvis, paracolic gutters and undersurface of the left hepatic lobe are not neglected. A 30° telescope is important to ensure adequate inspection of the dome of the liver, the subphrenic spaces and the anterior abdominal wall. Additional ports may be inserted to permit retraction of the stomach and transverse colon to facilitate inspection of the mesenteric root and to permit dissection of the gastrocolic or gastrohepatic omenta if formal exploration of the lesser sac is desired. Any abnormal or suspicious areas should be biopsied using standard laparoscopic scissors, cup biopsy forceps or toothed forceps. Exploratory laparotomy should never be denied to a patient on the basis of laparoscopic appearances alone, as granulomas, fibrotic areas, hamartomatous lesions and von Meyenburg's complexes commonly masquerade as metastases, especially on the hepatic capsule following the relief of obstructive jaundice.

Laparoscopic ultrasonography is performed alternately via both ports, gently sweeping, rotating and advancing the probe over the surface of the liver, hepatoduodenal ligament, stomach, duodenum and pancreatic head. In this way, detail regarding diffuse and focal abnormalities of the liver, gallbladder, common bile duct, lymph nodes of the paraaortic, celiac, portocaval and peripancreatic regions, pancreas and portal, superior mesenteric and splenic veins and arteries may be observed (Figs 3.4 and 3.5).[112,113] Until LapUS probes equipped with guided needle biopsy channels become available, laparoscopic and LapUS-guided needle biopsy must be performed by the free-hand technique through a separate needle puncture.[114]

LAPAROSCOPY FOR 'SECOND-LOOK' PROCEDURES

A putative case for laparoscopy in the evaluation of recurrent intra-abdominal malignancy has been made by some surgeons who would consider performing repeat tumor resections, an aggressive philosophy which would otherwise necessitate multiple laparotomies.[115] This concept has been considered mainly in the context of ovarian cancer, but has also been considered for colorectal cancer. The obvious limitation of laparoscopy under such circumstances is the adhesive obliteration and anatomical distortion frequently encountered following previous operations. Nevertheless, Marti-Vicente et al.[116] demonstrated the feasibility of this approach, performing 44 second-look and 28 third-look laparoscopies among a total of 205 staging laparoscopies for ovarian cancer. This technique was succesful in averting unnecessary second-look laparotomies due to the discovery of residual tumor in nearly half of such patients. Rosenhoff et al.[90] emphasized the utility of laparoscopy in obtaining good views of the upper abdominal cavity in patients previously operated for ovarian cancer, documenting metastatic spread in the subphrenic spaces in 77% of such patients. Canis et al.[117] reported their preliminary experience with second-look laparoscopy in 13 of 33 patients with previously treated ovarian cancer. Their retrospective analysis suggested a similar prognosis for patients who had undergone a negative examination, whether performed by laparoscopy or laparotomy, thus providing further support for the role of laparoscopy. However, a substantial false negative rate must be regarded as inevitable in such demanding circumstances, and this highlights the importance of obtaining widespread biopsy samples, including random samples from apparently normal areas of peritoneum.

Apart from staging laparoscopy in patients with potentially resectable hepatic metastases (see above), the case for second-look laparoscopy in the context of colorectal and other gastrointestinal cancers is even more controversial and is supported by little evidence. Nevertheless, some support for the feasibility of achieving laparoscopic access to the peritoneal cavity in such patients was provided by our experience of attempted laparoscopy in 52 patients with suspected liver tumors.[88] Although previous abdominal tumor resections had been undertaken in over three-quarters of these patients (usually proctocolectomies), laparoscopic access to the peritoneal cavity affording adequate views of the liver was achieved in 96% of cases with negligible morbidity. This reflects a routine policy of direct cutdown to the peritoneal cavity as a prelude to all laparoscopies, followed by careful adhesiolysis. Hemming et al.[21] reported success in documenting peritoneal recurrence of colorectal cancer in 2 of 3 laparoscopies in patients with rising tumor markers and normal radiologic investigations. Salky et al.[118] also attempted second-look laparoscopy in 7 patients with suspected recurrent colonic carcinoma, observing a positive yield in 1 with liver metastases, and avoiding surgery in all but 2. However, more work is clearly required in this area before such an approach can be supported.

REFERENCES

1. Kelling G. Zur Colioskopie und Gastroskopie. *Archive Klinische Chirurgie* 1923; **126**: 226-229.
2. Ott D. Die direkte Beluchtung der Bauchole, der Harnblase des Dickdarmes und des Uterous zu diagnostichen zwecken. *Rev Med Tcheu* 1909; **2**:27.
3. Gunning JE. The history of laparosocopy. *J Reprod Med* 1974; **12**: 223-231.
4. Jacobeus HC. Kurze Ubersicht uber meine Erfahrungen mit der Laparo-Thoracoskopie. *Münchener Medizinische Wochenschrift* 1911; **58**: 2017-2019.
5. Bernheim B. Organoscopy: cystoscopy of the abdominal cavity. *Ann Surg* 1911; **53**: 764-767.
6. Ruddock JC. Peritoneoscopy. *Surg Gynecol Obstet* 1937;**65**:523-539.
7. Benedict EB. Peritoneoscopy. *N Engl J Med* 1938;**218**:713-714.
8. Kalk H. Erfahrungen mit der Laparoskopie. *Zeitschrift Klinische Medezin* 1929;**111**: 303-348.
9. Fervers C. Die Laparoskopie mit dem Zystoscop. *Medizinische Klinik* 1933;**29**:1042-1045.
10. Veress J. Neues Instrument zur Ausführung von Brust oder Bauchpunktionen undPneumothoraxbehandlung. *Deutsche Medizinische Wochenschrift* 1938;**64**:1480-1481.
11. Berci G, Kont LA. A new optical system in endoscopy with special reference to cystoscopy. *Br J Urol* 1969;**41**:564.
12. Berci G, Shore JM, Panish J, Morgenstern L. The evaluation of a new peritoneoscope as a diagnostic aid to the surgeon. *Ann Surg* 1973;**178**:37-44.
13. Nezhat C. Videolaseroscopy: a new modality for the treatment of endometriosis and other diseases of reproductive organs. *Colposc Gynecol Laser Surg* 1986;**2**:221-224.
14. Cuesta MA, Meijer S, Borgstein PJ. Laparoscopy and the assessment of digestive tract cancer. *Br J Surg* 1992;**79**:486-487.
15. Cuschieri A. Diagnosis and staging of tumors by laparoscopy. *Sem Lap Surg* 1994;**1**: 3-12.
16. John TG, Garden OJ. Laparoscopic ultrasound: extending the scope of diagnostic laparoscopy. *Br J Surg* 1994;**81**:5-6.
17. Udwadia TE. Peritoneoscopy for surgeons. *Ann Roy Coll Surg Engl* 1986;**68**:125-129.
18. Nagy AG, James D. Diagnostic laparoscopy. *Am J Surg* 1989;**157**:490-493.
19. Easter DW, Cuschieri A, Nathanson LK, Lavelle-Jones M. The utility of diagnostic laparoscopy for abdominal disorders. *Arch Surg* 1992;**127**:379-383.
20. Schrenk P, Woisetschläger R, Wayand WU, Rieger R, Sulzbacher H. Diagnostic laparoscopy: a survey of 92 patients. *Am J Surg* 1994;**168**:348-351.
21. Hemming AW, Nagy AG, Scudamore CH, Edelman K. Laparoscopic staging of intra-abdominal malignancy. *Surg Endosc* 1995;**9**:325-328.
22. Weiss SM, Skibber JM, Mohiuddin M, Rosato FE. Rapid intra-abdominal spread of pancreatic cancer. *Arch Surg* 1985;**120**:415-416.
23. Gudjonsson B. Cancer of the pancreas. *Cancer* 1987;**60**:2284-2303.
24. de Rooij PD, Rogatko A, Brennan MF. Evaluation of palliative surgical procedures in unresectable pancreatic cancer. *Br J Surg* 1991;**78**:1053-1058.
25. Watanapa P, Williamson RCN. Surgical palliation for pancreatic cancer: developments during the past two decades. *Br J Surg* 1992;**79**:8-20.
26. Bramhall SR, Allum WH, Jones AG, Allwood A,

Cummins C, Neoptolemos JP. Treatment and survival in 13 560 patients with pancreatic cancer, and incidence of the disease, in the West Midlands: an epidemiological study. *Br J Surg* 1995; **82**: 111-115.

27. Bornmann PC, Harries-Jones EP, Tobias R, Van Stiegman G, Terblanche J. Prospective controlled trial of transhepatic biliary endoprosthesis versus bypass surgery for incurable carcinoma of head of pancreas. *Lancet* 1986; **i**: 69-71.

28. Shepherd AH, Royle G, Ross APR et al. Endoscopic biliary endoprosthesis in the palliation of malignant obstruction of the distal common bile duct: a randomised trial. *Br J Surg* 1988;**75**:1166-1169.

29. Andersen JR, Sorensen SM, Kruse A, Rollaer M, Matzen P. Randomised trial of endoscopic endoprosthesis versus operative bypass in malignant obstructive jaundice. *Gut* 1989;**30**:1132-1135.

30. Smith AC, Dowsett JF, Russell RCG, Hatfield ARW, Cotton PB. Randomised trial of endoscopic stenting versus surgical bypass in malignant low bile duct obstruction. *Lancet* 1994;**344**:1655-1660.

31. van den Bosch RP, van der Schelling GP, Klinkenbijl JHG, Mulder PGH, van Blankenstein M, Jeekel J. Guidelines for the application of surgery and endoprostheses in the palliation of obstructive jaundice in advanced cancer of the pancreas. *Ann Surg* 1994;**219**:18-24.

32. Cuschieri A, Hall AW, Clark J. Value of laparoscopy in the diagnosis and management of pancreatic carcinoma. *Gut* 1978;**19**:672-677.

33. Ishida H. Peritoneoscopy and pancreas biopsy in the diagnosis of pancreatic diseases. *Gastrointest Endosc* 1983;**29**:211-218.

34. Cuschieri A. Laparoscopy for pancreatic cancer: does it benefit the patient? *Eur J Surg Oncol* 1988;**14**:41-44.

35. Warshaw AL, Tepper JE, Shipley WU. Laparoscopy in the staging and planning of therapy for pancreatic cancer. *Am J Surg* 1986;**151**:76-80.

36. Warshaw AL, Gu ZY, Wittenberg J, Waltman AC. Preoperative staging and assessment of resectability of pancreatic cancer. *Arch Surg* 1990;**125**:230-233.

37. Fernández-del Castillo C, Warshaw AL. Laparoscopy for staging in pancreatic carcinoma. *Surg Oncol* 1993;**2**:25-29.

38. Bemelman WA, de Wit LT, van Delden OM et al. Diagnostic laparoscopy combined with laparoscopic ultrasonography in staging cancer of the pancreas head region. *Br J Surg* 1995;**82**: 820-824.

39. Fernández-del Castillo C, Rattner DW, Warshaw AL. Further experience with laparoscopy and peritoneal cytology in the staging of pancreatic cancer. *Br J Surg* 1995;**82**: 1127-1129.

40. John TG, Greig JD, Carter DC, Garden OJ. Carcinoma of the pancreatic head and periampullary region: tumor staging with laparoscopy and laparoscopic ultrasonography. *Ann Surg* 1995;**221**: 156-164.

41. Conlon KC, Dougherty E, Klimstra DS, Coit DG, Turnbull ADM, Brennan MF. The value of minimal access surgery in the staging of patients with potentially resectable peripancreatic malignancy. *Ann Surg* 1996;**223**:134-140.

42. Murugiah M, Paterson-Brown S, Windsor JA, Miles WFA, Garden OJ. Early experience of laparoscopic ultrasonography in the management of pancreatic carcinoma. *Surg Endosc* 1993;**7**:177-181.

43. Janes RH, Niederhuber JE, Chmiel JS et al. National patterns of care for pancreatic cancer: results of a survey by the commission on cancer. *Ann Surg* 1996;**223**: 261-272.

44. Gmeinwieser J, Feuerbach S, Hohenberger W et al. Spiral-CT in diagnosis of vascular involvement in pancreatic cancer. *Hepato-Gastroenterology* 1995;**42**: 418-422.

45. Meyer-Berg J. The inspection, palpation and biopsy of the pancreas. *Endoscopy* 1972; **4**:99.

46. Ishida H, Furukawa Y, Kuroda H, Kobayashi M, Tsuneoka K. Laparoscopic observation and biopsy of the pancreas. *Endoscopy* 1981;**13**:68-73.

47. Ishida H, Dohzono T, Furukawa Y, Kobayashi M, Tsuneoka K. Laparoscopy and biopsy in the diagnosis of malignant intra-abdominal tumors. *Endoscopy* 1984; **16**: 140-142.

48. Watanabe M, Takatori Y, Ueki K et al. Pancreatic biopsy under visual control in conjunction with laparoscopy for diagnosis of pancreatic cancer. *Endoscopy* 1989;**21**:105-107.

49. Strauch M, Lux G, Ottenjann R. Infragastric pancreoscopy. *Endoscopy* 1973; **5**: 30-32.

50. Meyer-Berg J, Ziegler U, Kirstaedter HJ, Palme G. Peritoneoscopy in carcinoma of the pancreas. Report of 20 cases. *Endoscopy* 1973;**5**:86-90.

51. Rosenbaum FJ. Laparoskopische Cholangiography. *Klinische Wochenschrift* 1955;**33**: 39.

52. Berci GB, Morgenstern L, Shore JM, Shapiro S. A direct approach to the differential diagnosis of jaundice. Laparoscopy with transhepatic cholecystocholangiography. *Am J Surg* 1973;**126**:372-378.

53. Martin JK, Goellner JR. Abdominal fluid cytology in patients with gastrointestinal malignant lesions. *Mayo Clin Proc* 1986;**61**:467-471.

54. Warshaw AL. Implications of peritoneal cytology for staging of early pancreatic cancer. *Am J Surg* 1991;**161**:26-30.

55. Lei S, Kini J, Kim K, Howard JM. Pancreatic cancer. Cytologic study of peritoneal washings. *Arch Surg* 1994;**129**:639-642.

56. Zerbi A, Balzano G, Bottura R, Di Carlo V. Reliability of pancreatic cancer staging classifications. *Int J Pancreatol* 1994;**15**:13-18.

57. Leach SD, Rose JA, Lowy AM et al. Significance of peritoneal cytology in patients with potentially resectable adenocarcinoma of the pancreatic head. *Surgery* 1995;**118**:472-478.

58. John TG, McGoogan E, Wigmore SJ, Paterson-Brown S, Carter DC, Garden OJ. Laparoscopic peritoneal cytology in the staging of pancreatic cancer. *Gut* 1995; **37**:A3.

59. Okita K, Kodama T, Oda M, Takemoto T. Laparoscopic ultrasonography. Diagnosis of liver and pancreatic cancer. *Scand J Gastroenterol* 1984;**19** (Suppl 94):91-100.

60. Jorgensen JO, McCall JL, Morris DL. Port site seeding after laparoscopic ultrasonographic staging of pancreatic carcinoma. *Surgery* 1995;**117**:118-119.

61. Siriwardena A, Samarji WN. Cutaneous tumor seeding from a previously undiagnosed pancreatic carcinoma after laparoscopic cholecystectomy. *Ann Roy Coll Surg Engl* 1993;**75**: 199-200.

62. Nduka CC, Monson JRT, Menzies-Gow N, Darzi A. Abdominal wall metastasis following laparoscopy. *Br J Surg* 1994;**81**:648-652.

63. van Dijkum EJMN, de Wit LT, Obertop H, Gouma DJ. Port-site metastases following diagnostic laparoscopy. *Br J Surg* 1996;**83**:1793-1794.

64. Sotnikov VN, Ermolov AS, Litvinof VI. The diagnosis of intrabdominal metastases of oesophageal cancer by means of laparoscopy. *Vaprosy Onkolgii* (Leningrad) 1973;**??**:35-38.

65. Cook AO, Levine BA, Sirinek KR, Gaskill HVI. Evaluation of gastric adenocarcinoma: abdominal computed tomography does not replace celiotomy. *Arch Surg* 1986;**121**:603-606.

66. Sussman SK, Halvorsen RA Jr., Illescas FF, et al. Gastric adenocarcinoma: CT versus surgical staging. *Radiology* 1988;**167**:335-340.

67. Geoghegan JG, Keane TE, Rosenberg IL, Dellipiani AW, Peel ALG. Gastric cancer: the case for a more selective policy in surgical management. *J Roy Coll Surg Edinb* 1993;**38**: 208-212.

68. Wanebo HJ, Kennedy BJ, Chmiel J, Steele G, Winchester D, Osteen R. Cancer of the stomach: a patient care study by the American College of Surgeons. *Ann Surg* 1993;**218**:583-592.

69. Gross E, Bancewicz J, Ingram G. Assessment of gastric carcinoma by laparoscopy. *Br Med J* 1984;**288**:1577.

70. Shandall A, Johnson C. Laparoscopy or scanning in oesophageal and gastric carcinoma. *Br J Surg* 1985;**72**:449-451.

71. Dagnini G, Caldironi MW, Marin G, Buzzaccarini O, Tremolada C, Ruol A. Laparoscopy in abdominal staging of esophageal carcinoma: report of 369 cases. *Gastrointest Endosc* 1986;**32**:400-402.

72. Possik RA, Franco EL, Pires DR, Wohnrath DR, Ferreira EB. Sensitivity, specificity, and predictive value of laparoscopy for the staging of gastric cancer and for the detection of liver metastases. *Cancer* 1986;**58**:1-6.

73. Kriplani AK, Kapur ML. Laparoscopy for pre-operative staging and assessment of operability in gastric carcinoma. *Gastrointest Endosc* 1991;**37**:441-443.

74. Bemelman WA, van Delden OM, van Lanschot JJB et al.Laparoscopy and laparoscopic ultrasonography in staging of carcinoma of the esophagus and gastric cardia. *J Am Coll Surg* 1995;**181**:421-425.

75. Molloy RG, McCourtney JS, Anderson JR. Laparoscopy in the management of patients with cancer of the gastric cardia and oesophagus. *Br J Surg* 1995;**82**:352-354.

76. Watt I, Stewart I, Anderson D, Bell G, Anderson JR. Laparoscopy, ultrasound and computed tomography in cancer of the oesophagus and gastric cardia: a prospective comparison for detecting intra-abdominal metastases. *Br J Surg* 1989;**76**:1036-1039.

77. Anderson DN, Campbell S, Park KGM. Accuracy of laparoscopic ultrasonography in the staging of upper gastrointestinal malignancy. *Br J Surg* 1996;**83** 1424-1428.

78. Lowy AM, Mansfield PF, Leach SD, Ajani J. Laparoscopic staging for gastric cancer. *Surgery* 1996;**119**:611-614.

79. Finch MD, John TG, Garden OJ, Allan PL, Paterson-Brown S. Laparoscopic ultrasonography for staging of gastroesophageal cancer. *Surgery* 1997;**121** (in press).

80. de Manzoni G, Macrì A, Borzellino G, Cordiano G. The value of *in vitro* ultrasonography in the intraoperative staging of gastric cancer. *Surg Endosc* 1994; **8**:765-769.

81. Bartlett DL, Conlon KCP, Gerdes H, Karpeh MS Jr. Laparoscopic ultrasonography: the best pretreatment staging modality in gastric adenocarcinoma. *Surgery* 1995;**118**:562-566.

82. Grimm H, Hamper K, Binmoeller KF, Soehendra N. Enlarged lymph nodes: malignant or not. *Endoscopy* 1992;**24**(Suppl 1):320-323.

83. Collier NA, Carr D, Hemmingway A, Blumgart LH. Preoperative diagnosis and its effect on the treatment of carcinoma of the gallbladder. *Surg Gynecol Obstet* 1984;**159**:465-470.

84. John TG, Carey FA, Anderson ID, Garden OJ. Abdominal wall metastases following laparoscopy. *Br J Surg* 1995;**82**:135-136.
85. Dagnini G, Marin G, Patella M, Zotti S. Laparoscopy in the diagnosis of primary carcinoma of the gallbladder. A study of 98 cases. *Gastrointest Endosc* 1984;**30**:289-291.
86. Kriplani AK, Jayant S, Kapur BM. Laparoscopy in primary carcinoma of the gallbladder. *Gastrointest Endosc* 1992;**38**:326-329.
87. Bleiberg H, Rozencweig M, Mathieu M, Beyens M, Gompel C, Gerard A. The use of peritoneoscopy in the detection of liver metastases. *Cancer* 1978;**41**:863-867.
88. John TG, Greig JD, Crosbie JL, Miles WFA, Garden OJ. Superior staging of liver tumors with laparoscopy and laparoscopic ultrasound. *Ann Surg* 1994;**220**:711-719.
98. Brady PG, Peebles M, Goldschmid S. Role of laparoscopy in the evaluation of patients with suspected hepatic or peritoneal malignancy. *Gastrointest Endosc* 1991;**37**:27-30.
99. Babineau TJ, Lewis WD, Jenkins RL, Bleday R, Steele GD, Forse RA. Role of staging laparoscopy in the treatment of hepatic malignancy. *Am J Surg* 1994;**167**:151-155.
100. Furukawa Y, Sakamoto F, Kanazawa H et al. A new method of B-mode ultrasonography under laparoscopic guidance. *Scand J Gastroenterol* 1982;**78** (Suppl 17):186 (Abstract).
101. Fornari F, Civardi G, Cavanna L et al. Laparoscopic ultrasonography in the study of liver diseases: preliminary results. *Surg Endosc* 1989;**3**:33-37.
102. Bönhof JA, Linhart P, Bettendorf U, Holper H. Liver biopsy guided by laparoscopic sonography. A case report demonstrating a new technique. *Endoscopy* 1984;**16**:237-239.
103. Fukuda M, Mima S, Tanabe T, Suzuki Y, Hirata K, Terada S. Endoscopic sonography of the liver - diagnostic application of the echolaparoscope to localize intrahepatic lesions. *Scand J Gastroenterol* 1984;**19** (Suppl 102):24-28.
104. Miles WFA, Paterson-Brown S, Garden OJ. Laparoscopic contact hepatic ultrasonography. *Br J Surg* 1992;**79**:419-420.
105. John TG, Madhavan KK, Redhead DN, Crosbie JL, Garden OJ. Laparoscopic ultrasonography in the staging of colorectal liver metastases: a prospective comparison with CT arterioportography. *Br J Surg* 1996;**83**:31.
106. Keate RF, Shaffer R. Seeding of hepatocellular carcinoma to peritoneoscopy insertion site. *Gastrointest Endosc* 1992;**38**:203-204.
107. John TG, Garden OJ. Needle track seeding of primary and secondary liver carcinoma after percutaneous liver biopsy. *HPB Surg* 1993;**6**:199-204.
108. Yamada N, Shinzawa H, Ukai K et al. Subcutaneous seeding of small hepatocellular carcinoma after fine needle aspiration biopsy. *J Gastroenterol Hepatol* 1993;**8**:195-198.
109. Russi EG, Pergolizzi S, Mesiti M et al. Unusual relapse of hepatocellular carcinoma. *Cancer* 1992;**70**:1483-1487.
110. Leuschner M, Leuschner U. Diagnostic laparoscopy in focal parenchymal disease of the liver. *Endoscopy* 1992;**24**:689-692.
111. Fornari F, Rapaccini GL, Cavanna L et al. Diagnosis of hepatic lesions: ultrasonically guided fine needle biopsy or laparoscopy. *Gastrointest Endosc* 1988;**34**:231-234.
112. Garden OJ. *Intraoperative and Laparoscopic Ultrasonography*. Oxford: Blackwell Science, 1995.
113. John TG, Garden OJ. Ultrasonography in laparoscopy. In: Brooks D (ed) *Current Review of Laparoscopy*; 2nd edn. Philadelphia: Current Medicine, 1995, pp. 77-95.
114. John TG, Garden OJ. Laparoscopic targeted liver biopsies. In: Tooulli J, Gossot D, Hunter JG (eds) *Endosurgery*. Edinburgh: Churchill Livingstone, 1996, pp455-462.
115. Attiyeh RR, Stearns MWJ. Second-look laparotomy based on CEA elevations in colorectal cancer. *Cancer* 1981;**47**:2119.
116. Marti-Vicente A, Sainz S, Soriano G et al. Utilidad de la laparoscopia como metodo de second-look en las neoplasias de ovario (Usefulness of laparoscopy as a second look method in neoplasms of the ovary). *Rev Esp Enf Digest* 1990;**77**:275-278.
117. Canis M, Chapron C, Mage G et al. Technique and preliminary results in second-look laparoscopy in epithelial malignant ovarian tumors. *Gynecol Obstet Biol Reprod* 1992;**21**:655-663.
118. Salky B, Bauer J, Gelernt I, Kreel I. Laparoscopy for gastrointestinal diseases. *Mt Sinai J Med* 1985;**52**:228-232.

4

Endoscopic Management of Gastrointestinal Malignancies

Frederick L. Greene

The recent advent of minimal access techniques, while in some ways overshadowing the traditional approach to endoscopy, has enhanced the need to continue a strong commitment to flexible endoscopic techniques by surgeons. Just as the rigid laparoscope did for diagnostic evaluation of the abdomen and pelvis in the early part of the 20th century, the flexible endoscope opened up new vistas in the late 1950's when introduced by Hirschowitz et al. for the evaluation of upper gastrointestinal pathology.[1] Utilizing principles of fiberoptic technology, evaluation and confirmation by photography of lesions in the esophagus, stomach and duodenum were made possible with a high degree of sensitivity and accuracy. Recently, the role of the fiberoptic bundle has given way to charged coupled devices (CCD) which give direct photographic feedback and allow routine application of video recording and high-resolution photography. In addition, videoendoscopy has created a wider role for the gastrointestinal assistant and other colleagues who wish to take part in procedures in the endoscopy suite. By viewing procedures in the endoscopy area as well as in remote areas, more individuals can participate in the consultative and learning process. These same electronic and engineering advances have created the environment for laparoscopic and thoracoscopic procedures to become routine. As pure technical entities, the laparoscope and flexible endoscope have become intertwined.

UPPER GASTROINTESTINAL FLEXIBLE ENDOSCOPY AND ITS RELATIONSHIP TO MINIMAL ACCESS SURGERY

Using flexible upper endoscopes, the esophagus, stomach and entire duodenum can be visualized and biopsied. Although endoscopes have been developed for manipulation throughout the small intestine,[2] they have not become commercially available or successful and have not allowed the small bowel to be routinely investigated per the oral route.

The principles of upper endoscopy created the technology for the introduction of endoscopic retrograde cholangiopancreatography (ERCP) in the late 1960's[3] and endoscopic sphincterotomy in the mid 1970's.[4]

As in ERCP, gastrointestinal endoscopy is predominately used in symptom resolution. Esophagogastroduodenoscopy (EGD) is primarily recommended in patients with abdominal pain, dysphagia, melena or unexplained weight loss. Studies have shown the increased sensitivity of endoscopic techniques when compared to conventional radiography of the upper gastrointestinal tract.[5] Small lesions may be identified routinely through endoscopy and may be biopsied or studied cytologically. In addition to symptom resolution, screening of the upper gastrointestinal tract is an important consideration when head and neck carcinoma is diagnosed because of the greater likelihood of finding squamous cell carcinoma of the esophagus or pulmonary tree in association with similar lesions in the head and neck area. In addition, early evaluation and screening of patients with caustic stricture due to lye or acid burns have proved valuable in identifying early cancer related to continuing inflammation caused by these agents. Similarly, the evaluation of patients with longstanding achalasia or reflux esophagitis and stricture has shown a small but definite increase in the finding of adenocarcinoma in the distal esophagus.[6] Annual screening with random biopsy has proven beneficial in these patients and should be continued even when surgical procedures have been performed to reverse both achalasia and reflux peptic disease.

ESOPHAGEAL ENDOSCOPY

The most important use of flexible endoscopy, relative to the esophagus, is to identify early neoplasia in patients who present with dysphagia. It is obvious that identification of both squamous cell carcinoma and adenocarcinoma is important before patients present with symptoms. Early identification of cancer will enhance the chances of cure. When patients present with dysphagia or odynophagia it is likely that mediastinal lymphatic seeding and submucosal spread of disease have already occurred. Routine biopsy, both at the level of the lesion and at proximal and distal intervals, will be helpful for the surgeon or radiotherapist who is called upon to provide primary resection or radiotherapeutic control of the mucosal tumor. A further use of endoscopy for this disease process is to identify trancheoesophageal fistulae in patients who present with coughing or evidence of pulmonary infiltrate along with dysphagia. Palliative techniques may be employed for esophageal carcinoma and may be facilitated by endoscopic application. These include dilatation with either rigid or balloon devices, application of laser energy for ablation and placement of devices which allow for high-dose radiation directly to the tumor area.[7]

Flexible esophagoscopy has also been extremely useful in the therapeutic management of benign esophageal stricture which is primarily due to esophageal reflux of acid or secondary to previous alkali or acid ingestion. These procedures may be accomplished under general anesthesia or local anesthetic techniques and may require re-application if the fibrotic and inflammatory process continues. As mentioned previously, early biopsy and brush cytology are important in ruling out dysplasia or early cancer associated with benign stricture.

The technical aspects of esophagoscopy have been described in several atlases and monographs.[8,9] Since the esophagus is a straight tube, once peroral intubation is achieved and the upper constrictors are traversed by getting the patient to swallow, general examination is relatively easy except when large bulky lesions or stenosis are present. As in any endoscopic procedure, the endoscopist must always have a clear view of the lumen of the esophagus before advancing the endoscope. The major difficulty of esophagoscopy is the interpretation of the findings. For the surgical endoscopist, the primary differential is between inflammatory and neoplastic lesions and the presence or absence of varices.

Adjunctive techniques, such as biopsy and brush cytology, are especially important and should be readily available when esophagoscopy is performed. Small lesions, when thought to be suspicious, should be routinely biopsied since these may be the earliest forms of squamous or adenocarcinoma. If stenotic lesions are found or large bulky lesions are noted which may require additional therapeutic maneuvers, it is best to perform these procedures at a separate setting if they have not already been discussed with the patient.

It is important to note certain landmarks in the esophagus which will help in localizing any lesions. One readily reproducible landmark is the Z-line which is produced by the interface of the squamous and columnar mucosa of the stomach. This is readily apparent because of the pale appearance of esophageal mucosa when compared to the hyperemic or salmon-colored mucosa of the stomach cardia. In most adults, the Z-line or gastroesophageal junction is 40-42 cm from the upper incisors. This landmark should certainly be quantified during routine endoscopy, especially if a hiatus hernia is noted which will tend to shift the gastroesophageal junction to a more proximal location. In addition, specific distances from the upper incisors should be recorded for any lesions that are noted.

FLEXIBLE GASTROSCOPY

As is true with the esophagus, one of the main uses of early endoscopic gastroscopy is the identification of cancer associated with symptoms of pain, weight loss and unexplained gastrointestinal bleeding. For many years, gastric ulceration was thought to be a precancerous event which, if left unchecked, would eventually develop into an adenocarcinoma. Routine gastrointestinal endoscopy has shown that most gastric ulcers are in fact benign and show no greater risk of developing into cancer. The importance of early endoscopy is in the evaluation of carcinomas of the stomach which present as early ulcerations rather than polypoid or exophytic lesions.

The use of flexible endoscopy has also been important in patients who have undergone previous gastric resection for benign ulcer disease. These patients have a propensity to develop marginal ulcer, reflux bile gastritis, anastomotic narrowing and carcinoma in the remaining gastric pouch many years after previous gastric resection.[10] The use of endoscopy in these patients is more challenging because of the unusual anatomy and the need for greater experience and interpretive skills in identifying lesions and biopsying difficult areas of the gastric or small bowel anatomy. Use of endoscopic screening has led to applications of local therapy for small gastric cancer, especially in areas of the world where gastric carcinoma has a high incidence.[11]

Since the surgical endoscopist is performing gastroscopy mainly to differentiate neoplastic from inflammatory or acid-peptic disease, biopsy techniques are important. All tumors tend to have a superficial inflammatory exudate and therefore the small biopsy forceps that are readily utilized through flexible endoscopes may in fact not give representative biopsies of underlying tissue. It is important to biopsy aggressively beneath the surface of exophytic masses in the stomach in order to achieve appropriate tissue sampling. Three to four biopsies should be routinely performed in multiple areas and should accompany biopsies of the mucosa in the surrrounding, but apparently normal, mucosa. If ulcers are obvious, biopsy of the rim and not the base of the ulcer crater should be routinely performed. This will minimize the chances of a diagnosis of 'inflammation only' when an ulcer is in fact neoplastic.

One of the most difficult diagnoses to make endoscopicaly is in the patient with suspected gastric lymphoma. Generally, gastric lymphoma presents with widened gastric rugae which are infiltrated by the lymphomatous process (Fig. 4.1). Here again, unless aggressive biopsy is performed deep into the mucosa and submucosa, the diagnosis will be missed. Some have advocated snare biopsy of large areas of the mucosa in order to make the diagnosis of gastric lymphoma.[12] This may be necessary when small pinch biopsies are non-diagnostic.

Gastrointestinal malignancy remains a significant worldwide health problem causing millions of deaths each year. In the United States, approximately 250 000 people are diagnosed each year as having cancer of the digestive tract and almost half die of their disease, which represents 25% of all cancer deaths.[13] Since 80% of these lesions arise from the mucosal surface of the gastrointestinal tract, early surveillance and detection may be appropriate for identifying a population of patients who will benefit from early treatment.

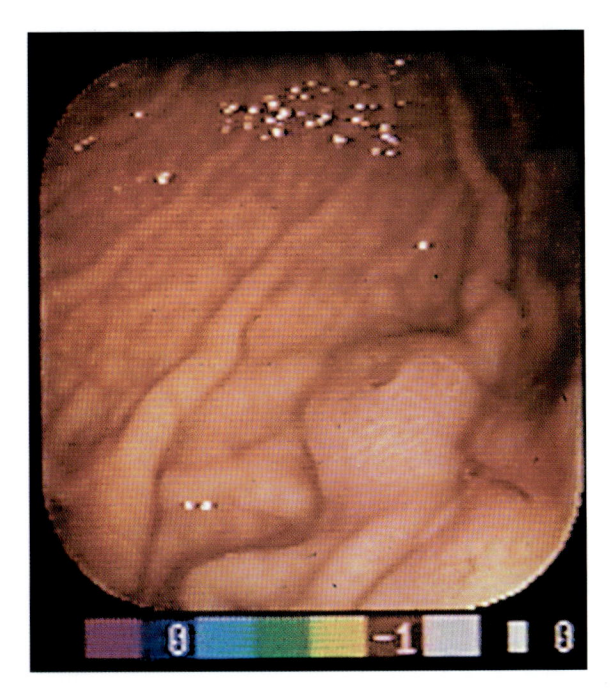

Figure 4.1 – Gastric lymphoma presenting with widened gastric rugae and prominent mass.

Endoscopic studies of the upper and lower gastrointestinal tract serve as an ideal mechanism for early detection since visual inspection, biopsy and photographic documentation are possible using these techniques. Radiologic methods have been shown to be less sensitive and specific in the early detection of gastrointestinal cancer for both upper and lower gastrointestinal lesions. Although endoscopic studies do have their advantages, the significant cost of these procedures and the defined risks, although low when done by recognized experts, preclude their use in mass screening surveillance. The problems of cost may be lessened when specific entities are approached endoscopically and defined algorithms are developed for appropriate utilization of screening techniques.

SCREENING

Upper gastrointestinal lesions

Approximately 25 000 cases of gastric cancer and 12 000 case of esophageal cancer were expected in the United States in 1996.[13] Although the overall incidence of gastric cancer continues to fall in the United States, worldwide this disease continues to be of significant epidemiologic importance. Small bowel cancer is much less of a health threat worldwide, although approximately 3000 cases were expected in 1996 in the United States.[13]

For most of the US population, there is no benefit from mass screening to offset the risks, discomfort and costs of periodic endoscopic inspection of the upper gastrointestinal mucosa. Polypoid disease, such as found in the lower gastrointestinal tract and which is potentially premalignant, is not a factor when upper gastrointestinal cancer is considered. Therefore, removal of premalignant lesions from the proximal gastrointestinal tract will not reduce overall cancer rates. For these reasons, mass endoscopic screening of asymptomatic people for early detection of cancers of the upper gastrointestinal tract is not warranted in the United States.[14] In regions of the world where esophageal and gastric cancer are more significant, such as Southeast Asia, the Middle East and certain parts of South America, surveillance may be warranted.

There is, however, an indication for surveillance of high-risk groups. Most high-risk groups are defined by environmental factors, genetic screening or associated previous lesions or procedures that may make the gastrointestinal tract more susceptible to neoplasia. As

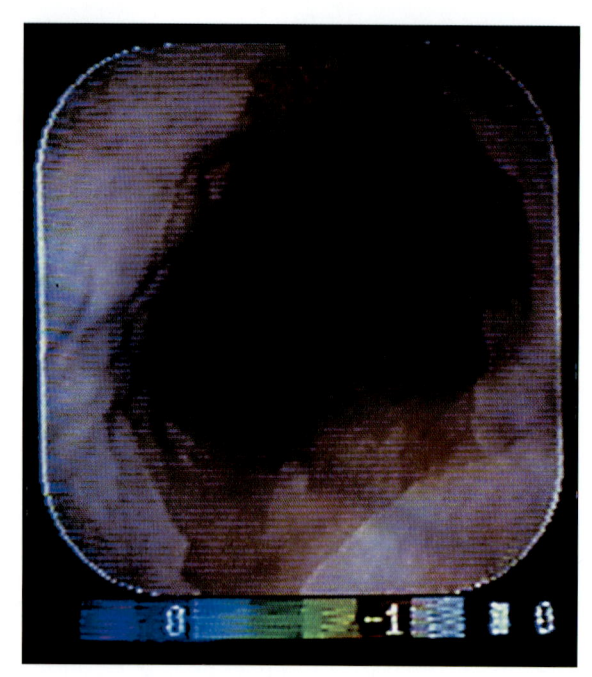

Figure 4.2 – Barrett's metaplasia.

disease processes undergo greater scrutiny, changing concepts regarding endoscopic surveillance for certain potentially premalignant lesions or prior procedures may need re-thinking and inclusion in screening strategies in the future.

Achalasia

Achalasia is a physiologic disease of the esophagus induced by the inability of the lower esophageal sphincter to relax with eventual reduction in overall peristalsis and stasis of food products in the esophagus. Squamous carcinoma develops in 1.7-8.2% of patients with untreated achalasia after an average 17-20 years from the onset of symptoms.[15] This represents a risk that is approximately 7 times that of the general population. Treatment of achalasia, which includes dilatation of the lower esophageal sphincter or surgical myotomy, may reduce the risk of eventual cancer to that of the general population. Patients who have treatment late in the course of their disease may have continuing dysplasia or risk of esophageal carcinoma and therefore should be included in surveillance programs on an annual basis. Since the lower esophageal sphincter may be rendered incompetent, columnar (Barrett's) changes may be found in patients with achalasia. Approximately 4-5% of patients with achalasia may in fact have Barrett's changes following treatment.[16] This is further indication for surveillance in these patients, even after treatment for achalasia, and yearly surveillance is recommended.

Barrett's esophagus

This represents an acquired condition in which the esophagus becomes lined by columnar epithelium secondary to chronic injury from exposure usually to gastric acid. It is important to recognize that the process is not limited to the distal esophageal mucus and the mid or proximal esophagus may also be involved. Reflux of bile and pancreatic enzymes may hasten the changes seen in Barrett's esophagus and this process may continue even after appropriate anti-reflux surgical procedures are performed. It has been estimated that metaplasia and columnar epithelium occur in 10-18% of patients with chronic gastroesophageal reflux.[17] It is appropriate to look carefully for this entity when patients who have symptoms of esophageal reflux disease are endoscoped (Fig. 4.2).

The major clinical significance of this condition is its predisposition to the development of adenocarcinoma in 8-10% of patients.[18] This propensity toward neoplasia may not be reduced even after anti-reflux procedures. Squamous carcinoma associated with Barrett's esophagus is unusual but can occur. This is seen most often in patients who have alcohol and tobacco abuse co-existent with their reflux esophagitis.

There is adequate evidence that progression to adenocarcinoma occurs in areas of columnar epithelium that first develop dysplasia. This adds a rationale for utilizing endoscopic evaluation and biopsy in the routine surveillance of patients with Barrett's esophagus. Follow-up studies show that survival in patients whose carcinoma is noted by endoscopic surveillance is twice as high as in those who develop adenocarcinoma identified as part of a surveillance program.[19] Patients who are found to harbor adenocarcinoma associated with Barrett's changes should undergo esophagectomy. Controversy exists as to whether esophagectomy should be offered to patients with dysplasia alone associated with Barrett's changes. It is important to obtain adequate biopsies when Barrett's change is identified since sampling errors may occur and associated malignancy may be missed. Biopsies should be done in four separate quadrants and should be obtained to a level of at least 6 cm above the gastroesophageal junction or the level of obvious gross Barrett's changes. Even using this technique, large areas will not be biopsied and, therefore, additional sampling errors may occur. Brush cytology may allow wider sampling and should be considered when biopsies are utilized. Staining with vital dye is not helpful since adenocarcinoma may not take up vital stains, as is seen with squamous cell carcinoma of the esophagus. The use of flow cytometry may be important to look for aneuploid cells associated with dysplasia.

It is important to enter patients with Barrett's changes into an appropriate endoscopic screening program but the frequency of examination may be controversial. Recommendations have varied from twice yearly endoscopic examination to performing the procedure ever 1-2 years. Men may be at a greater risk for development of adenocarcinoma associated with Barrett's changes and, therefore, should be surveyed more frequently perhaps than women.[20] Once dysplasia is recognized, endoscopic examination should probably be performed every 6 months. If severe dysplasia or evidence of carcinoma *in situ* is recognized, esophagectomy should be strongly considered.

Cancer of the aerodigestive tract

Cancers of the upper digestive tract are associated with alcohol and tobacco abuse. These tumors may affect multiple sites in the head and neck region and it has been estimated that 8-16% of patients with squamous cell carcinoma of the head or neck may have synchronous second primary tumors of the upper aerodigestive tract which includes the esophagus. Approximately 0.6-5.1% of patients with previous head and neck cancer may develop esophageal tumors.[21] It is recommended that routine esophagoscopy should be performed when head and neck tumors are identified and patients with prior head and neck cancer should be screened for the development of cancer. The use of vital dyes, such as Lugols' solution, may show early tumors in the esophagus.

Patients who have had previous resection for esophageal cancer and who have a portion of the esophagus remaining may also be appropriate candidates for endoscopic surveillance but the frequency of this examination has not been established. Because of the 'field theory' concept, the remaining esophagus is at risk from the environmental effects of tobacco and alcohol abuse. Patients who undergo resection for esophageal cancer should be endoscoped 6 months after the procedure and annually thereafter. As is true with head and neck carcinomas, patients with squamous cell cancer of the esophagus, may be at risk for subsequent aerodigestive tumors and careful head and neck examination and chest X-ray should be performed routinely in these patients.

Caustic injury

Squamous cell carcinoma of the esophagus may develop in areas of stricture produced by injury, most commonly from lye. This may develop years after the injury and, therefore, lifelong follow-up is mandatory. The most common site of chronic inflammatory injury is at the level of the tracheal bifurcation. The incidence of carcinoma in these patients ranges from 0.8 to 5.5%.[22] Resection may be appropriate in patients who have continued evidence of stricture and should be considered for patients who are at least 15-20 years post lye injury if inflammation is still present.

Chronic atrophic gastritis

Chronic atrophic gastritis may be classified into two major types. Type A may be autoimmune in origin and shows diffuse gastric involvement with antral sparing. Pernicious anemia is associated with this type of atrophic gastritis but carcinoma is unusual. Type B, more commonly than Type A, may be related to environmental factors and is associated with antral involvement and focal changes within the gastric body. The intestinal metaplasia which occurs with Type B atrophic gastritis may progress to dysplasia and carcinoma in 5-10% of patients. *Helicobacter pylori* infection may promote this form of gastritis[23] and may potentially be associated with subsequent gastric carcinoma. Patients who have Type B gastritis should undergo yearly endoscopic surveillance and surveillance ever 6 months if dysplasia is apparent. Type B atrophic gastritis is usually asymptomatic and, therefore, these patients should have routine screening whether they have symptoms or not. Patients with Type A gastritis or associated pernicious anemia probably do not need surveillance since carcinoma only develops in a small fraction of these.

Familial polyposis

Patients with a genetic disposition to develop familial polyposis coli and Gardner's syndrome may have associated gastric and duodenal polyps which are

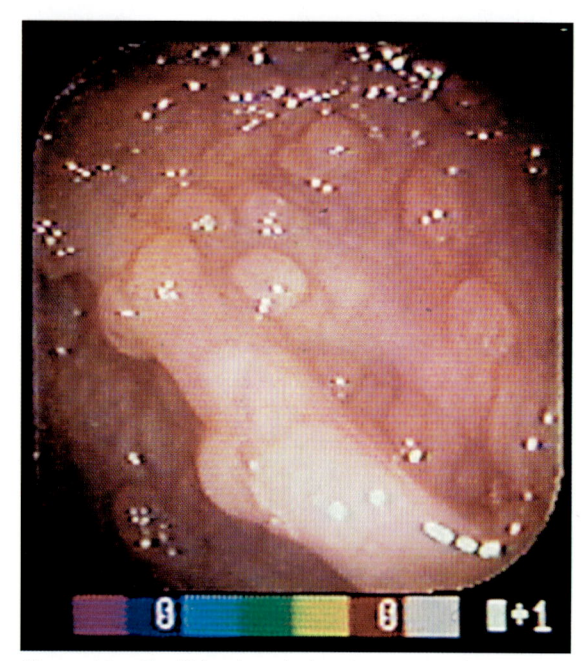

Figure 4.3 - Familial polyposis showing associated gastric and duodenal polyps.

premalignant (Fig. 4.3). Although these gastric polyps may be adenomatous or hyperplastic and occur with higher frequency, few patients develop gastric cancer. Duodenal polyps may occur in 46-93% of patients with familial polyposis, are usually adenomatous and more frequently lead to carcinoma (approximately 4%).[24] It is recommended that patients with familial polyposis, who have undergone previous colon resection, should be entered into a screening program to identify gastric and duodenal polyps. Periampullary cancers are seen in a significant number of this population and, therefore, the second or third portion of the duodenum should be carefully inspected in endoscopic studies. Once these tumors develop and are associated with symptoms, the chance of cure is low.

Gastric polyps

Gastric mucosal polyps are uncommon and usually asymptomatic. Although discovered mostly as incidental findings, larger polyps may cause obstruction and bleeding. Approximately 25% of gastric polyps are adenomatous and the remainder are hyperplastic. Adenomatous polyps in the stomach are neoplastic and carry a risk of malignancy which is related to size. Hyperplastic polyps have been associated with carcinomas elsewhere in the stomach in 4-28% of patients.[25]

It is recommended that gastric polyps be routinely biopsied and should be removed if pedunculated or symptomatic. Hyperplastic polyps should be documented but routine surveillance is not recommended. For patients with adenomatous polyps in the stomach, polypectomy and surveillance is recommended and should be done on a yearly basis or at least until no additional polyps are found in two consecutive yearly endoscopic examinations.

Previous gastrectomy for benign conditions

Since the early 1920's, it has been recognized that patients who have undergone gastric resection for benign peptic ulcer disease may be at risk for subsequent development of adenocarcinoma of the gastric remnant (Fig. 4.4).[26] Cancer has been reported in 2-8.7% of patients over an interval of 15-28 years post resection, which is higher than the 1-1.7% incidence estimated for the general population in the United States. Gastric carcinoma may develop after Billroth I and Billroth II reconstruction. Generally, patients are asymptomatic at the time of development of these tumors which supports the concept that yearly endoscopic screening should begin at least 15 years post resection for benign disease. Several prospective screening studies have supported the concept that annual endoscopic evaluation with biopsy may disclose both dysplasia and early adenocarcinoma.[27] Patients who have undergone completion gastrectomy following detection adenocarcinoma by routine screening will enjoy a much greater survival rate than patients who present with symptomatic disease from gastric remnant cancer. It is recommended, therefore, that gastroscopy with random biopsies should begin 15 years after previous gastric resection.[27] If severe dysplasia is noted, surveillance endoscopy should be performed every 6 months or completion gastrectomy be considered because of severe dysplasia alone.

ENDOSCOPIC PALLIATION OF GASTROINTESTINAL MALIGNANCY

Flexible upper endoscopy plays a major role currently in the diagnosis of malignant esophageal stricture and is now favored over radiographic studies. The ability to assess the size of an esophageal cancer, its distance

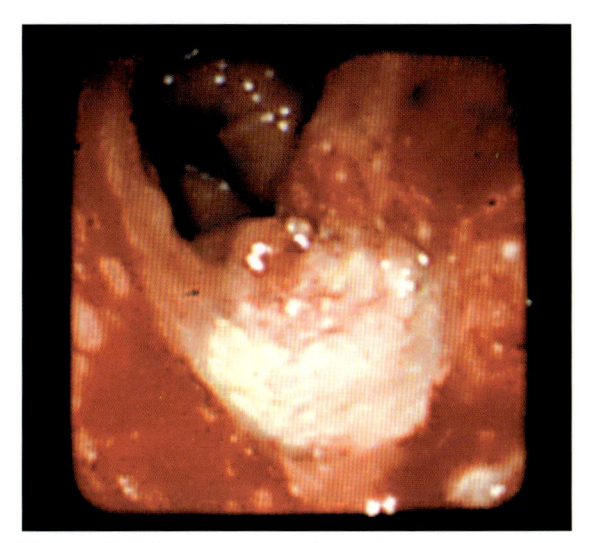

Figure 4.4 - Adenocarcinoma of the gastric remnant.

from the upper incisors and to utilize photography and videoscopic data-keeping make flexible endoscopic assessment mandatory in the investigation of patients complaining of dysphagia. Aside from a diagnositic tool, the flexible upper endoscope may be used as a palliative vehicle for many patients who may eventually undergo surgical resection or who are treated non-surgically using combinations of radiation or chemotherapy.

The initial, and still most important, role for endoscopic palliation is in the application of bouginage to relieve significant dysphagia. The principle of dilating an esophageal stricture with bougie was introduced in the 16th century. The initial technique was to use a wax taper blindly to dilate the narrowed area of the esophagus. The word 'bougie' is derived from the Arabic name of Boujiyah, Algeria, a medieval center known for its wax candle trade.[28] Current principles of endoscopic treatment were developed more than 100 years ago when the English physician J.C. Russell introduced a balloon dilator in the late 1880's that was similar to those used today. Samuel Mixter of Boston developed the concept of passing a bougie over a string which served as a guide to avoid perforation. The patient would initially swallow the string and once the string became anchored in the small intestine, a dilating bougie was passed. Sir Arthur Hurst introduced the mercury-filled flexible bougie in 1915. Utilizing these ancient and more modern concepts, the introduction of both rigid and flexible endoscopy embraced the technique of bouginage and served to make it safer.

Since the main complaint of patients with esophageal cancer is unrelenting dysphagia, dilatation of the stricture segment may be accomplished using balloon techniques or tapered bougies which can be safely passed over a guidewire (Savary-Guillard bougies). Stricture may occur in any area of the esophagus but is commonest in the middle and distal segments which correspond to common locations of both squamous cancer and adenocarcinoma. Utilization of dilating techniques is also appropriate in patients who have been previously treated with external beam radiation or current intracavitary techniques using high-dose rate brachytherapy (HDRB), which may result in a nonmalignant stricture. The flexible endoscope serves as an excellent tool to facilitate follow-up biopsy in patients who have been treated.

A popular method of esophageal dilatation is to employ a hydrostatic balloon system which may be passed directly through the instrument channel of most flexible esophagoscopes. These systems are graduated from diameters of 8-15 mm and are much safer than bougies that are placed blindly or with the assistance of guidewires. Contrast agents may be instilled into the balloons to confirm the location of these devices either radiographically or flouroscopically. Repeat dilatation may be needed for patients with stricture secondary to tumor as well as secondary to the effects of radiotherapy.

Upper endoscopy employing flexible endoscopes is frequently used as a vehicle for both laser application and the delivery of contact irradiation to segmental areas of the esophagus which harbor cancer. Contact laser application using neodymium-YAG has been efficacious in relieving malignant obstruction if the patient has an identifiable lumen through which the laser fiber may be passed.[29] In this situation, dilatation of the esophagus may be needed prior to laser treatment.

More recently, both external beam radiation and intraluminal radiation utilizing flexible endoscopic techniques have enabled treatment of malignant esophageal strictures. Patients generally are treated in an outpatient setting. Initially, a guidewire is placed through the flexible endoscope to allow passage of a plastic tube which will serve as an afterloading receptacle for either iridium or cesium seeds which may generate 500-1000 rads of radiation energy in a small area of tumor.[30] This technique has the advantage of avoiding effects on lung and surrounding tissue which may be affected by external beam therapy. The endoscopist must work in close

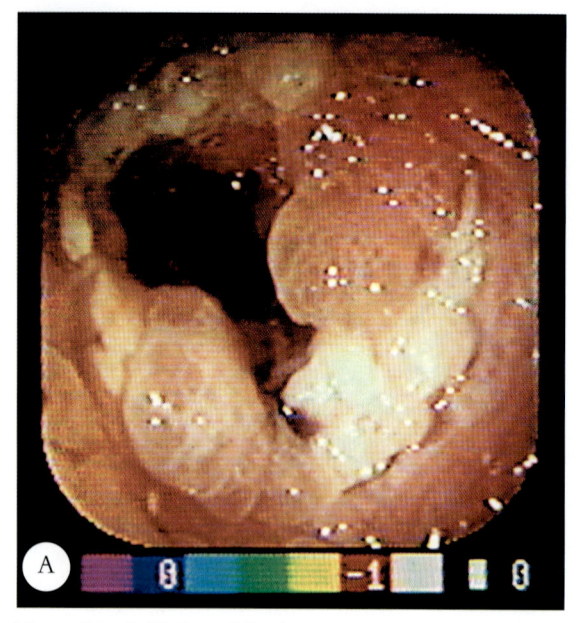

Figure 4.5 - Palliation of dysphagia in a patient with advanced esophageal carcinoma. The endoscopically-placed expandable metallic stent is visible (A) in its most proximal part (B).

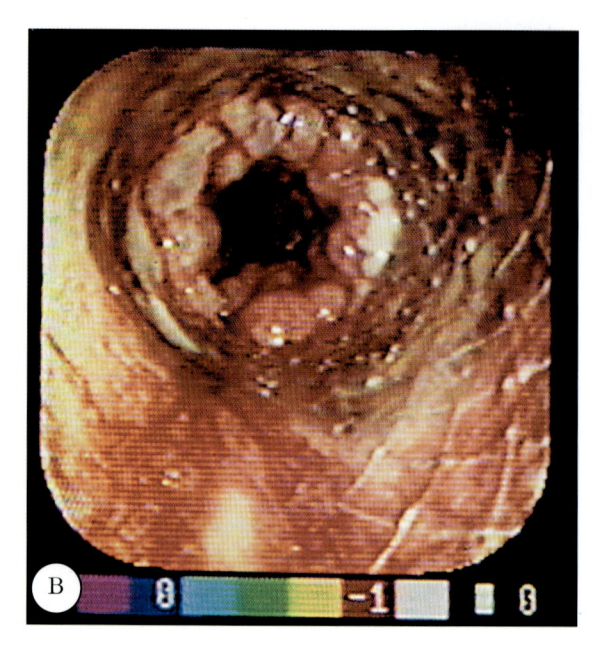

association with the radiation oncologist to ensure that the afterloading device is placed at the appropriate level in order to encompass the entire length of the esophageal tumor. A postendoscopic chest X-ray prior to application of radiation ensures appropriate placement of the afterloading device.

More recently, intraluminal stents have been developed which allow for safe placement utilizing flexible endoscopic techniques (Fig 4.5).[31] These stents are collapsible but when placed into the esophagus, expand to create a lumen which allows the patient to eat a soft diet. These stents are made in a variety of lengths ranging from 7 to 15 cm. The endoscope serves as a vehicle for proper placement of the stent and may be utilized for dilatation of strictures once the stent is in place. Stents may be placed to palliate an intraluminal tumor as well as obstruction caused by extraluminal disease. Even patients with tracheoesophageal fistulae may have solid stents placed to serve as a buttress between the esophagus and trachea in order to allow the patient some protection from chronic aspiration. The long-term effect of these expandable stents has not been realized but most early experiences suggest that they are better tolerated than older techniques of operative placement of thick rubber or solid stents. Treatment can be carried out in an outpatient setting and this improves the overall quality of life in these patients who may have only a few more months to live.

Palliation of carcinoma of the esophagus using endoscopic techniques, while safely performed by those with significant experience, may be fraught with significant complications including perforation and bleeding. Passage of flexible endoscopes through an area of narrowed friable tumor may itself lead to perforation unless direct visualization is maintained at all times. Use of the laser and various types of bougies may cause acute perforation of the esophagus into the mediastinum or pleural space and a chest film must be obtained following these procedures to exclude this complication. These principles also apply to the newer techniques of endoscopic stent placement. Use of fluoroscopy during the procedure and X-ray confirmation following placement of the stent with or without dilatation is mandatory in order to assure that stricture is not a result of recurrent tumor.

The flexible endoscope has served as an important diagnostic and therapeutic maneuver in assessing patients with esophageal cancer and in palliating the stricture caused by this disease. In patients who have undergone esophageal resection, endoscopic surveillance of the remaining esophagus or the esophagogastric or esophagocolic anastomosis is appropriate and may identify early recurrent disease. Application of dilatation may also be used if anastomotic strictures occur and this serves as a further method to palliate patients with this significant malignant process.

ENDOSCOPIC MANAGEMENT OF LOWER GASTROINTESTINAL MALIGNANCY

Since 1966, when the first complete flexible examination of the large bowel was performed,[32] the advent and introduction of colonoscopy has been of tremendous value in both the diagnosis and follow-up of patients with benign and malignant diseases of the large bowel. The colonoscope is also a vehicle for performing polyp resection, control of bleeding and laser ablation of a variety of lesions (Figs 4.6 and 4.7). While routinely used by gastroenterologists, it should become an extension of preoperative evaluation and follow-up by the surgeon who has been trained to provide both open abdominal treatment of colonic lesions and, now, minimal access procedures through the laparoscope. One of the important issues for any surgeon is to confirm the presence of specific abnormalities that require resection and to rule out additional lesions which may change the operative intervention (Figs 4.8-4.10). The colonoscope, more than barium studies, can serve as a method of confirmation and decision-making prior to surgical intervention.

Currently, videoendoscopy, using the chip camera, has largely replaced traditional fiberoptic colonoscopy. The instrumentation, however, is basically unchanged in that the surgeon-endoscopist must develop coordination, both as it pertains to flexible motion of the tip and the rotational concepts which require practise and expertise to ensure the safe introduction of the scope. Introduction of the colonoscope is more difficult than upper endoscopy in that the length and mobility of the colon create a situation where skill is required to traverse the many folds of the colon and to provide fixation of the tip during advancement of the endoscope toward the ileum. Preparation of the colon is also of importance since remaining fecal material or other debris may reduce the optical quality as well as affect the endoscopist's ability to introduce the scope safely. Colon preparation by both mechanical and antibiotic means may be appropriate to reduce the bacterial content and to create a safer environment for the application of laser or electrocautery.

Classically, the colon has been evaluated with barium contrast studies which continue to be utilized and which may serve as valuable imaging studies, especially in patients with diverticulosis and carcinoma. It is generally believed, however, that direct vision utilizing colonoscopy will detect small lesions and mucosal abnormalities which may be missed by barium studies.

Colonoscopy is generally performed following an abnormal or indeterminate barium enema and certainly must be performed when patients with chronic rectal bleeding are found to have a 'normal' barium enema. Because of the magnification and excellent optical quality provided by videoendoscopy, small mucosal abnormalities such as arteriovenous

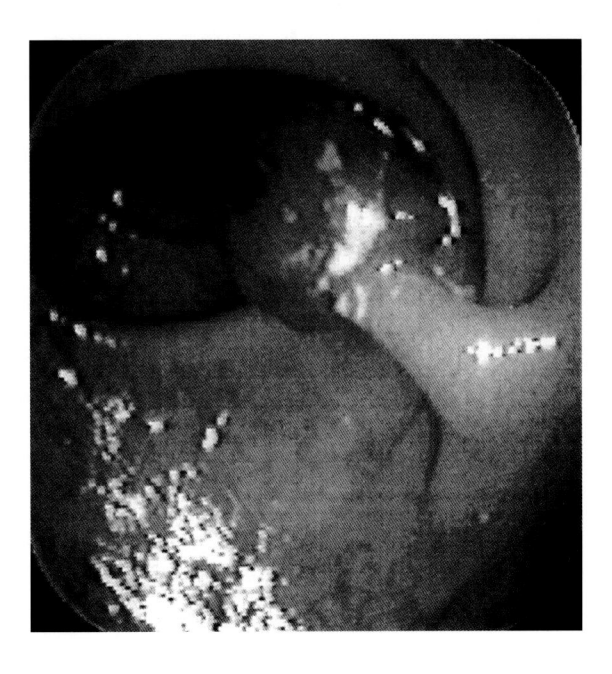

Figure 4.6 - Pedunculated colonic polyp.

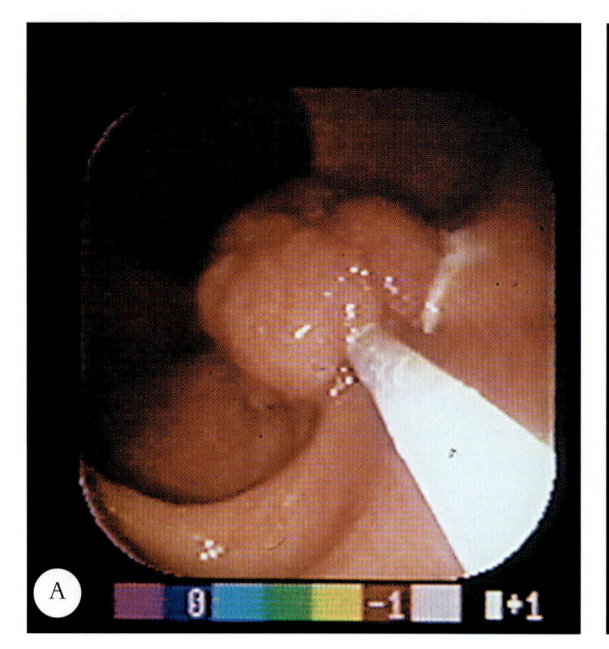

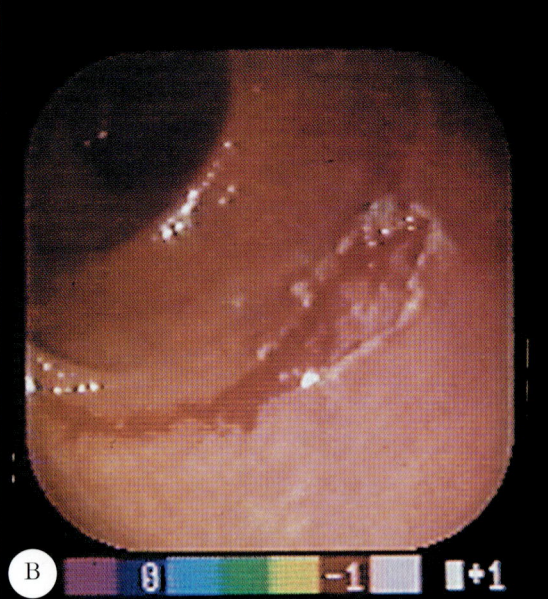

Figure 4.7 - Polyp resection. After the base of the polyp is enclosed in a wire snare (A), electrocautery is used for its removal and concomitant hemostasis (B).

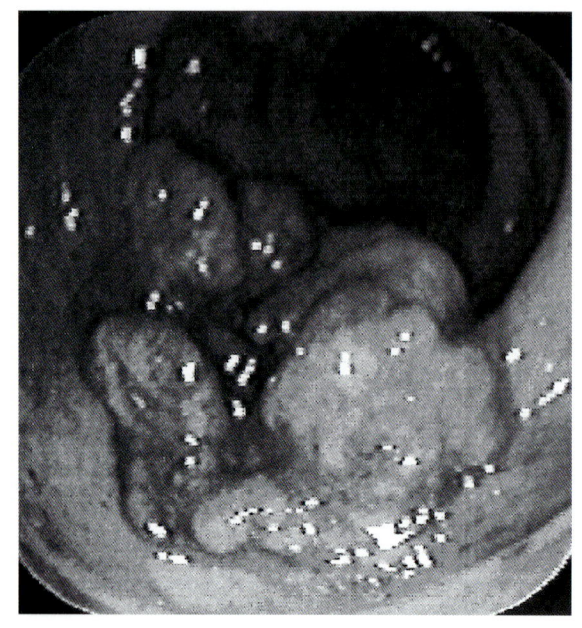

Figure 4.8 - Adenocarcinoma of the colon.

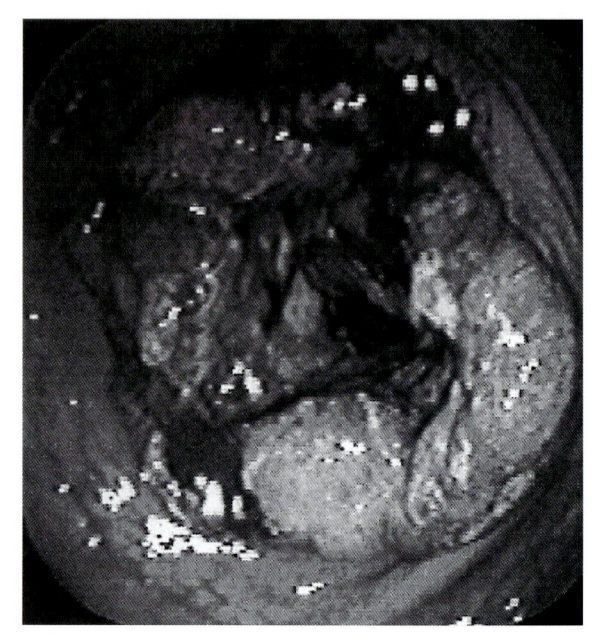

Figure 4.9 - Carcinoma of the entire circumference of the rectum.

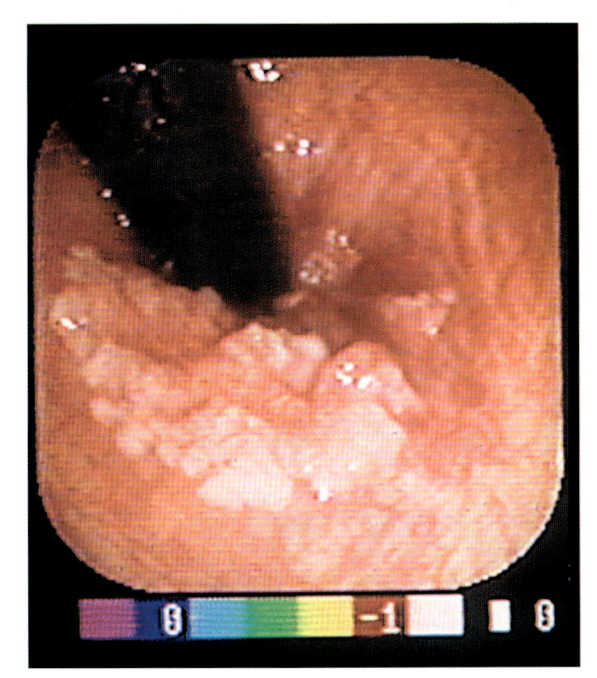

Figure 4.10 – Resection of dentate-line tumors using a transanal approach.

malformations may be clearly seen and documented with color photography or video footage. Significant bleeding from the colon is still a relative contraindication to the performance of colonoscopy since the endoscopist's ability to visualize the colonic lumen is reduced and may ultimately lead to perforation.

The colonoscopic evaluation is especially useful in determining the presence and extent of inflammatory bowel disease, which is limited to or involves the colon. In the presence of chronic ulcerative colitis, which heightens the incidence of adenocarcinoma of the colon, repeated colonic examinations with biopsy may be required to follow patients who are not being evaluated for surgical resection. Repeat biopsy is especially important for multiple areas in patients with ulcerative colitis to identify early dysplasia which may require total abdominal colectomy. In patients who are being actively evaluated for complete colectomy, colonoscopy is important to rule out the synchronous association of adenocarcinoma and fully to evaluate the distal ileum, if possible, for evidence of 'backwash ileitis'. The most important application of colonoscopy is to help in the differentiation between Crohn's disease and ulcerative colitis which require completely different operative approaches, especially if sphincter preservation is generally limited to patients with chronic ulcerative colitis. Long-standing Crohn's disease may in fact be associated with adenocarcinoma and patients with Crohn's colitis should be re-evaluated.

The most important group of patients to be evaluated with colonoscopy are those at risk of developing adenocarcinoma and who may require surgical resection. Patients over the age of 50, especially those with a family history of colon cancer, should undergo total colonoscopy if melena is noted or there is altered bowel habit. It is only through the application of early endoscopy that positive interpretation with biopsy can be achieved and this may prompt resection and cure. Although a small percentage of patients will have synchronous cancers at the time of discovery of an adenocarcinoma of the colon,[33] additional benign lesions in the form of tubulovillous polyps may reach an incidence of 40-50% in patients with documented cancer and may change the length of the colon to be resected.[34] The therapeutic potential of the colonoscope allows polyps, especially those that are pedunculated, to be resected using a snare wire prior to definitive colectomy providing they are isolated to a segment which would not be routinely removed during the treatment procedure. This type of approach will be extremely important as early cancers are treated using minimal access techniques. The surgeon managing patients with colorectal carcinoma must have a clear understanding of the luminal and transperitoneal endoscopic techniques that are used.

TRANSANAL ENDOSCOPIC MICROSURGERY

Transanal endoscopic microsurgery (TEM) was initially introduced in 1983 by Buess for the resection of rectal adenomas.[32] The indications have been extended to include the local resection of well-to-moderately differentiated rectal carcinoma stage pT_1 and even pT_2 in elderly patients with multiple risk factors, and palliative excision of pT_3 carcinomas.[33]

The advantages of the procedure include the precise excision made possible by a magnified, stereoscopic image through a 40 mm rectoscope, the constant gas dilatation of the rectum and the minimal postoperative pain, short hospitalization stay and low complication rate as compared to the classic laparotomy approach.[34] TEM allows dissection of lesions located up to 25 cm from the anal verge.

Complications from TEM include suture dehiscence (3%), rectovaginal fistula (2%), postoperative bleeding (2%) and perineal phlegmon (1%).[34-37] Oncologic results from TEM, although preliminary, include a local recurrence rate of only 4-5% for pT_1 tumors but up to 66% for poorly differentiated pT_1 lesions.[34]

REFERENCES

1. Hirschowitz B, Curtiss LE, Peters CW, Pollard H. Demonstration of a new gastroscope - the "fiberscope". *Gastroenterology* 1958;**35**:40.
2. Lewis BS, Waye JD. Total small bowel enteroscopy. *Gastrointest Endosc* 1987;**33**:435.
3. McCune WS, Shorb PE, Moscovitz H. Endoscopic cannulation of the ampulla of Vater: a preliminary report. *Ann Surg* 1968;**167**:753.
4. Zimmon DS, Falkenstein DB, Kessler RE. Endoscopic papillotomy for choledocholithiasis. *N Engl J Med* 1975;**293**:1181-1182.
5. Ichikawa H. *Screening in Cancer.* Geneva: UICC Publications, 1978.
6. Tytgat G. Diagnosis and differential therapy of malignant esophageal stenosis. *Internist* 1982;**23**:251.
7. Kiefhaber P. Indications for endoscopic Neodymium-YAG laser treatment in the gastrointestinal tract. Twelve years experience. *Scand J Gastroenterol* 1987;**139**(Suppl):53.
8. Greene FL. Esophagogastroduodenoscopy - indication, technique and interpretation. In: Greene F, Ponsky J (eds) *Endoscopic Surgery*. Philadelphia, WB Saunders, 1994, pp. 27-35.
9. Cotton PB, Williams CB. *Practical Gastrointestinal Endoscopy*, 3rd edn. Oxford: Blackwell Scientific, 1990.
10. Greene FL. Neoplastic changes in the postgastrectomy stomach. *Prob Gen Surg* 1990;**7**:55-64.
11. Kamiya T, Morishita T, Asa Kura H et al. Long term followup study on gastric adenomas. *Cancer* 1982;**50**:2496.
12. Donohue JH, Haberman TM. The management of gastric lymphoma. *Surg Oncol Clin NA* 1993;**2**:213-232.
13. Wingo PA, Tong T, Bolden S. Cancer statistics, 1995. *CA Cancer J Clin* 1996;**45**:8-30.
14. Reed WP, Greene FL. Endoscopic screening and surveillance for gastrointestinal malignancy. In: Greene FL, Ponsky JL (eds) *Endoscopic Surgery*. Philadelphia: WB Saunders, 1994, pp. 70-88.
15. Wychulis AR, Woolam GL, Anderson HA et al. Achalasia and carcinoma of the esophagus. *JAMA* 1971;**215**:1638-1641.
16. Agha FP, Keren DF. Barrett's esophagus complicating achalasia after esophagomyotomy: a clinical radiologic and pathologic study of 70 patients with achalasia and related motor disorder. *J Clin Gastroenterol* 1987;**9**:232-237.
17. Dent TL, Kukora JS, Buinewicz BR. Endoscopic screening and surveillance for gastrointestinal malignancy. *Surg Clin NA* 1989;**69**:1205-1225.
18. Haggitt RC. Adenocarcinoma in Barrett's esophagus: a new epidemic? *Hum Pathol* 1992;**23**:475-476.
19. Duhaylongsod FG, Wolfe WG. Barrett's esophagus and adenocarcinoma of the esophagus and gastroesophageal junction. *J Thorac Cardiovasc Surg* 1991;**102**:36-42.
20. Blot WJ, Devesa SS, Kneller RW et al. Rising incidence of adenocarcinoma of the esophagus and gastric cardia. *JAMA* 1991;**265**:1287-1289.
21. Shiozaki H, Tahara H, Kobayashi K et al. Endoscopic screening of early esophageal cancer with the Lugol dye method in patients with head and neck cancers. *Cancer* 1990;**66**:2068-2071.
22. Goldman LP, Weigert JM. Corrosive substance investigation: a review. *Am J Gastroenterol* 1994;**79**:85-90.
23. Kuipers EJ. Atrophic gastritis and *Helicobacter pylori* infection in patients with reflux esophagitis treated with ameprazole or fundoplication. *N Engl J Med* 1996;**334**:1018-1022.
24. Kurtz RC, Sternberg SS, Miller HH et al. Upper gastrointestinal neoplasia in familial polyposis. *Dig Dis Sci* 1991;**32**:459-465.
25. Tomasulo J. Gastric polyps: histologic types and their relationship to gastric carcinoma. Cancer 1971;27:1346-1355.
26. Greene FL. Neoplastic changes in the stomach after gastrectomy. *Surg Gynecol Obstet* 1971;**171**:477-480.
27. Greene FL. Gastric remnant carcinoma based on the results of a 15-year endoscopic screening program. *Ann Surg* 1996; **223**:701-708.
28. Adams DB. Endoscopic management of esophageal stricture. In: Greene FL, Ponsky JL (eds) *Endoscopic Surgery*. Philadelphia: WB Saunders, 1994, pp.36-54.
29. Fleischer D. Endoscopic laser therapy for carcinoma of the esophagus. *Endosc Rev* 1984;**1**:37-49.
30. Greene FL, Boulware RJ, Bianco J. Role of esophagogastroscopy in application and follow-up of high-dose rate brachytherapy for treatment of esophageal carcinoma. *Surg Lap Endosc* 1995;**5**:425-430.
31. Wu WC. Silicone-covered self expanding metallic stents for the palliation of malignant esophageal obstruction and esophagorespiratory fistulas: Experience in 32 patients and a review of the literature. *Gastrointest Endosc* 1994;40:22-33.

32. Buess G, Hutterer F, Theiss J et al. Das System fur die transanale endoskopische rectumoperation. *Chirurg* 1984;**55**:677-680.
33. Buess G, Kipfmuller K, Hack D et al. Technique of transanal endoscopic microsurgery. *Surg Endosc* 1988;**2**:71-75.
34. Mentges B, Buess G, Schafer D et al. Local therapy of rectal tumors. *Dis Colon Rectum* 1996;**39**:886-892.
35. Buess G, Mengtes B, Manncke K et al. Technique and results of transanal endoscopic microsurgery in early rectal cancers. *Am J Surg* 1992;**163**:63-70.
36. Saclarides TJ, Smith L, Ko ST et al. Transanal endoscopic microsurgery. *Dis Colon Rectum* 1992;**35**:1183-1191.
37. Said S, Chiavellati L, Pichlmaier H. Transanal endoscopic microsurgery: technique and clinical results. *Minerva Chir* 1992;**47**:1055-1064.

5

Laparoscopic Cholecystectomy: Lessons Learned from Gallbladder Cancer

Frank H. Chae and Jonathan M. Sackier

*L*aparoscopic cholecystectomy has become the procedure of choice for removal of the diseased gallbladder. With cancer of the gallbladder to be expected in 1-2% of all biliary tract operations, it is likely that surgeons will be confronted with increasing numbers of unsuspected gallbladder carcinoma during the course of their laparoscopic experience.[1] Unfortunately, gallbladder carcinoma is rarely diagnosed before operative intervention. The limitations of ultrasonography or other imaging methods as diagnostic tools for this type of cancer are well known.[2] Approximately 10-30% of the cancer cases are confined to the gallbladder wall and are not diagnosed until their histologic appearance is identified on postoperative microscopic examination. Although a minority, this group has the best prognosis since gallbladder carcinoma overall is associated with a poor overall outcome. Carcinoma of the gallbladder is the fifth commonest malignancy of the gastrointestinal tract in the United States after carcinoma of the colon, pancreas, stomach and esophagus, and despite being relatively uncommon, about 5000 new cases are diagnosed each year.[3]

Contraindications to laparoscopic cholecystectomy are few but there are growing concerns about port-site implantation and peritoneal spreading of tumor cells after the laparoscopic procedure in the face of unsuspected gallbladder cancer. The general consensus is that laparoscopic cholecystectomy should not be used for gallbladder cancer; however, the problem lies in the occult nature of this tumor since the majority are discovered only after the operation. Also, the effect of the laparoscopic procedure on the long-term prognosis of gallbladder cancer is unknown. This chapter addresses the issues and concerns about performing laparoscopic cholecystectomy in cases of gallbladder carcinoma.

INDICATIONS FOR CHOLECYSTECTOMY

Adenocarcinoma represents about 90% of reported gallbladder carcinomas reported. The rest include squamous, undifferentiated, carcinoid, and clear cell types. The most common presenting signs are those of advanced disease as the tumor spreads by direct local extension usually into segments IV and V of the liver. About 50% of patients present with jaundice, reflecting common duct involvement and up to 10% present with acute cholecystitis as a result of cystic duct obstruction from tumor.[4,5] Nevin et al.[6] established a staging system (Table 5.1) based on the level of tumor infiltration in the gallbladder wall. The American Joint Committee on Cancer followed and instituted the TNM classification to take into account the size and extension of the tumor as well as the nodal groups involved (Table 5.2).[7]

Gallbladder cancer prognosis is poor, with an average survival of just 6 months. The fact that as high as 90% of gallbladder cancer patients present with stage V disease reduces 5-year survival rate to <5%. If

Table 5.1 – Stages of gallbladder cancer

Stage	Depth of invasion
I	Mucosa only
II	Muscularis involvement
III	Subserosal involvement
IV	All layers and lymph node
V	Local invasion or distant metasasis

Table 5.2 – TNM classification

T: Size of tumor	Stage
Tis: Carcinoma *in situ*	I: T1, N0, M0
T2: perimuscular invasion	II: T2, N0, M0
T1: mucosa invasion	III: T1, T2/T3, N0/N1, M0
T3: one adjacent organ (> 2 cm Liver)	IVA: T4, N0/N1, M0
T4: >2 organs or >2 cm into Liver	IVB: any T, N2, M0 or any T, any N, M1

N: Region Lymph Nodes

N0: no nodal involvement
N1: Cystic duct, Pericholedochal or Hilar lymph node involvement
N2: Peripancreatic, Periduodenal, Periportal, Celiac or Superior Mesenteric nodal involement

there is no transmural extension of the tumor, 5-year survival increases to 20%. Despite radical resection, the tumor tends to be locally aggressive and usually invades regional liver and portal areas. Over the past 50 years, there has been no appreciable improvement in survival from gallbladder carcinoma.[4,8,9]

If the diagnosis is suspected, whether from clinical signs or abnormal gallbladder ultrasonography, a CT scan should be done to evaluate the liver parenchyma as well as the adjacent structures such as the stomach, duodenum, omentum or colon for metastatic involvement. These findings if present, would of course preclude the possibility of cure.[4,5,9-11]

Carcinoma limited to the mucosa offers the best chance of cure with cholecystectomy and such a procedure is deemed adequate therapy with excellent survival; these cases are most often found incidentally at the time of cholecystectomy for gallbladder disease or in patients found to have gallbladder polyps.[5,12] If the tumor spreads beyond the mucosa, the prognosis is poor and there is high recurrence; therefore, a second-stage operation is required to resect the gallbladder bed along with lymph node dissection. This step is referred to as radical or extended cholecystectomy.[3,4,8-11]

Local invasion of the skin or metastasis to the subcutaneous tissues has not been recognized as a typical mode of spread in gallbladder carcinoma. Only isolated case reports are found describing manifestations to the head, neck, extremities and umbilicus.[13,14] Unfortunately, most reports describing gallbladder cancer spread after laparoscopic cholecystectomy involve tumor growth out of cannula sites or diffuse peritoneal metastasis. Furthermore, these recurrences are associated with the more aggressive tumor stages not discovered until after pathological examination and hence preclude the option of conversion to the open approach which may apparently reduce the risk of spread.

COMPLICATIONS OF THE LAPAROSCOPIC APPROACH

Laparoscopic procedures have been adapted for the surgery of an increasing number of malignant diseases. As more laparoscopic procedures are performed for tumor resection, there are a growing number of reports available dealing with cannula-site metastasis following the laparoscopic technique. This complication also appears to be more frequent than metastatic spread following conventional open techniques. The physiological explanation for this tendency has not been explained.

Although gallbladder carcinoma remains a rare entity, the growing number of cases describing occult carcinoma discovered postoperatively is not surprising given the increasing number of laparoscopic cholecystectomies being performed. A prospective analysis of 1518 laparoscopic cholecystectomies by the Southern Surgeons Club revealed only 4 cases (0.3%) of gallbladder carcinoma with no mention of tumor recurrence.[15]

There has been growing alarm about the spread of tumor cells to trocar sites following laparoscopic cholecystectomy for unsuspected gallbladder cancer discovered only after the operation. Most reports are case presentations documenting the occurrence of cannula site metastasis. However, this has raised enough concern to convince many that carcinoma of the gallbladder should be considered a contraindication to laparoscopic resection. Moreover, a calcified or 'porcelain' gallbladder is associated with carcinoma in 15-20% of cases and contraindicates a minimal access procedure (Fig. 5.1). A retrospective analysis of 928 patients who underwent elective cholecystectomy reports only 9 cases (0.97%) of gallbladder carcinoma.[16] Although a relatively small study, the paper revealed several interesting trends. When compared to patients without gallbladder cancer, the patients with carcinoma were older, had thicker gallbladder walls and had more external gallbladder abnormalities detected intraoperatively. Interestingly, for gallbladder carcinoma in advanced stages, the recurrences seem to occur more rapidly after laparoscopy than the open method, resulting in diffuse spread to peritoneum and cannula sites. Laparoscopy, however, was found to be effective when the disease was confined to the gallbladder mucosa and removed intact without spillage of bile. If the gallbladder is torn during dissection, the risk of spread appears to increase even if the original tumor is a carcinoma *in situ*. Large studies are needed to confirm these findings.

An alarming feature of cannula site metastasis from gallbladder carcinoma is the short period of time required for the tumor growth to reach clinically significant size. The usual reported time period is between 2 and 4 months. In cases requiring a second stage laparotomy for extended wedge resection of the gallbladder bed because of the advanced stage of

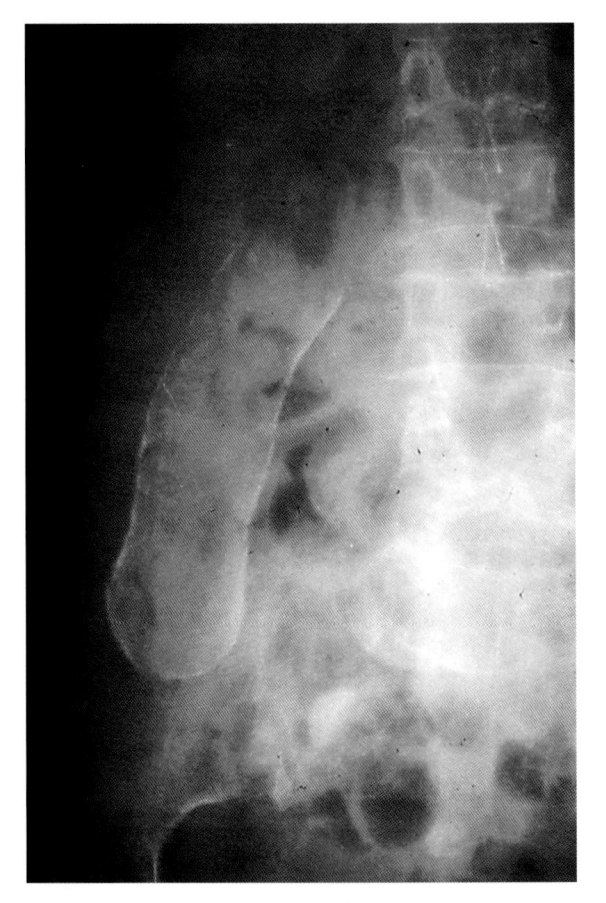

Figure 5.1 – X-ray of a porcelain gallbladder

gallbladder cancer, microscopic implantation of viable tumor cells from the cannula sites has been demonstrated only weeks after the original operation.[17-21]

Port-site metastasis appears to occur more frequently than laparotomy incisional metastasis; however, if laparoscopy is conducted for diagnostic purposes only rather than for resection, there appears to be minimal associated risk of spread.[17] In 1 case of laparoscopic cholecystectomy in a patient with undetected colon cancer presenting with bowel obstruction, a cutaneous metastasis developed in a trocar site only 9 months after colon resection.[22] In cases where laparoscopic dissection has been abandoned and converted to the open technique, tumor implantation has occurred in trocar sites while sparing the laparotomy wound. Certainly for most umbilical port-site recurrences, direct seeding from the exposed gallbladder as it is removed from the abdomen may explain the mechanism, but questions remain as to recurrences in other auxiliary port sites as well as the umbilical wound which will never come into contact with the gallbladder specimen. Although most studies report umbilical port-site recurrence, the other port sites are also more at risk of development of tumor implants than is a concomitant laparotomy wound. If the gallbladder contents are spilled, there appears to be an increased incidence of port metastasis.[22-27]

Most cases of advanced tumor spread to areas adjacent to the gallbladder are as a result of direct extension of the original tumor and are unlikely to be related to the laparoscopic procedure. There has been no reported link between recurrence of gallbladder carcinoma to adjacent organs and the use of laparoscopy. Also, excluding cannula site metastasis, substantial risk of diffuse peritoneal seeding after laparoscopy has yet to be demonstrated.

Why are laparoscopic trocar sites highly susceptible to tumor recurrences? One speculation might be because the peritoneal layers of the cannula sites are mostly left unclosed. The peritoneal layer is usually apposed after laparotomy and this may play a deterrent role in tumor recurrence.[18] In the process of wound healing, there is a high rate of cell proliferation in this area and peritoneal closure may be the limiting factor in preventing or minimizing tumor seeding.[28] Despite the well recognized tendency of intraabdominal malignancies to spread toward the umbilicus - the classic Sister Mary Joseph's nodules - the unprecedented short time required for recurrence, as little as 2 months for clinical detection, clearly points to the alarming propensity of gallbladder carcinoma for metastatic seeding to laparoscopic puncture sites.

If gallbladder carcinoma is discovered after laparoscopic cholecystectomy, the patient must be followed closely to detect recurrence of tumor implants, particularly in the umbilical wound site. Any abnormal wound healing must be investigated with CT scan and, if in doubt, a local wound excision should be performed. Other than excising the recurrent spread, the options remain unclear. The therapeutic effects of preventive radiation or local application of chemotherapy are still speculative. One case has been reported of 11-month tumor free survival after subjecting the patient to a trial of extended cholecystectomy, including prophylactic excision of the umbilical cannula site used in the initial laparoscopy, followed by adjuvant radiotherapy to the gallbladder bed and umbilical scar.[21] The stage involved was lymph node-free gallbladder carcinoma (T2N0M0) extending through the muscular layer. Interestingly, microscopic examination of the umbilical wound sample revealed gallbladder cancer cells even though there was no clinical manifestation 18 days following the initial laparoscopy. The remaining port sites were free of clinically detectable tumor.

Another study also reports tumor implantation near the umbilical port site only 21 days after laparoscopic cholecystectomy for unsuspected gallbladder carcinoma. This patient underwent extended resection and received adjuvant chemotherapy and radiotherapy leading to 17 month tumor free follow-up.[17]

Aside from containing leakage of bile or gallstones from the gallbladder, an additional benefit for the use of a protective bag could be the minimization of iatrogenic cancer cell spillage and thereby reduced seeding. No paper published thus far has addressed this step definitively, but as this extra precaution may prevent devastating consequences, some have proposed its adoption in all laparoscopic cholecystectomies even though an encounter with gallbladder carcinoma is rare.[17,21,24]

These examples emphasize the need carefully to evaluate the gallbladder preoperatively in the hope of detecting gallbladder carcinoma. The suggestive signs of tumor on ultrasonography of the gallbladder are a fungating mass, a fixed lesion filling the lumen, smoothed raised mucosa or mucosal thickening.[2] Nevertheless, preoperative detection of early stage and therefore curable gallbladder carcinoma remains elusive. One suggestion is that any patient with a questionable preoperative sonogram should undergo open cholecystectomy, although this recommendation is unsubstantiated.[5,9,21,25]

Despite reports from Japan[11] that gallbladder cytology is of significant prognostic value, it does not distinguish invasive from the noninvasive tumors in gallbladder carcinoma. Studies demonstrating its advantage over histologic evaluation of the gallbladder tumor depth have yet to be performed.[5,17]

An important point to stress is the difference between diagnostic and therapeutic laparoscopy in gallbladder carcinoma. As yet, there is no clear demonstrable risk of tumor spread or its effect on the prognosis of gallbladder carcinoma with the use of laparoscopy for diagnostic evaluation. The minimally invasive nature of laparoscopy remains advantageous over conventional open laparotomy when evaluated in terms of operative morbidity and mortality rates. It is particularly ideal in compromised patients who would not be able to tolerate or recover from full laparotomy. Laparoscopic evaluation allows visualization of the gallbladder and its surroundings to stage gallbladder tumor involvement accurately and is far superior to either ultrasound or CT examinations.[8,25,29] This may prevent unnecessary exploratory laparotomies for incurable gallbladder cancer and allow expedient initiation of alternative palliative procedures such as endoscopic biliary endoprosthesis.[30] On the other hand, rapid malignant seeding has been reported after diagnostic laparoscopy in the presence of malignant gynecologic epithelial tumors and hence the true behavior of gallbladder cancer spread even after a diagnostic laparoscopic evaluation remains speculative.[26]

CONCLUSION

Cancer of the gallbladder has always been associated with an unfavorable prognosis. Despite recent improvements in diagnostic imaging modalities and a better understanding of the natural history of gallbladder cancer, the majority of cases present in advanced stages with poor prognosis. Unfortunately, most cases of gallbladder carcinoma are not discovered until after its removal for gallbladder disease. It is this scenario of unsuspected gallbladder carcinoma that is associated with tumor seeding reported after laparoscopic cholecystectomy. The definitive management of occult gallbladder carcinoma remains elusive due to the paucity of data. The long-term effect of laparoscopic cholecystectomy in the management of occult gallbladder carcinoma and the implications for metastatic seedings on the long term survival rate will only be clarified with time.

Based on available data, several guidelines regarding laparoscopic cholecystectomy should be followed. If gallbladder carcinoma is suspected in the preoperative evaluation, open cholecystectomy should be performed and if permissible, an extended cholecystectomy with regional lymph node dissection should be added. If there is any suspicion of malignancy during laparoscopic cholecystectomy, the case should be converted to an open procedure. The port sites should be excised if any manipulation of the gallbladder occurs with the laparoscopic instruments and all peritoneal openings should be closed, including the 5 mm port sites. The issue of using bags routinely to retrieve the gallbladder has yet to be resolved and should be left to the surgeon's discretion

Once removed, all gallbladder specimens should be examined grossly during the procedure for presence of tumor. If there is any suspicion of mucosal abnormality, a frozen section should be sent for confirmation and all port sites should be excised if pathology confirms carcinoma. With gallbladder carcinoma confined to the muscular wall and not involving the margin of the cystic duct, laparoscopic cholecystectomy alone appears to be adequate therapy. However, for more advanced disease, the risk of tumor implantation during laparoscopic dissection is convincing enough to warrant conversion to the open technique. When the carcinoma discovered after laparoscopic cholecystectomy involves deep invasion of the gallbladder wall, a complete metastatic workup involving CT scans of the chest, abdomen and pelvis is necessary. This should be followed by wide resection of the gallbladder bed along with the cannula sites.

Prudence would also dictate that patients with any evidence of gallbladder carcinoma who have undergone laparoscopy, should be followed closely for recurrence of tumor around the cannula sites. Any abnormal healing of the port sites should be investigated for tumor growth. For tumor recurrences, wide excision of the wound sites should be performed. The role of radiation and chemotherapy in laparoscopically associated tumor recurrence still remains to be determined. Finally, the long term effect of initial laparoscopic cholecystectomy on gallbladder cancer morbidity and mortality needs to be followed. Furthermore, more research is required to explain the apparent propensity of tumor cells for port-site metastasis.

REFERENCES

1. Bergdahl L. Gallbladder carcinoma first diagnosed at microscopic examination of gallbladders removed for presumed benign disease. *Ann Surg* 1980;**191**:19-22.
2. Tsuchiya Y. Early carcinoma of the gallbladder: macroscopic features and US findings. *Radiology* 1991;**179**:171-175.
3. Piehler J, Crihlow R. Primary carcinoma of the gallbladder. *Surg Gynecol Obstet* 1978;**147**:929
4. Silk YN, Douglas HO, Nava HR, Driscoll DL, Tartarian G. Carcinoma of the gallbladder; the Roswell Park experience. *Ann Surg* 1989;**210**:751-757.
5. Donohue JH, Nagorney DM, Grant CS, Tsushima K, Ilstrup DM, Adson MA. Carcinoma of the gallbladder. *Arch Surg* 1990;**125**:237-241.
6. Nevin JE, Moran TJ, Kay S, King R. Carcinoma of gallbladder: staging, treatment and prognosis. *Cancer* 1976;**37**:141-148
7. Beahars OH. Gallbladder. In: Beahars OH, Henson DE, Hutter RV, Kennedy BJ (eds) *Manual for Staging of Cancer*, 3rd edn. Philadelphia: JB Lippincott, 1988, pp. 93-98.
8. Cubertafond P, Gainant A, Cucchiaro G. Surgical treatment of 724 carcinomas of the gallbladder: results of the French Surgical Association Survey. *Ann Surg* 1994;**219**:275-280.
9. Ouchi K, Suzuki M, Saijo S, Ito K, Matsuno S. Do recent advances in diagnosis and operative management improve the outcome of gallbladder carcinoma? *Surgery* 1993;**113**:324-329.
10. Chijiwa K, Tanaka M. Carcinoma of the gallbladder: an appraisal of surgical resection. *Surgery* 1994;**115**:751-756.
11. Ouchi K, Owada Y, Matsuno S, Sato T. Prognostic factors in the surgical management of gallbladder carcinoma. *Surgery* 1987;**101**:731-737.
12. de Aretxabala X, Roa I, Burgos L et al.. Gallbladder cancer in Chile. *Cancer* 1992;**69**:60-65.
13. Rousselot R. Tumeur ombilicele, metastase revelatrice d'un cancer vesiculaire. *Bull Soc Fr Derm Syph* 1964;**71**:670-672.
14. Padilla RS, Jermillo M, Dao A, Chapman W. Cutaneous metastatic adenocarcinoma of gallbladder origin. *Arch Dermatol* 1982;**118**:515-517.
15. The Southern Surgical Club. A prospective analysis of 1518 laparoscopic cholecystectomies. *N Engl J Med* 1991;**324**:1073-1078.
16. Wibbenmeyer LA, Wade TP, Chen RC, Meyer RC, Turgeon RP, Andrus CH. Laparoscopic cholecystectomy can disseminate in situ carcinoma of the gallbladder. *J Am Coll Surg* 1995;**181**:504-510.
17. Wade TP, Comitalo JB, Andrus CH, Goodwin MN, Kaminski DL. Laparoscopic cancer surgery: lessons from gallbladder cancer. *Surg Endosc* 1994;**8**:698-701.
18. Jacobi CA, Keller H, Monig S, Said S. Implantation metastasis of unsuspected gallbladder carcinoma after laparoscopy. *Surg Endosc* 1995;**9**:351-352.
19. Ng JW, Lee KK, Chan AY. Documentation of tumor seeding complicating laparoscopic cholecystectomy for unsuspected gallbladder carcinoma. *Surgery* 1994;**115**:530-531.
20. Dubronte F, Wittman T, Karacsony G. Rapid development of malignant metastases in the abdominal wall after laparoscopy. *Endoscopy* 1978;**10**:127-130.
21. Kim HJ, Roy T. Unexpected gallbladder cancer with

cutaneous seeding after laparoscopic cholecystectomy. *S Med J* 1994;**87**:817-820.

22. Ugarte F. Laparoscopic cholecystectomy port seeding from a colon carcinoma. *Am Surg* 1995;**61**:820-821.

23. Nally C, Preshaw RM. Tumor implantation at umbilicus after laparoscopic cholecystectomy for unsuspected gallbladder carcinoma. *Can J Surg* 1994;**37**:243-244.

24. Copher JC, Rogers JJ, Dalton ML. Trocar-site metastasis following laparoscopic cholecystectomy for unsuspected carcinoma of the gallbladder. *Surg Endosc* 1995;**9**:348-350.

25. Clair DG, Lautz DB, Brooks DC. Rapid development of umbilical metastases after laparoscopic cholecystectomy for unsuspected gallbladder carcinoma. *Surgery* 1993;**113**:355-358.

26. Gershman A, Daykhovsky L, Chandra M, Danoff D, Grundfest WS. Laparoscopic pelvic lymphadenectomy. *J Laparoendosc Surg* 1990;**1**:63-68.

27. Merz BJ, Dodge GG, Abellera RM, Kisken WA. Implant metastasis of gallbladder carcinoma in situ in a cholecystecomy scar: a case report. *Surgery* 1993;**114**:120-124.

28. Eggermont AM, Steller EP, Sugarbaker PH. Laparotomy enhances intraperitoneal tumor growth and abrogates the anti-tumor effects of interleukin-2 and lymphokine-activated killer cells. *Surgery* 1987;**102**:71-78.

29. Bhargava DK, Sarin S, Verma K. Laparoscopy in carcinoma of the gallbladder. *Gastrointest Endosc* 1983;**29**:21-25.

30. Vij JC, Govil A, Chaudhary A, Gulati R, Mehta S, Ganguli S. Endoscopic biliary endoprosthesis for palliation of gallbladder carcinoma. *Gastrointest Endosc* 1996;**43**:121-123.

6

Laparoscopic Colectomy: The Concerns and the Benefits

Steven D. Wexner and Eric G. Weiss

No one could have predicted the tremendous impact on surgery of the introduction of laparoscopic cholecystectomy. Not only has the procedure become the treatment of choice for the majority of patients with biliary colic or cholecystitis, but the laparoscope has been applied to nearly every surgical specialty and procedure.

The unbridled enthusiam emanates from the remarkable results that have occurred with laparoscopic cholecystectomy and has been extrapolated to other forms of surgery. However, the results of improved cost, less pain, shorter hospitalization and convalescence, as well as other benefits, have not been universally borne out in other forms of laparoscopic surgery.

LAPAROSCOPIC COLORECTAL SURGERY VERSUS OTHER LAPAROSCOPIC PROCEDURES

Specifically, in laparoscopic colorectal surgery, the benefits mentioned above have not been universally realized. It is unclear why laparoscopic colorectal procedures are different from other laparoscopic procedures and why some or all of the benefits seen in other procedures are not found with laparoscopic colorectal surgery. There are five fundmental differences between laparoscopic colorectal surgery and almost all other laparoscopic procedures.

1. Laparoscopic colorectal surgery is typically a multi-quadrant procedure. Most segmental colectomies require mobilization of the colon in at least two quadrants and sometimes more if a subtotal colectomy or another procedure is being performed. Therefore, it is often necessary to move personnel as well as to change the position of instruments, monitors and the patient to access these quadrants. These maneuvres are in marked contrast to laparoscopic cholecystectomy, fundoplication, herniorrhaphy or appendectomy where the target organ lies in a single quadrant. In these latter scenarios, once the trocars are placed and the instruments inserted, there is no need to reposition and little need to change specific instruments.

2. Vascular ligation is relatively easy in cholecystectomy as the singly small artery is readily, safely, rapidly and inexpensively controlled with several clips. Similarly, appendectomy requires only minor and hernia repair no vessel ligation. In fundoplication the dispute about short gastric ligation rages on, but the vessels are largely accessible, although this is sometimes challenging. It may require a great deal of time to secure these vessels and even with extreme caution, impressive hemorrhage can occur.

   Obviously, the colon has numerous arcades of branching vessels that need to be ligated. These vessels are often large and at times embedded in a thick, fatty mesentery. It therefore becomes a tedious and often time-consuming process to ligate vessels when performing a colectomy. Typically, either numerous clips, ties or more commonly, vascular staplers are used for this ligation. Although the latter method is quicker, it certainly adds to the cost of the procedure. One must balance cost against time in this scenario. The recent introduction of the harmonic scalpel device may expedite this phase of the operation.

3. Specimen retrieval can be easily accomplished through a standard trocar site for most cholecystectomies or appendectomies, and no specimens are produced during herniorrhaphy or fundoplication. However, an enlarged trocar site or a formal, albeit 'small', incision is necessary to remove specimens in laparoscopic colorectal surgery, unless the anus, or in the case of abdominoperineal resection, the perineum, can be used as the exit route.

4. Once the specimen has been removed or the defect repaired, these other laparoscopic procedures are complete, whereas an anastomosis needs to be performed in the majority of colorectal procedures. The increased complexity and time needed to perform a well vascularized, tension free, circumferentially intact anastomosis is very different from the removal of a gallbladder.

5. Most importantly, the major indication in most series of laparoscopic colorectal surgery is malignancy.[1,2] Whether similar short-term and long-term outcomes for cancer utilizing laparoscopic approaches are achievable is debatable and are the focus of this chapter.

LAPAROSCOPIC VERSUS OPEN COLECTOMY

In comparing laparoscopic and open procedures, numerous parameters must be considered. Any new procedure should be safer with a lower procedural related mobility and mortality than the standard procedure. Numerous series of laparoscopic colorectal surgery show that the morbidity and mortality in performing laparoscopic colorectal surgery is similar to that reported in open series.[3,4]

In evaluating the theoretical benefits of laparoscopic surgery over open surgery, it is important to assess length of stay, postoperative pain, cosmesis, resolution of ileus and cost.

Length of stay

Length of stay continues to be one of the most closely scrutinized parameters in this comparison. Although length of stay would appear to be an inherently easy parameter to compare, the definition and criteria used for discharge vary greatly between institutions, which makes comparison between series very difficult. A collective series by Wexner and Reissman[6] compiled data on 486 patients with a mean hospitalization of 7.1 days. This length of stay is not significantly different from that for many colectomies performed in the United States; however, length of stay is longer in Europe and other countries. Some series show a remarkably shorter length of stay than 7.1 days but not all patients may have been discharged on a regular diet - some may have been discharged on clear liquids and told to advance their diets at home. Furthermore, patients have been discharged home prior to the first bowel movement. In the series reported by Phillips et al.,[4] the mean length of hospitalization of 4.1 days may in large part be attributable to the fact that many patients did not undergo resectional surgery, but rather colotomy and polypectomy. We recently reviewed our initial 140 laparoscopic colectomies[7] and found a remarkably similar hospital stay for our non-resectional procedures.

Allowing patients earlier *ad lib* oral intake, even after laparotomy, has been shown to decrease length of stay. Two prospective randomized trials confirm that patients can tolerate early oral intake after laparotomy.[8,9] In these two studies, between 0.6 and 1.3 days of hospitalization were gained by allowing patients clear liquids immediately postoperatively and advancing diets as tolerated to solid food. The average length of stay was 6 days. Therefore, it does not appear that laparoscopy exerts a significant effect on postoperative stay after colectomy. However, practice patterns are changing and hopefully even shorter stays will be possible.

Postoperative pain

Several series have evaluated the pain associated with laparoscopic colon surgery as compared to laparotomy. Ramos et al.[10] showed that patients undergoing standard surgery used patient-controlled analgesia for 6.2 days postoperatively versus 2.9 days if the procedure was performed laparoscopically. More recently, Pfeifer et al.[11] analyzed two matched groups of patients who had undergone either open or laparoscopic colorectal surgery. There were no statistically different responses when patients were asked to compare the pain of the laparoscopic procedure either to previous 'open' operation or their own expectations. Others, however, support the view that laparoscopic procedures are associated with less postoperative pain.[12]

Cosmesis

Improved cosmesis is another proposed benefit of laparoscopic surgery. Pfeifer et al.[11] asked patients to compare their incisions to those either of previous surgery or their own perceptions. There was no statistically significant difference in the responses between the open and laparoscopic groups.

Laparoscopic colorectal surgery is feasible and is associated with procedural mobility and mortality similar to laparotomy and colectomy. The ability to tolerate oral intake, day of discharge and cosmesis do not appear to significantly differ between the procedures. In some series, there may be less postoperative pain associated with laparoscopic procedures. However, these parameters are all secondary when the pathology is malignant. Parameters such as long-term survival and tumor recurrence need to be considered. Unfortunately, more time is needed to evaluate the long-term outcome in respect to cancer survival and recurrence. As the first laparoscopic colon resection was performed in 1991, only minimal 5-year follow-up data are available. To address the advisability of the technique for cure of colorectal carcinoma, a question can be posted. Suppose a hypothetical patient with a Dukes' B rectal adenocarcinoma is a candidate for a curative laparoscopic colectomy. The patient has the procedure and the intracorporeal resection and anastomosis takes only 90 min. The procedure is performed in the outpatient setting and the patient is discharged home tolerating a regular diet, moving her bowels and pain free. Although she is not disabled like the vast majority of patients with colorectal carcinoma, she is elderly and therefore retired from the workforce. So far, the procedure sounds like a resounding triumph. However, 6 months later, the patient develops an unresectable pelvic recurrence. No data are available to answer the question as to whether the recurrence could have been avoided by an 'open' resection. In retrospect, in the absence of a scientifically valid answer to the question, were the extra few meals and few days at home a fair trade to this patient who will now die from what was a potentially curable disease?

ONCOLOGICAL PRINCIPLES OF LAPAROSCOPIC COLORECTAL SURGERY

Despite this apparent paucity of long-term data, parameters that may indicate adequate oncological operations have been described. Comparisons of the number of lymph nodes harvested during resection, length of bowel removed, distance to the margins and the level of vascular ligation have all been reported.

The most commonly reported variable in considering the oncologic adequacy of a colon resection is the number of lymph nodes found by the patholgist. One must remember that the actual number of lymph nodes harvested has never been shown to correlate either with survival or recurrence. Moreover, Scott and Grace[13] have shown that lymph node harvest must consist of at least 13 lymph nodes to allow adequate staging. A similar number may be retrieved by performing a vascular ligation close to the bowel wall for a long distance, as when performing a shorter bowel resection with a higher ligation, so even the number of lymph nodes harvested does not guarantee proper staging. The method of isolating lymph nodes is also important in determining the actual number. The number of lymph nodes found in any given specimen is dependent on the diligence of the pathologist and whether any techniques are used to increase the number of lymph nodes found.[14]

Despite these potential shortcomings, many series have presented the number of lymph nodes harvested (Table 6.1). The mean number of nodes found in open and laparoscopic procedures is typically less than

Table 6.1 – Lymph node harvest

Reference	Year	Number of nodes (range)	
		Open	Laparoscopic
Bleday et al.[15]	1993	9.5	10.57
Darzi et al.[16]	1995	11.0	8.0
		6.0 (4-14)	9.5 (6-19)
Dodson et al.[17]	1993	7.0	4.2
Fine et al.[18]	1995	N/A	9.1
Franklin et al.[19]	1995	14.7	15.8
Hoffman et al.[20]	1994	8.0	6.1
Larach et al.[21]	1993	–	9.8 (0-22)
Lord et al.[22]	1996	8.9	7.8
Musser et al.[23]	1994	7.9	10.6
Peters and Bartels[24]	1993	8.5	7.9
Tate et al.[12]	1993	10 (2-14)	13 (2-18)
Tucker et al.[25]	1995	6.4	8.7
Van Ye et al.[26]	1994	–	–
Wexner et al.[27]	1993	–	19 (3-84)
Zucker et al.[28]	1994	–	7.3 (5-11)

N/A = not available

the 13 recommended by Scott and Grace.[13] However, there are essentially no differences in the number of lymph nodes harvested by open and laparoscopic procedures.

Milsom et al.[29] reviewed lymph node harvest in a slightly less traditional venue. They performed laparoscopic proctosigmoidectomy on 9 'fresh' cadavers. The entire specimen was mobilized and divided laparoscopically with intracorporeal high ligation of the inferior mesenteric artery. After the specimen was removed, an autopsy was performed and only 1 node remained in the inferior mesenteric artery pedicle in 1 of the 9 cadavers; otherwise a complete lymph node harvest was obtained with this technique. This single remaining lymph node probably does not jeopardize an oncologic operation as there is considerable controversy whether high ligation offers any survival advantage. This excellent technical exercise in cadavers supports the feasibility of the procedure in living patients.

The length of specimen removed as well as the distance to the proximal and distal margins have also been studied. Generally, proximal margins have not been a problem. The distal margin is much more variable and in procedures such as low anterior resection, the margins must be at least 2 cm in every case.[30] In fact, during laparotomy it is exceedingly rare not to have margins of at least 5 cm. In the laparoscopic literature, there is considerably less data available with respect to margins. Table 6.2 shows three series, one comparing 'open' versus laparoscopic procedures[12] and the other reviewing a variety of laparoscopically performed colectomies.[19] In the former, both the open and laparoscopic margins were small (mean 2.0-2.5 cm). However, in the laparoscopic group in which the mean tumor height was 2.0 cm, the minimum margin was only 5 mm. It is clearly inappropriate to offer a patient hope of a curative sigmoid colectomy if a distal margin of only 5 mm is obtained.

Radial margins play a particularly important role in rectal cancer. Quirke et al.[31] have shown that if the radial margin of the mesorectum is involved with the tumor, then there is an extremely high rate of pelvic recurrence of rectal cancer. The complete removal of the mesorectum championed by Heald and Ryall[32] supports this theory. In a study of 12 patients who underwent laparoscopic-assisted abdominoperineal resections for rectal cancer, Darzi et

Table 6.2 – Distal margins in reported series for laparoscopic surgery for malignacy

Reference	Distal margin (cm)	Laparoscopic	Open
Tate et al.[12]	Length of bowel (cm)	2.0 (0.5)	2.5 (2-5)
	Mean distal margin (cm) (range)	14 (11-21)	15 (7-25)
		17	
Franklin et al.[19]	Right distal margin (cm)	17	
	Anterior distal margin (cm) (range)	13	
	LAR distal margin (cm)	5	
	APR distal margin (cm)	2	
Lord et al.[22]	Distal margin (cm)	3.5	6.1

N/A = not available; APR = Abdominoperineal resection; LAR = Low anterior resection

al.[16] reported a radial margin of only 0.5 cm (0.1-1.5 in laparoscopic cases compared to 0.9 cm (0.1-3.6) in open cases. The 50% reduction in the average laparoscopic margin compared to laparotomy may be a result of 'coning down' in the pelvis. Despite reports that rectal dissection is 'perfect' for laparoscopy, these smaller radial margins may be a potential problem.

Combining the above data regarding lymph node harvest, radial and distal margins and the length of bowel suggests that technically a similar oncologic operation is achieved by open and laparoscopic procedures. Nonetheless, these theoretical parameters may not correlate with long-term disease-free survival.

COMPLICATIONS

Several unique problems associated with laparoscopy need to be discussed.

Loss of tactile sensation

Laparoscopy causes impairment of tactile sensation and hinders the ability to palpate the bowel. There have been several reports of resection of a segment of bowel supposedly containing a tumor or polyp only to discover that the suspected lesion remained in a segment of bowel not resected. [21,33] Similarly, there have been several cases reported in which postoperative bowel obstruction requiring laparotomy was due to an unrecognized synchronous proximal tumor.[34,35] The interference with tactile sensation also makes identification of certain anatomic structures more difficult. Ureteral stents are rarely placed for 'simple' procedures and intraoperative colonoscopy is not routine in an open setting. However, due to difficulty in visualizing and feeling the ureter or feeling a small intraluminal mass, 25% and 53%, respectively of colorectal surgeons questioned routinely added these techniques for safety to their laparoscopic procedure. [33]

Port-site metastases

An increasing number of port-site recurrences have been reported, a problem only reported in two series prior to laparoscopy. Hughes et al.[36] reported 13 cases of wound recurrence of cancer in 1603 patients, 50% of which were not isolated and were associated with intraabdominal carcinomatosis. Thus, the total incidence of isolated wound recurrence was 0.4%. Sistrunk[37] earlier reported the dangers of expressing the colon through a small incision to remove a cancer or polyp and then returning the bowel to the adominal cavity. A prohibitively high rate of wound recurrences was noted with this technique, which in many respects parallels the delivery and treatment of some cancers removed laparoscopically. The problems with this technique also highlight why laparoscopic colotomy and polypectomy are unacceptable.[38] In a series of 1711 patients with Astler-Coller B_2 or C colorectal cancer operated on for cure and treated with adjuvant chemotherapy, 623 developed local and/or distant recurrences, of whom 26 had recurrences involving the wound.[39] However, only in 3 (0.2%) patients was wound recurrence isolated and it was more commonly associated with either disseminated disease or carcinomatosis. The prognosis in this group of patients was extremely poor as 20 of 26 patients had died at the last follow-up.

Port-site recurrences have been reported for numerous cell types and organs (Tables 6.3 and 6.4). Although the grand total of cases and therefore the true incidence is not known, this is disturbing. Port-site recurrences seem aggressive in that they often occur early and in many instances are the only source of recurrent disease. Port-site recurrences have developed not only after an advanced stage tumor was removed but also after curative resection of early lesions such as Dukes' A carcinoma. Some surgeons have advocated the use of bags or wound protectors to seal the open trocar sites from coming into contact with potential cancer cells.[96] However, the use of a bag does not safeguard against port-site recurrences as these have also been found at 'remote' ports used in manipulation, dissection and cautery.

Table 6.3 – Port-site recurrences by organ

Organ system	Reference	Total number of cases
Colon	35, 38, 40-55	45
Gallbladder	40, 42, 56-75	25
Genitourinary	76, 77	2
Gyneacology	76, 78-84	8
Pancreatic	85-87	3
Lung	88-91	4
Other	92-95	6
Total		93

Table 6.4 – Interval port site recurrences

Reference	Year	Duke's stage	Interval to recurrence (months)
Alexander et al.[43]	1993	C	3
Walsh et al.[46]	1993	C	6
Fusco and Paluzzi[44]	1993	C	10
Guillou et al.[47]	1993	C	N/A
O'Rouke et al.[40]	1993	B	2.5
Cirocco et al.[50]	1994	C	9
Wilson et al.[51]	1994	N/A	N/A
Nduka et al.[42]	1994	C	3
Prasad et al.[41]	1994	B	6
		A	26
Berends et al.[48]	1994	B	N/A
		C	N/A
		D	N/A
Lauroy et al.[38]	1994	A	9
Boulez and Herriot[52]	1994	3 stages N/A	N/A
Ramos et al.[49]	1994	C	N/A
		C	N/A
		C	N/A
Ngoi (pc)	1994	C	N/A
Gionnone (pc)	1994	B	2
Gould (pc)	1994	N/A	4
Newman et al. (pc)	1994	C	6
Cohen and Wexner[53]	1994	B	3
(postal surrvey)		B	6
		C	6
		C	9
		C	12
Fingerhut[35]	1995	A	N/A
		B	N/A
		B	N/A
Jacquet et al.[45]	1995	C	1
		B	10
		B	9
Drouard et al.	1995	A	9
(pc)		B	6
		B	6
		C	5
		C	1
		C	9
		D	2
Ugarte[54]	1995	C	10
Beck (pc)	1995	N/A	N/A
Lumley et al.[55]	1996	D	N/A

There are numerous theories to explain these localized recurrences. Technical problems with grasping forceps causing microperforations of the bowel near the tumor may allow exfoliated cells to access the periotoneal cavity. The pneumoperitoneum may aerosolize tumor cells and allow implantation in the 'puncture' type wounds created by trocars. Extraction of the specimen via small opening may similarly exfoliate cells into the trocar sites. There may also be an immunologic process that allows cancer cells to remain viable and grow in port sites. Some surgeons cite the simple explanation that Dukes' A and B lesions recurring at port sites are in fact Dukes' C lesions that have been improperly staged due to inadequate nodal harvest. Two alternative explanations have been postulated by proponents of laparoscopy for cure of carcinoma. First, direct contact between the tumor and wound due to failure to use a specimen extraction bag or wound protector, and secondly, failure intracorporeally to divide the vessels prior to transfascial tumor delivery. However, Montorsi et al.[97] noted a port-site recurrence after a completely intracorporeal curative resection of a Dukes' B lesion in which 28 nodes had been sampled, and the specimen extracted in a plastic bag. This one case soundly refutes the three aforementioned series.

The role of the pneumoperitoneum in the enhancement of tumor growth during laparoscopy has also been studied. Jones et al.[98] reported an experimental hamster model of the effect of the pneumoperitoneum on port-site recurrences. Two sets of hamsters were inoculated with human colon cancer cells at various concentrations. One group had trocars placed without a pneumoperitoneum being established while in the other group a pneumoperitoneum was established for 10 min. In the latter, there was an almost twofold increase in tumor implantation suggesting that the pneumoperitoneum may independently influence port-site recurrences. Jacobi et al.[99] studied colon adenocarcinoma in rats using cell kinetics as well as tumor cell weight). The number of tumor cells increased with insufflation compared to controls. Similarly, subcutaneous tumor growth was enhanced by laparoscopy and laparotomy, and more so in the former. Intraperitoneal tumor growth was unaffected.

The process by which tumor cells are spread to potential port sites is unclear. Thomas et al.[100] and Kockerling (presented at SAGES Scientific Session, March 1996) in separate centers, recently found that during laparoscopy, the gas did not include viable tumor cells, whereas both the instruments and the ports did. Therefore, it may not be the pneumoperitoneum aerosolizing tumor cells but rather the instruments with subsequent contamination of port sites

Ugarte[54] reported the peculiar case of a 79-year-old woman undergoing a laparoscopic cholecystectomy. One month postoperatively, she presented with a bowel obstruction which was found to be due to a transverse colon neoplasm. She underwent a right hemicolectomy for a Dukes' C lesion. At the time of laparoscopy, there was no evidence of metastic or peritoneal disease. Nine months after laparotomy, she developed a painful mass at one of the laparoscopic gallbladder port sites which was subsequently biopsied and found to be consistent with metastic adenocarcinoma of colonic origin. There was no evidence of tumor implantation to the midline wound. A similar report (DE Beck, personal communication) supports the view that the pneumoperitoneum may be directly involved in port-site recurrences. Port-site recurrences have been reported after laparoscopic cholecystectomy in at least 2 patients without seeding of the laparotomy incision.[99,101]

Regardless of the cause, certain unique problems, at least in the short term, have occurred with laparoscopic treatment of colorectal malignancies. Early port-site recurrence is a problem that, although not universally seen, should cast caution on performing curative procedures for these conditions. Long-term outcome can only be addressed by randomized controlled trials, designed to study both short- and long-term outcomes. Such studies are currently underway. Conversely, it seems reasonable to consider laparoscopically-guided surgery for those patients requiring a palliative operation.

ADHESION FORMATION

Adhesion formation after abdominal surgery with resultant small bowel obstruction continues to be one of the major long-term complications associated with open surgery. It has been thought that laparoscopic techniques inherently should decrease postoperative adhesion formation given their minimally invasive nature. Little literature exists to support this hypothesis.

Bessler et al.[102] reported a porcine model comparing adhesion formation after laparotomy versus laparoscopic-assisted colon resections. Fourteen days after the initial procedure, the animals were sacrificed and adhesions were identified. Adhesions were only identified in 1 of the laparoscopic-assisted animals (9%) compared to 9 (82%) of the laparotomy animals. A similar study was performed at our institution.[103] Based on this porcine model, laparoscopy may decrease postoperative adhesion formation and thus postoperative small bowel obstructions. Again, however, only long-term results obtained through randomized trials with large numbers of patients will ultimately answer this question.

Recently, as part of a multi-institutional trial, our institution looked at postoperative adhesion formation using a hyaluronidase membrane.[104] Patients undergoing a two-stage ileoanal J-pouch were randomized to have their wounds 'lined' with a hyaluronidase membrane. At the time of ileostomy closure 6 weeks to 3 months later, laparoscopy was performed through the stoma site to access adhesion formation to the midline wound. The number and severity of adhesions was significantly less when the hyaluronidase membrane was used compared to controls. At follow-up there was no statistical decrease in small bowel obstruction between the groups. However, with longer follow-up a decrease in small bowel obstructions may be seen due to decreased adhesion formation. The combination of this type of membrane with laparoscopy may even further decrease the incidence of adhesions.

COST CONSIDERATIONS

Cost contributes an increasingly important role in health care decisions. Arguably, cost should not necessarily dictate or influence care but it should be taken into account when new techniques or procedures are being offered to patients.

Cost is an extremely difficult issue to examine. It is difficult to determine the cost of an intervention as the costs and charges, as well as the reimbrusement, vary widely. If charges compared to costs are reviewed, the former will usually be inflated. It is also difficult to dissect cost into its specific components.[4] There are short-term costs associated with hospitalization and the actual procedures as well as cost savings associated with shorter convalesence and earlier return to work. The latter two factors are extremely important potential long-term cost savings should the theoretical benefits of laparoscopy prove to be true.

Most studies have concentrated on the short-term costs associated with the procedures and hospitalization. Typically laparoscopic procedures will involve more 'technology'. This includes reusable and disposable instruments, monitors, extra personnel and stapling devices. Studies usually neglect to include an amortized cost for the laparoscopic hardware and such calculations, although meaningful, are fraught with problems. In addition to these 'extras', the time to perform the procedure can be longer, at least early in the learning curve.[105] Typically, the increased time does not alter the surgeons' costs, however operating room time and anesthesia time are significantly affected. Conversely, the trend toward shorter hospitalization with less intensive postoperative care may offset these costs. Several series have tried to determine the costs of laparoscopic colon resections compared to the standard open procedure (Table 6.5). Several trends can be seen in this data. First, in almost all the series the cost of a converted procedure was more than that either of a laparoscopic or an open procedure. Patients may require conversion because of more advanced disease, more difficult surgery or both. Thus, these patients are relatively sicker and potentially require longer hospitalization. Secondly,

Table 6.5 – Cost considerations of laparoscopic colon resection

Author	Laparoscopic	Open	Converted
Falk et al.[3]	12 000★	12 500★	15 000★
Reiver et al.[16]	23 294	19 384	0
Senagore et al.[107]	12 131	14 496	17 583
Musser et al.[23]	9811	N/A	11 207
Hoffman et al.[20]	12 464	10 213	13 956
Vayer et al.[108]	26 662	22 938	13 956
Pfeifer et al.[11]	26 626	26 903	19 702

★★ All costs in US $; ★Estimated cost for right hemicolectomy

there is a trend in all but 2 of the series for the overall cost of a laparoscopic procedure to be more than that of the open procedure. Pfeiffer et al.[11] categorized costs into 10 groups including room, pharmacy, surgery, anesthesia, laboratory, physical therapy, respiratory and radiology costs for laparoscopic, open and converted procedures. Although there were no statistically significant differences in cost among any group, the overall increase in the cost of the laparoscopic procedure was due to increased operating room costs including anesthesia.

CONCLUSION

Laparoscopic colorectal surgery is feasible and procedural mobidity and mortality are similar or in many cases superior to those seen after open procedures. Oncologically, it is premature either to condemn or condone the procedure because of port-site recurrences, as short-term variables such as lymph node harvest, margins and level of ligation are generally similar to those noted after open procedures. Certainly in terms of financial issues, there do not appear to be any significant cost savings in performing a laparoscopic colectomy for carcinoma. However, if consideration of long-term disability costs are included in this equation, the balance may shift in favor of laparoscopy. At present, laparoscopic colon resections for cancer do not offer significant benefits compared to open procedures. Long-term, critical evaluation of large numbers of patients in a prospective randomized trial will hopefully define any differences in long-term outcome, morbidity and mortality. Laparoscopy for colorectal malignancy should be offered with curative intent only to patients enrolled in a prospective randomized trial. Conversely, it is perfectly appropriate for a well-trained surgeon to offer it to patients with metastatic malignancy or benign disease.

REFERENCES

1. Ortega AE, Beart RW, Steele GD et al. Laparoscopic bowel surgery registry. Preliminary results. Dis Colon Rectum 1995;38:681-686.
2. Ballantyne GH. Laparoscopic assisted colorectal surgery. Review of results of 752 patients. Gastroenterologist 1995;3:75-89.
3. Falk PM, Beart RW Jr, Wexner SD et al. Laparoscopic colectomy: a critical appraisal. Dis Colon Rectum 1993;36:28-33.
4. Phillips EH, Franklin M, Carrell BJ et al. Laparoscopic colectomy. Ann Surg 1993;216:703-707.
5. Deen PA, Beart RW Jr, Nelson H et al. Laparoscopic assisted segmental colectomy: early Mayo Clinic experience. Mayo Clin Proc 1994;69:834-840.
6. Wexner SD, Reissman P. Laparoscopic colorectal surgery: a provocative critique. Int Surg 1994;79:235-239.
7. Wexner SD, Reissman P, Pfeifer J, Bernstein M, Geron N. Laparoscopic colorectal surgery: analysis of 140 pateints. Surg Endosc 1995;10:133-136.
8. Binderow SR, Cohen SM, Wexner SD, Nogueras JJ. Must early oral postoperative intake be limited to laparoscopy? Dis Colon Rectum 1994;37:584-589.
9. Reissman P, Teoh TA, Cohen SM, Weiss EG, Nogueras JJ, Wexner SD. Is early oral feeding safe after elective colorectal surgery? Ann Surg 1995;222:73-77.
10. Ramos JM, Beart RW, Goes R, Ortega AE, Schlinkert RT. Role of laparoscopy in colorectal surgery. A prospective evaluation of 200 cases. Dis Colon Rectum 1995;38:494-501.
11. Pfeifer J, Wexner SD, Reissman P et al. Laparoscopic versus open colon surgery: cost and outcome. Surg Endosc 1995;9:1322-1326.
12. Tate JJ, Kwok S, Dawson JW et al. Prospective comparison of laparoscopic and conventional anterior resection. Br J Surg 1993;80:1396-1398.
13. Scott KW, Grace RH. Detection of lymph node metastases in colorectal carcinoma before and after fat clearance. Br J Surg 1989;76:1165-1167.
14. Cohen SM, Wexner SD, Schmitt SL, Noguras JJ, Lucas FV. Effect of xylene clearance on mesenteric fat on harvest of lymph nodes after colonic resection. Eur J Surg 1994;160:693-697.
15. Bleday R, Babineau T, Force RA. Laparoscopic surgery for colon and rectal cancer. Sem Surg Oncol 1993;9:59-64.
16. Darzi A, Lewis C, Menzies-Gow N, Guillou PJ, Monson JRT. Laparoscopic abdominoperineal resection of the rectum. Surg Endosc 1995;9:414-417.
17. Dodson RW, Cullado M, Tangen LE et al. Laparoscopic assisted abdominoperineal resection. Contemp Surg 1993;42:42-44.
18. Fine AP, Lanasa S, Gannon MP, Cline CW, James R. Laparoscopic colon surgery: report of a series. Am Surg 1995;61:412-416.
19. Franklin ME, Rosenthal D, Norem RF. Prospective evaluation of laparoscopic colon resection versus open colon resection for adenocarcinoma. Surg Endosc 1995;9:811-816.
20. Hoffman GC, Baker JW, Fitchett CW, Vansant JH. Laparoscopic assisted colectomy: initial experience. Ann Surg 1994;219:732-743.

21. Larach SW, Salomon MC, Williamson PR, Goldstein E. Laparoscopic assisted colectomy: experience during the learning curve. *Coloproctology* 1993;**1**:38-41.

22. Lord SA, Larach SW, Ferrara A, Williamson PR, Lago CP, Lube MW. Laparoscopic resections for colorectal carcinoma: a three year experience. *Dis Colon Rectum* 1996;**39**:148-154.

23. Musser PJ, Boorse RC, Madera F, Reed FJ III. Laparoscopic colectomy: at what cost? *Surg Laparosc Endosc* 1994;**4**:1-5.

24. Peters WR, Bartels TL. Minimally invasive colectomy: are the potential benefits realized. *Dis Colon Rectum* 1993;**36**:751-756.

25. Tucker JG, Ambroze WL, Orangio GR, Duncan TD, Mason EM, Lucas GW. Laparoscopic assisted bowel surgery. *Surg Endosc* 1995;**9**:297-300.

26. Van Ye TM, Cattery RP, Henry LG. Laparoscopic assisted colon resections compare favorably with open technique. *Surg Laparosc Endosc* 1994;**4**:25-31.

27. Wexner SD, Cohen SM, Johnansen OB *et al.* Laparoscopic colorectal surgery: a prospective assessment and current perspective. *Br J Surg* 1993;**80**: 1602-1605.

28. Zucker KA, Pitcher DE, Ford RS. Laparoscopic assisted colon resection. *Surg Endosc* 1994;**8**:12-18

29. Milsom JW, Bohm B, Deconini C, Fazio VW. Laparoscopic oncologic proctosigmoidectomy with low colorectal anastomosis in a cadaver model. *Surg Endosc Surg Endosc* 1994;**8**:1117-1123.

30. Orkin B. Rectal carcinoma: treatment. In: Beck DE, Wexner SD (eds). *Fundamentals of Anorectal Surgery.* New York, McGraw-Hill, 1992, pp.261-369.

31. Quirke P, Durdey P, Dixon MF, Williams NS. Local recurrence of rectal adenocarcinoma due to inadequate surgical resection. *Lancet* 1986;**i**:996-998.

32. Heald RJ, Ryall RDH. Recurrence and survival after total mesorectal excision for rectal cancer. *Lancet* 1986;1479-1482.

33. Wexner SD, Cohen SM, Ulrich A, Reissman P. Laparoscopic colorectal surgery: are we being honest with our patients? Dis Colon Rectum 1995;**38**:1-5.

34. McDermott J, Devereaux D, Caushaj P. Pitfall of laparoscopic colectomy: an unrecognized synchronous cancer. *Dis Colon Rectum* 1994;**37**:602-603.

35. Fingerhut A. Laparoscopic colectomy. The French experience. In: Jager R, Wexner SD (eds) *Laparoscopic Colorectal Surgery.* New York: Churchill Livingstone, 1995, pp. 253-257.

36. Hughes ES, McDermott FT, Poliglase AI, Johnson WR. Tumor recurrence in the abdominal wall scar after large bowel cancer surgery. *Dis Colon Rectum* 1983;**36**:571-572.

37. Sistrunk WE. Mikulicz operation for resection of the colon. Its advantages and dangers. *Ann Surg* 1928;**88**:577.

38. Lauroy J, Champault G, Risk N, Boutelier P. Metastatic recurrence at the cannula site: should digestive carcinomas still be managed by laparoscopy. *Br J Surg* 1994;**81**(Suppl):31(Abstract).

39. Reilly WT, Nelson H, Schroeder G, Wieand HS, Bolton J, O'Connell MJ. Wound recurrence following conventional treatment of colorectal cancer: a rare but perhaps underestimated problem. *Dis Colon Rectum* 1996;**39**:200-207.

40. O'Rourke N, Price PM, Kelly S, Sikora K. Tumour innoculation during laparoscopy (letter). *Lancet* 1993;**342**:368.

41. Prasad A, Avery C, Foley RJE. Abdominal wall metastases following laparoscopy (letter). *Br J Surg* 1994;**81**(Suppl):31.

42. Nduka CC, Monson JRT, Menzies-Gow N, Darzi A. Abdominal wall metastases following laparoscopy. *Br J Surg* 1994;**81**:648-652.

43. Alexander RJ, Jacques BC, Mitchell KG. Laparoscopically assisted colectomy and wound recurrence (letter). *Lancet* 1993;**341**:249-250.

44. Fusco MA, Paluzzi MW. Abdominal wall recurrence after laparoscopic assisted colectomy for adenocarcinoma of the colon. *Dis Colon Rectum* 1993;**36**: 858-861.

45. Jacquet P, Averbach AM, Stephens AD, Sugarbaker PH. Cancer recurrence following laparoscopic colectomy. *Dis Colon Rectum* 1995;**38**:1110-1114.

46. Walsh DC, Wattehow DA, Wilson TG. Subcutaneous metastases after laparoscopic resection of malignancy. *Aust NZ J Surg* 1993;**63**:536-565.

47. Guillou PJ, Carzi A, Monson JRT. Experience with laparoscopic colorectal surgery for malignant disease. *Surg Oncol* 1993;**2**(Suppl):43-49.

48. Berends FJ, Kazemier G, Bonjer HJ, Lange JF. Subcutaneous metastases after laparoscopic colectomy. *Lancet* 1994;**344**:58.

49. Ramos JM, Gupta S, Anthone GJ, Ortega AE, Simons AJ, Beart JW. Laparoscopy and colon cancer: is the port site at risk? *Arch Surg* 1994;**129**:897-900.

50. Cirocco WC, Schwartzman A, Golub RW. Abdominal wall recurrence after laparoscopic colectomy for colon cancer. *Surgery* 1994;**116**:842-846.

51. Wilson JP, Hoffman GC, Baker JW, Fitchett CW, Vansant JH. Laparoscopic assisted colectomy. Initial experience. *Ann Surg* 1994;**219**:732-734.

52. Boulez J, Herriot E. Multicentric analysis of laparoscopic colorectal surgery in FDCL group: 274 cases. *Br J Surg* 1994;**81**:527.

53. Cohen SM, Wexner SD. Laparoscopic colorectal surgery: are we being honest with our patients? *Dis Colon Rectum* 1994;**37**:858-861.

54. Ugarte F. Laparoscopic cholecystectomy port seeding from a colon carcinoma. *Am Surg* 1995;**61**:820-821.

55. Lumley JW, Fielding GA, Rhodes M, Nathanson LK, Siu S, Stitz RW. Laparoscopic-assisted colorectal surgery: lessons learned from 240 consecutive patients. *Dis Colon Rectum* 1996;**39**:155-159.

56. Sailer M, Debus S, Fuchs KH, Thiede A. Peritoneal seeding of gall bladder cancer after laparoscopic cholecystectomy. *Surg Endosc* 1995;**9**:1298-1300.

57. Clair DG, Lactz DB, Brooks DC. Rapid development of umbilical metastases after laparoscopic cholecystectomy for unsuspected gallbladder carcinoma. *Surgery* 1993;**113**:355-358.

58. Drouard F, Delamarre J, Capron JP. Cutaneous seeding of gallbladder cancer after laparoscopic cholecystectomy. *N Engl J Med* 1991;**325**:1316.

59. KeBler T, Michaljevic L. Implantations metastase eines Gallenblasencarcinoms am Nabel nach laparoskopischer cholecystektomie. *Chirug* 1994;**65**:564-565.

60. Nally C, Pizohaut RM. Tumor implantation at umbilicus after laparoscopic cholecystectomy for unsuspected gallbladder carcinoma. *Can J Surg* 1994;**37**:243-244.

61. Pezet D, Fondrinier E, Rotman N et al. Parietal seeding of carcinoma of the gall bladder after laparoscopic cholecystectomy. *Br J Surg* 1992;**79**:230.

62. Targarena EM, Pons MJ, Viella P, Trias M. Unsuspected carcinoma of the gall bladder. A laparscopic dilemma. *Surg Endosc* 1994;**8**:211-213.

63. Weiss SM, Wengert PA, Horkauy SE. Incisional recurrence of gall bladder cancer after laparoscopic cholecystectomy. *Gastrointest Endosc* 1994;244-246.

64. Barsoum GH, Windsor SW. Parietal seeding of carcinoma of the gall bladder after laparoscopic cholecystectomy. *Br J Surg* 1992;**79**:846.

65. Foruta K, Yoshimoto H, Watonabe R, Herohimoto M, Iwashita A. Laparoscopic cholecystectomy for a suspected case of gall bladder carcinoma. *Am J Gastroenterol* 1991;**86**:1851.

66. Gornish AL, Averbach D, Schwartz MR. Carcinoma of the gall bladder found during laparoscopic cholecystectomy: a case report and review of the literature. *J Laparoendosc Surg* 1991;**1**:361-367.

67. Paraskevopoulos JA, Pechliverides G. Parietal seeding of carcinoma of the gall bladder after laparoscopic cholecystectomy. *Br J Surg* 1992;**79**:845.

68. Swaroop VS, Udwacha TE. Laparoscopic cholecystectomy for gall bladder cancer. *Am J Gastroenterol* 1992;**87**:1522-1523.

69. Luccironi P, Konigsrainer A, Eberl T, Margreiter R. Tumour innoculation during laparoscopic cholecystectomy. *Lancet* 1993;**342**:59.

70. Berthet B, LeTreut YP, Assadounon R. Metastase sur le site d'extraction laparoscopique des cancers de la vesicle de diagnostic postoperatoire. *Lyon Chirugicale* 1993;**89**:50-51.

71. Bethet B, LeTreut YP, Blanc AP. Cholecystecomie por coeliochirugie et cancer de la vesicle. *Gastroenterol Clin Biol* 1992;**16**:724.

72. Landen S, Hymons V, Wibin E. Essaimage parietal d'un carcinome vesiculaire apres chirugie coeliscopie. *Ann Chir* 1993;**47**:455-456.

73. Fligelstone L, Rhodes M, Flock D, Puntis M, Crosby D. Tumour innoculation during laparoscopy (letter). *Lancet* 1993;**342**:368.

74. Fong Y, Brennon MF, Turnbull A, Colt D, Blumgart LH. Gall bladder cancer discovered during laparoscopic surgery. *Arch Surg* 1993;**128**:1054-1056.

75. Kim HJ, Roy T. Unexpected gallbladder cancer with cutaneous seeding after laparoscopic cholecystectomy. *S Med J* 1994;**87**:817-820.

76. Stolla V, Ross D, Bladow F, Rather C, Ayuso D, Serment G. Subcutaneous metastases after coelioscopic lymphadenectomy for visical urothelial carcinoma. *Eur Urol* 1994;**36**:342-343.

77. Andersen JR, Stoen K. Implantation metastases after laparoscopic biopsy of bladder cancer. *J Urol* 1995;**153**:1047-1048.

78. Patsner B, Damien M. Umbilical metastases from a stage IB cervical cancer after laparoscopy: a case report. *Fertil Steril* 1992;**88**:1248-1249.

79. Dobrente, Wittmann T, Karacsony G. Rapid development of malignant metastases in the abdominal wall after laparoscopy. *Endoscopy* 1978;**10**:127-130.

80. Stockdale AD, Pocock J. Abdominal wall metastases following laparoscopy: a case report. *Eur J Surg Oncol* 1985;**11**:373-375.

81. Hsui J, Gluen FT, Kemp GM. Tumor implantation after diagnostic laparoscopic biopsy of serous ovarian tumors of low malignant potential. *Obstet Gynecol* 1986;**68**:90-95.

82. Gleeson NC, Nicosia SV, Mark JE, Hoffman MS, Cavanagh D. Abdominal wall metastases from ovarian carcinoma after laparoscopy. *Am J Obstet Gynecol* 1993;**169**:522-523.

83. Childers JM, Aqua KA, Surwit EA, Hallum AV, Hatch KD. Abdominal wall tumor implantation after laparoscopy for malignant conditions. *Obstet Gynecol* 1994;**84**:765-769.

84. Shepherd JH, Carter PG. Wound recurrence by implantation of a borderline ovarian tumour following

laparoscopic removal. *Br J Obstet Gynecol* 1994; **101**:265-266.

85. Siriwardena A, Samarji WN. Cutaneous tumour seeding from a previously undiagnosed pancreatic carcinoma after laparoscopic cholecystectomy. *Ann R Coll Surg Engl* 1993;**75**:199-200.

86. Watson DJ. Abdominal wall metastases after laparoscopic gastroenterostomy. *Med J Aust* 1995; **163**:106-107.

87. Jorgensen JO, McCull JL, Morris DL. Port site seeding after laparoscopic ultrasonographic staging of pancreatic carcinoma. *Surgery* 1995;**117**:118-119.

88. Fry WA, Siddiqui A, Pensler JM, Mustafavi H. Thoracoscopic implantation of cancer with a fatal outcome. *Ann Thorac Surg* 1995;**59**:42-45.

89. Fhurer RL. Video-assisted thoracic surgery (letter). *Ann Thorac Surg* 1993;**56**:199-200.

90. Walsh GL, Nesfitt JC. Tumor implants after thoracoscopic resection of a metastatic sarcoma. *Ann Thorac Surg* 1995;**59**:215-216.

91. Zim APC. Port site recurrence following video-assisted thoracoscopic surgery. *Surg Endosc* 1995;**9**: 1133-1135.

92. Cole SJ, Rogers J, Williams NS. Laparoscopic surgery for colorectal cancer. *Br J Surg* 1994;**81**:775.

93. Russi EG, Pergolizzi S, Mesiti M et al. Unusual relapse of hepatocellular carcinoma. *Cancer* 1992;**70**: 1483-1487.

94. Keate RF, Shuffer R. Seeding of hepatocellular carcinoma to pentenoscopy insertion site. *Gastrointest Endosc* 1992;**38**:203.

95. Cava A, Ramon J, Gonzalez-Quintella A, Martin F, Aramburo P. Subcutaneous metastasis following laparoscopy in gastric adenocarcinoma. *Eur J Surg Oncol* 1990;**26**:63-67.

96. Wexner SD, Cohen SM. Port site metastases after laparoscopic colorectal surgery. *Br J Surg* 1995;**82**: 295-298.

97. Montorsi M, Fumagalli U, Rosati R, Bona S, Chella B, Huscher C. Early parietal recurrence of adenocarcinoma of the colon after laparoscopic colectomy. *Br J Surg* 1995;**82**:1036-1037.

98. Jones DB, Guo LW, Reinhard MK et al.Impact of pneumoperitoneum trocar site implantation of colon cancer in hamster model. *Dis Colon Rectum* 1995;**38**: 1182-1188.

99. Jacobi CA, Ordermann J, Bohm B, Zieren HU, Volk HD, Muller JM. Increased tumor growth after laparoscopy with air vs CO_2. *Surg Endosc* 1996;**33**: 551(Abstract).

100. Thomas WM, Eaton MC, Hewett PJ. A proposed model for the movement of cells within the abdominal cavity during CO_2 insufflation and laparoscopy. *Aust NZ J Surg* 1996;**66**:105-106.

101. Wade TP, Comitalo JB, Andrus CH et al. Laparoscopic cancer surgery: lessons from gall bladder carcinoma. *Surg Endosc* 1995;**8**:698.

102. Bessler M, Whelan RL, Halverson A, Allendorf JDF, Nowygrod R, Treat MR. Controlled trial of laparoscopic-assisted vs. open colon resection in a porcine model. *Surg Endosc* 1996;**10**:732-735.

103. Reissman P, Teoh T-A, Skinner K, Burns JW, Wexner SD. Adhesion formation after laparoscopic anterior resection in a porcine model: a pilot study. *Surg Laparosc Endosc* 1996;**6**:136-139.

104. Becker JM, Dayton MT, Fazio VW et al. Prevention of postoperative abdominal abscesses by a sodium hyaluronate-based bioresorbable membrane: A prospective randomized double-blind multicenter study. *J Am Coll Surg* (in press).

105. Reissman P, Cohen S, Weiss EG, Wexner SD. Laparoscopic colorectal surgery: ascending the learning curve. *World J Surg* (in press).

106. Reiver D, Kmiot WA, Cohen Sm, Weiss EG, Nogueras JJ, Wexner SD. A prospective assessment of laparoscopic versus open procedures in colorectal surgery. *Dis Colon Rectum* 1994;**37**:22(Abstract).

107. Senagore AJ, Luchtefeld MA, MacKeigan JM, Mazier WP. Open colectomy versus laparoscopic colectomy: are there differences? *Am Surg* 1993;**59**:549-554.

108. Vayer Aj, Larach SW, Williamson PR et al. Cost effectiveness of laparoscopic colectomy. *Dis Colon Rectum* 1993;**36**:34.

7

Role of Video-Assisted Thoracic Surgery in the Management of Pulmonary Cancer and Tumors of the Mediastinum

Joseph S. Friedberg and Larry R. Kaiser

Minimal access surgery, specifically video-assisted thoracic surgery (VATS), has had a profound impact on the current practice of thoracic surgery. This chapter addresses the role VATS has assumed in the diagnosis and treatment of cancers in the pulmonary parenchyma as well as masses in the mediastinum. Potential advantages, disadvantages and controversies are discussed.

The thoracic cavity is, in some respects, ideally suited for minimal access surgery. Placement of a double lumen endotracheal tube allows selective pulmonary collapse and visualization of the greater portion of the desired hemithorax. The chest has the advantage, as compared to the abdomen, of being a rigidly supported cavity. This obviates the need for airtight seals and gas insufflation to maintain a working environment. Unlike conventional laparoscopy, the surgeon is not restricted to using instruments which can fit through a port with a valve or gasket. Not only does this allow the introduction of larger or even standard non-thoracoscopic instruments, but it also affords the surgeon the opportunity to place a finger in the chest for digital inspection of the lung parenchyma. The drawback of the thoracic cavity is that all manipulations must take place via rib interspaces which should be traumatized as little as possible to maintain the potential benefits of minimally invasive surgery. Given that thoracotomy is one of the more morbid incisions, there are substantial theoretical advantages to any approach which may decrease postoperative pain and loss of function.

HISTORY

The history of thoracoscopy can be traced to Hans Christian Jacobaeus, a professor of internal medicine at the Serafimerlasarettet Hospital in Stockholm, who in 1910 proposed introducing a cystoscope into the chest cavity to aid in the diagnosis and treatment of pulmonary tuberculosis.[1,2] Approximately 10 years later he reported lysing pleural adhesions under local anesthesia as an adjunct to collapse therapy and also the use of pleuroscopy in the localization and diagnosis of both pleural and pulmonary lesions. From that time until the introduction of video technology in the 1980's 'thoracoscopy' was predominantly limited to 'pleuroscopy', most frequently for diagnostic purposes in cases of effusion of unknown etiology. Most commonly, a mediastinoscope was introduced into the pleural cavity for inspection and biopsy.[3] This remains a simple and useful technique, but has very little utility in the treatment of diseases within the pulmonary parenchyma. In addition to the superior visualization afforded by advanced video optics, VATS offers the significant advantage of allowing the surgeon to operate with both hands through strategically placed ports. Traditional thoracoscopy or pleuroscopy is very much like mediastinoscopy in that the surgeon is committed to using one hand to control the scope, thereby leaving only one hand free to operate an instrument. Generally this instrument is a biopsy forceps or a thin suction device which is manipulated through the scope with minimal range of motion.

PROCEDURE

Most patients are candidates for VATS, the exceptions being those with extensive and tenacious pleural adhesions and those unable to tolerate single lung ventilation. No attempt is made to give a detailed description of VATS techniques, but it is important to have a general understanding of the procedure in order to understand both its potential and limitations.

The patient is positioned and draped for a standard thoracotomy. It is important to have all of the instruments at the ready for an expeditious conversion to an open procedure. This may be required if life-threatening hemorrhage occurs or if the surgeon feels the operation is being compromised by utilization of minimally invasive techniques.

Guided by the preoperative plain films and computed tomography (CT) scans, the initial incision is usually made in the 7th or 8th intercostal space along the line of the anterior superior iliac spine. The technique employed in creating a port site is the same as for placement of a thoracostomy tube and, indeed, it is generally via this site that such a tube is placed at the conclusion of the procedure. (Fig. 7.1) It is important, as when placing a chest tube, always to place a digit into the chest to identify or create an adequate pleural space and to assure safe entry for the thoracoscopic port. The low chest incision allows a panoramic view of the thoracic cavity and strategic positioning of the remaining ports. After introduction of the scope and camera through the first port, safe entry into the chest for the remaining ports can be viewed on the monitors. For most procedures, two more ports are created and are placed in a triangular configuration and, if convenient, placed in the line of a standard thoracotomy incision. For small biopsies it

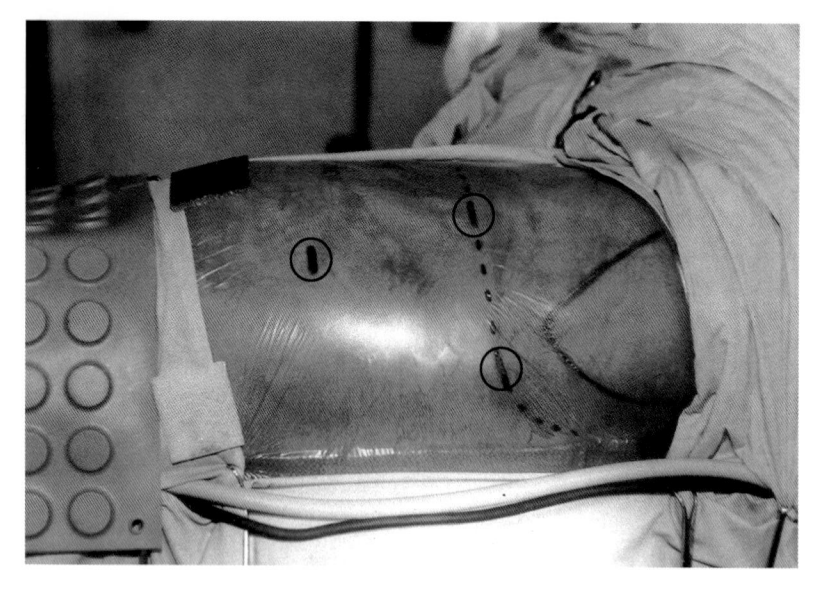

Figure 7.1 – Patient positioned for thoracoscopy. The standard posterolateral thoracotomy incision is outlined and the three thoracoscopy incision sites are denoted by circles. The inferior line marks the location of the insertion of the videothoracoscope. The patient is in the lateral decubitus position.

is frequently the anterior port site through which specimens are withdrawn as the interspaces are larger in this part of the rib cage.

Depending on the operation performed, it may become necessary to enlarge one of the port sites into a 6-10 cm 'utility' or 'access' incision which may be placed in one of several potential locations. The utility incision is a standard feature for VATS lobectomy, and the use of a rib spreader varies according to exposure and the surgeon's preference.[5] Specimen bags should be used for withdrawal of potentially malignant or infected tissues from the chest cavity following the same principles applied in laparoscopic surgery.

Most authors report using a combination of conventional and specialized endoscopic instruments to perform the procedures. The instrumentation designed specifically for VATS includes an ever expanding armamentarium of devices which perform the same functions as those used in open operations, but are designed to be manipulated from outside the chest cavity and are easier to introduce through small openings. Specialized linear staplers in several sizes and configurations are also available. Most thoracic surgeons employ the 0° thoracoscope, but the angled telescopes are also very useful and enable the operator better to 'see around' the lung.

Finally, almost all authors recommend that the goal of VATS must be to perform the same procedure through limited access as would be performed through a standard thoracotomy. There are, however, some who feel VATS is a different type of thoracic surgery and requires completely different techniques (see below).[11]

VIDEO-ASSISTED THORACIC SURGERY FOR BENIGN PULMONARY PATHOLOGY

Although this chapter is devoted to the role of VATS in dealing with thoracic tumors, it is worth briefly noting that VATS is well suited for a number of other pulmonary processes. These include, but are not limited to: treatment of spontaneous pneumothorax, diagnosis of interstitial lung disease and the emerging field of reduction pneumoplasty. In a recent review of more than 1300 VATS cases, treatment of spontaneous pneumothorax was the most common application for pulmonary VATS.[6] With respect to diagnosis of interstitial lung disease in the critically ill patient, however, it remains our bias, as well as that of others, to perform a wedge resection through a small anterior thoracotomy. Although this technique may not yield as much visual information as a VATS biopsy, it will provide tissue for diagnosis, does not subject the patient to the potential hazards of changing from a single to a double lumen endotracheal tube and it does not require single lung ventilation.

For diagnosis of interstitial pulmonary disease in the nonacute setting, there have been retrospective studies advocating the superiority of VATS over open biopsy, citing better lung visualization, access to all areas of the lung, and decreased length of hospital stay.[7]

VIDEO-ASSISTED THORACIC SURGERY IN THE DIAGNOSIS OF INDETERMINATE PULMONARY NODULES AND STAGING OF LUNG CANCER

Video-assisted thoracic surgery versus other diagnostic modalities

VATS technology has significantly affected the practice of thoracic surgery and pulmonary medicine with respect to its use in the diagnosis of the solitary pulmonary nodule. Most pulmonary nodules require a prompt diagnosis, the exceptions being those which have been radiographically stable for 2 years, display a benign pattern of calcification, or occur in a young nonsmoker without any previous history of cancer or outstanding risk factors.

The options for establishing a tissue diagnosis of a nodule include transbronchial biopsy, transthoracic needle biopsy and VATS biopsy. Transbronchial biopsy at the time of fiberoptic bronchoscopy for tumors without endobronchial disease provides a yield of 20-80% with a specifically benign diagnosis established only 10% of the time.[8]

Transthoracic needle biopsy results are slightly better with the diagnostic yield for malignant lesions in the range of 85%, but with a 10% false negative rate reported.[9] Viewed critically, this technique is also unreliable for making definitive benign diagnoses.[10,11]

A recent modification of transthoracic needle aspiration is the transthoracic core biopsy technique utilizing a 20 gauge coaxial needle. In a retrospective study comparing these two transthoracic needle modalities, the core biopsies yielded a statistically significant higher diagnosis rate for benign nodules, with an overall specific benign diagnosis yield of 91%. Of note, this technique was complicated by a 54% incidence of pneumothorax which is considerably higher than that usually reported.[12]

The sensitivity and specificity of VATS biopsies approach 100% for both malignant and benign lesions.[3,13-15] The reason for this, quite simply, is that the entire nodule is excised with a rim of surrounding lung parenchyma for pathologic examination (Fig. 7.2). Any yield less than 100% would result from an inability to locate or excise the nodule. The superiority of VATS as a diagnostic modality is supported by a recent study directly comparing VATS biopsies to transthoracic needle biopsies.[14] As in other studies, the weakness of the transthoracic aspiration technique was in making benign diagnoses. In this series, comparing over 300 patients in each group, the transthoracic needle biopsy group contained 47 patients with a 'nonspecific benign' diagnosis of which 32 (68%) were subsequently found to be malignant. The VATS group yielded a specific malignant or benign diagnosis in 292 of the 301 patients (96%). The authors concluded that VATS is a safe and accurate method of evaluating a pulmonary nodule.

The staging and diagnostic capabilities for VATS in lung cancer extend beyond wedge resection of the indeterminate pulmonary nodule. In addition, VATS offers an opportunity to view the visceral and parietal pleural surfaces which may reveal previously undetected metastatic disease (Fig. 7.3). Such findings may prevent unnecessary thoracotomy.[15] Furthermore, although mediastinoscopy is a relatively simple procedure with a low complication rate, there is an approximately 10% incidence of false negative findings in the best of hands. Accurate staging is important not least because neoadjuvant chemotherapy has been shown significantly to improve survival in stage IIIa non-small cell lung cancer and may well come to play a role in lesser stage cancers as well.[16,17] It has been suggested that VATS may play a role in improving staging, particularly with respect to evaluating adenopathy in the aortopulmonary window, a site not accessible by standard cervical mediastinoscopy.[13,18,19]

Nodule localization techniques

Different techniques have been developed to assist the surgeon in locating pulmonary nodules. The preoperative CT scan may be all that is needed to localize most lesions, particularly those that are peripherally

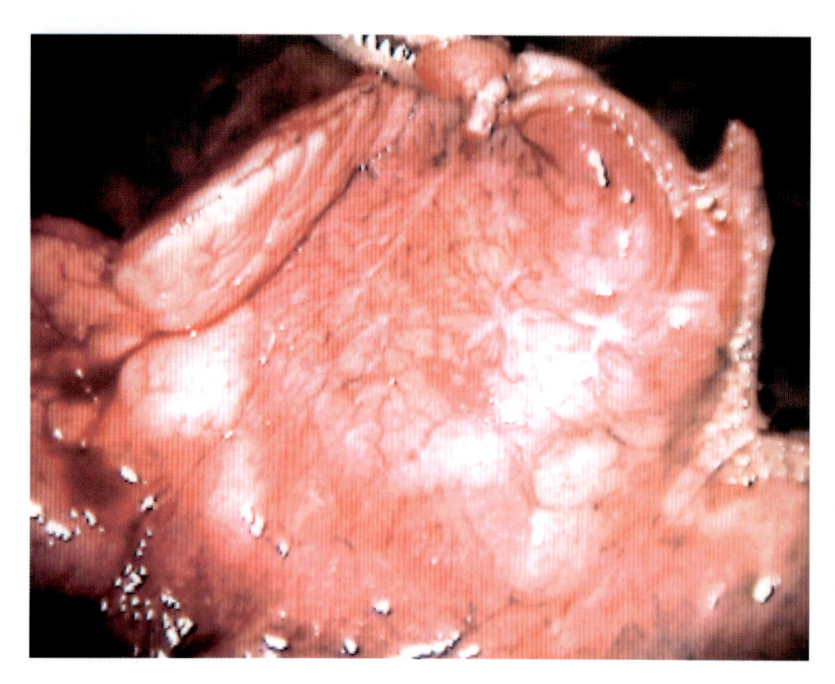

Figure 7.2 – A solitary pulmonary nodule being excised along with a wedge of lung parenchyma. The parenchyma is grasped with a specially modified ring forceps and several firings of the endoscopic stapler are necessary to complete the wedge.

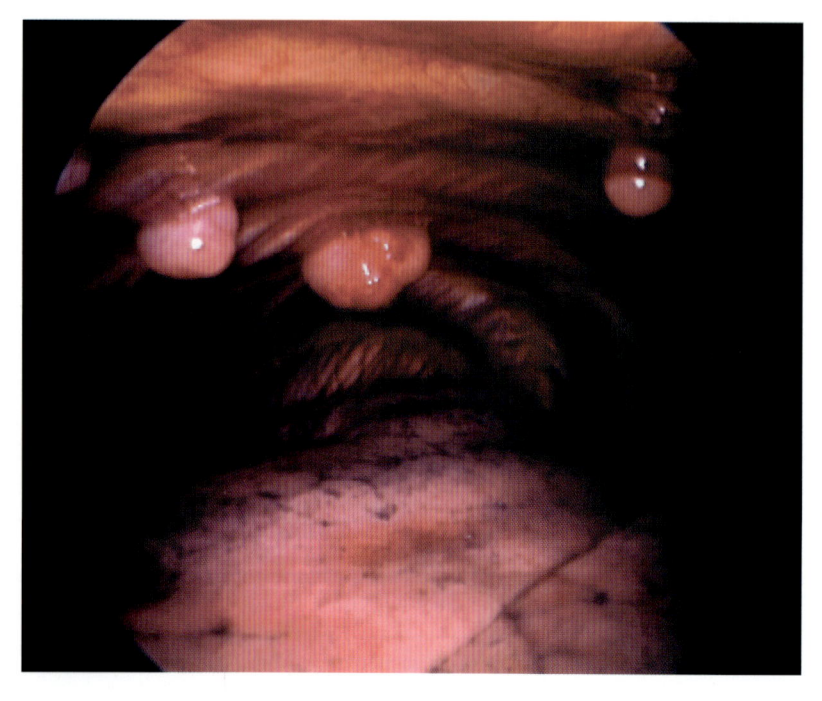

Figure 7.3 – Diffuse areas of metastatic disease involving the parietal pleura. These small nodules, not appreciated on the CT scan, are well visualized at videothoracoscopy. A biopsy of one of the nodules confirms metastatic carcinoma. The visceral pleural surface in this case is remarkably free of disease.

located. If there are no visual cues, the surgeon can introduce a finger through one incision while moving the lung to the examining finger with an atraumatic grasping instrument through the other port. With practice and experience, essentially all nodules may be located by palpation no matter where they are located in the lung. The narrow posterior interspaces sometimes make digital palpation difficult or at least uncomfortable (Fig. 7.4) Other techniques for localizing nodules for a VATS excision have been reported and include CT-guided needle localization similar to the technique used in breast biopsies, CT-guided methylene blue injections and intraoperative ultrasound.[20,21] Recently, a modified version of a tactile sensor originally designed to provide the sense of touch for robots has been reported to accurately detect tumor nodules as small as 2 mm which had escaped visualization in preoperative CT scanning.[22]

Video-assisted thoracic surgical lobectomy

VATS has, in many centers, changed the algorithm for evaluation of the solitary pulmonary nodule. The use of VATS in the diagnosis of the indeterminate pulmonary nodule is widely practised. Controversy exists, however, as to the appropriate course of action should the VATS-excised nodule prove to be a non-small cell lung cancer on the frozen section.

It has been established with confidence that anything less than a lobectomy is not optimal treatment for stage I non-small cell lung cancer.[23] Thanks to improvements in pain control and intensive care, even patients with borderline pulmonary function are often better able to tolerate a pulmonary resection. Any surgeon who has had the opportunity to treat patients undergoing a lung volume reduction procedure has surely been impressed at how well most tolerate the operation when their pulmonary function tests are only a fraction of what is generally accepted as adequate to undergo surgery. Even in extremely high-risk surgical candidates, an operative mortality of <1% can be achieved for pulmonary resections using a standard thoracotomy.[24] Therefore, given the advisability of performing a lobectomy even for a stage I non-small cell lung cancer, and the ability of most patients to tolerate such an operation, a wedge resection should only be performed under exceptional circumstances as the definitive treatment for a known primary lung cancer.

Thus, confronted with a stage I non-small cell lung cancer at the time of a thoracoscopic excisional biopsy, the question is whether to proceed with a VATS lobectomy or to convert to an 'open' thoraco-

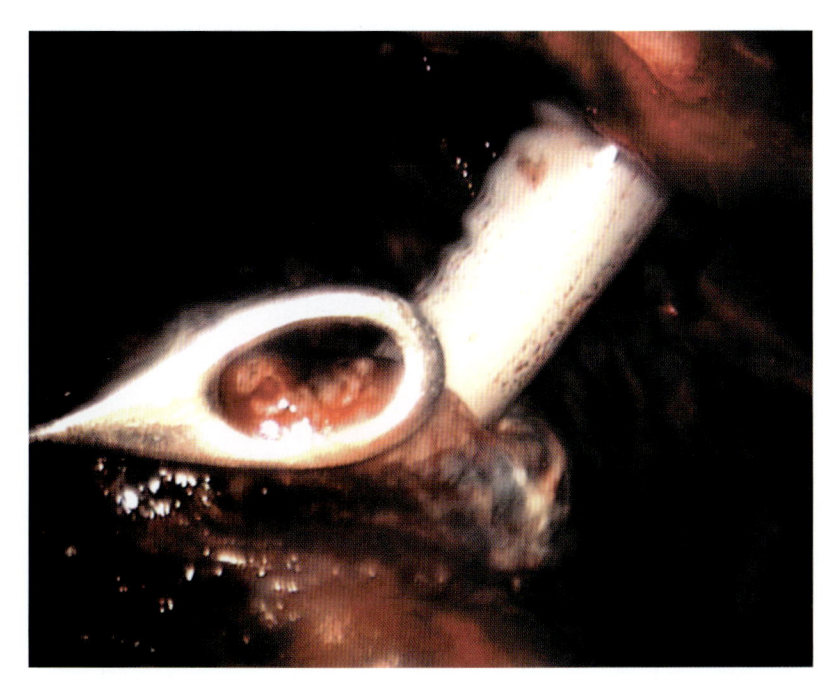

Figure 7.4 – The lung is grasped with a ring forceps and moved to the examining finger inserted through an opposing incision. Palpation of the lung in this fashion allows even deep-seated pulmonary nodules to be located. There is no better technique for locating nodules than the one illustrated here.

tomy. Many patients are candidates for a VATS lobectomy, but the current contraindications to VATS lobectomy include inability to tolerate single-lung ventilation, an underdeveloped fissure, extensive pleural adhesions, lymph nodes which appear adherent to major vessels, chest wall or endobronchial involvement, large tumors (generally >5 cm), bulky hilar or mediastinal adenopathy and following the use of neoadjuvant chemotherapy.[19,25-27]

The safe performance of an anatomic dissection by the VATS approach and extraction of the specimen without excessive rib spreading requires a 6-10 cm. 'utility incision' in addition to the other thoracoscopy ports. This is clearly a compromise between a completely 'closed' three-port thoracoscopic procedure and a standard "open" thoracotomy and the benefits are not clear cut. The proponents of VATS lobectomy feel the smaller incision and lack of rib spreading lead to less postoperative pain and quicker recovery.[19] Others feel that VATS may be a suboptimal approach for a cancer operation and that the benefits with respect to less postoperative pain may be minimal compared to a standard or modified thoracotomy incision.[24,28,29]

One of the more interesting controversies to arise has dealt with the performance of the procedure itself. Essentially all authors, regardless of the incisions or instruments employed, perform a classic anatomic individual ligation procedure. The bronchovascular structures are dissected individually and divided using either staplers, sutures or a combination of both. According to the majority of surgeons, the goal of VATS is to perform the same 'open' operation, but with smaller incisions, video visualization and special instrumentation. Lewis,[11] however, actually performs an operation different from that in the standard open thoracotomy. He reports excellent results using a 'simultaneously stapled' technique. Using this technique he isolates the bronchovascular root of the lobe being resected and staples and divides it en masse. In a series of 16 patients on whom he had performed lobectomies using this technique, he reported no major complications and concluded that simultaneous stapling is a safe technique that is actually better suited to the VATS approach than extensive hilar dissection with individual ligation. He contends that individual isolation of the pulmonary vessels from outside the chest is the most likely culprit in causing a hemorrhagic complication and that his technique helps to prevent this. Long-term follow-up is not yet available.

To date there is only one study that directly compares VATS and open lobectomies in a randomized fashion. Patients with stage I non-small cell lung cancer were randomized to either VATS lobectomy (25 patients) or muscle-sparing thoracotomy and lobectomy (30 patients).[4] The VATS lobectomy was accomplished through a 6-8 cm utility incision without rib spreading. The authors found that between the two groups there was no significant difference in operating time, intraoperative blood loss, duration of chest tube drainage, length of hospital stay, postoperative pain or recovery time. They demonstrated the safety and feasibility of the VATS approach for lobectomy, but failed to identify any short-term advantages of the minimally invasive approach. Furthermore, although they had no major complications, they voiced concern about the ability to rapidly control a major hemorrhage during a VATS procedure. Finally, they noted that the ultimate comparison between the two groups, 5-year survival, will not be available for several more years.

Generally, the intraoperative complications and blood loss are reported to be similar for both VATS and open lobectomies. The operative time for VATS lobectomy compared to open lobectomy, however, is variably reported to be shorter,[30] longer[25,31] or not significantly different.[18] The reason for this is not completely clear, but probably reflects the different approaches and techniques of the different operators.

Most authors emphasize eliminating or minimizing rib spreading during VATS procedures as this is felt to contribute to postoperative pain. Reduction of postoperative pain is one of the driving forces behind VATS as well as most other minimally invasive surgical techniques. The results, however, are inconclusive. Some feel that there is a definite decrease in postoperative pain which translates into shorter hospital stays and quicker recovery[19,30] Others find that VATS results in significantly less postoperative pain compared to standard or muscle-sparing thoracotomy, but hospital stay is not significantly decreased.[25,31] Finally, as previously stated, others have found no significant difference in postoperative pain, length of hospital stay or time to recovery when comparing VATS lobectomy against open lobectomy done via a muscle-sparing incision.[18]

One retrospective study focused on the issue of chronic pain after VATS pulmonary resections by comparing it to similar resections performed through a posterolateral thoracotomy.[32] Patients were asked to assess discomfort on the operated side using a visual analog scale. Their use of analgesics and the presence or absence of any residual shoulder dysfunction was also quantitated. A total of 343 patients were studied between 3 and 31 months after operation. There were 142 VATS and 97 thoracotomy patients in the "<1 year postoperative group," and 36 VATS and 68 thoracotomy patients in the ">1 year post-operative group." The VATS patients in the "<1 year post-operative group" had less pain and shoulder dysfunction but a similar pain medication requirement when compared to the thoracotomy group. In the ">1 year postoperative group", there were no significant differences between the VATS patients and the thoracotomy patients.

Video-assisted thoracic surgical pneumonectomy

Little has been written about VATS pneumonectomy. One group reported a series of 6 VATS pneumonectomies as part of a larger series including 56 VATS lobectomies. They resected stage I and stage II non-small cell lung cancers utilizing a 6 cm submammary access port. They divided all vessels with staplers and reported placing a vascular clamp on the proximal pulmonary artery prior to application of the stapler. The specimen was placed in a bag prior to withdrawal from the chest cavity. They claimed to have noticed less postoperative pain in this group of patients than their 'usual' thoracotomy patients and conclude that this is a safe technique for removal of early stage lung cancers less than 6 cm in diameter and without mediastinal involvement.[33]

Another study reported 2 VATS pneumonectomies in a series of 20 major pulmonary resections.[34] There is relatively little discussion pertaining to the VATS pneumonectomies, but essentially the same techniques were used and observations made as in the previous study.

Cost

The cost of VATS remains an area of controversy. A retrospective study compared the cost of thoracoscopic wedge resections to wedge resections performed via a standard thoracotomy. The findings were generally favorable for the VATS approach with an approximately US$600 greater cost for disposable instruments, but a 20-min reduction in operating time which made the overall operating room costs similar. The anesthesia cost was essentially equal for both groups. However, the length of hospital stay for the VATS group was 4.4 days compared to 6.5 days for the open group and the VATS groups spent an average of 0.14 day in the intensive care unit compared to 1.17 days for the thoracotomy group. The total average cost for the VATS patients was US$12, 129 versus US$16, 042 for the thoracotomy group. It should be noted that these values were not statistically significant ($p = 0.48$). The authors reported, however, that they planned to use fewer disposable thoracoscopic instruments to further decrease cost. They also felt their VATS patients experienced less postoperative pain.[35]

Another retrospective study compared the cost of VATS biopsies to wedge resections performed through limited posterolateral thoracotomies.[36] Thirty-seven patients had elective biopsies for diagnosis of interstitial lung disease: 16 had VATS procedures and 21 open procedures. Between the two groups no significant difference was reported in operative mortality, length of operation, number of specimens obtained, chest tube output, day of chest tube removal or the amount of postoperative analgesics required. There was, however, a US$2663 higher operating room cost for the VATS group compared to the thoracotomy group which was statistically significant ($p = 0.04$). The authors noted that they did not use disposable equipment. The total hospital cost was also higher: US$6491 for VATS and US$5575 for thoracotomy ($p = 0.05$). The authors concluded that VATS is a safe, reliable technique for wedge biopsies, but incurs higher costs. These findings are in accordance with a cost analysis comparing VATS and open lung biopsies for diagnosis of interstitial lung disease.[37] This analysis is based on a 5-7 day hospital stay for the open procedure and a 4 day stay for the VATS procedure. In addition, the author assumes a greater operating room cost for the VATS group and 1 day in the intensive care unit for both groups. Given these assumptions the author estimated a cost of approximately US$6500 for the open biopsy and US$10 400 for the VATS wedge.

COMPLICATIONS

There are numerous complications which VATS shares with open thoracic surgery, such as persistent air leaks, intercostal neuralgia, wound infections, cardiac arrhythmias and respiratory failure. Overall, it appears that the rates of these complications are not significantly different from those seen with a standard open procedure, generally in the range of 5-15%. Prolonged air leak is the most frequently cited complication. Similarly, the mortality rate is also low (1% or less).[6,26,38,39] There are, however, complications specific to VATS which include tumor seeding of port sites and intrathoracic hemorrhage without immediate direct access to the bleeding vessel.

Bleeding

In a series of more than 1300 patients, 6 bleeding complications were reported, 2 hemorrhages after decortication, neither of which required surgical intervention, 2 intercostal hemorrhages at port sites which were controlled thoracoscopically, 1 subclavian artery injury during lysis of adhesions, 1 segmental pulmonary artery injured during lobectomy dissection and 1 hilar hemorrhage secondary to a stapler malfunction. The arterial injuries all required immediate conversion to open thoracotomy for repair.[6,40]

In another series of 57 VATS lobectomies, 2 patients required emergent thoracotomy for control of vascular injuries, 1 for a pulmonary artery injury, the other for a pulmonary venous problem.[41] Both injuries occurred because of staple malfunction. The authors tallied a total of 243 firings of the endoscopic stapler used in their 57 cases and calculated a stapler failure rate of 0.82%. They emphasized the need for careful examination and loading of all staplers and the ability of the surgeon to handle such a situation should it arise.

In another series of more than 900 VATS procedures, which included 41 lobectomies, there were 18 conversions to open procedures to control intraoperative bleeding.[39] The authors state that these injuries occurred, "mainly during lobectomies for cancer and occurred either during vessel division or during stapling". They also report one emergency conversion to control "massive" pulmonary venous hemorrhage from a stapler misfire which cut, but did not staple.

Pulmonary arterial injuries have the advantage of occurring in a low pressure system and can usually be controlled with pressure using a sponge stick. It can easily be imagined, however, that a major vascular injury could occur during a procedure which is being performed without a utility incision. If the surgeon were unable immediately to introduce an appropriate instrument to tamponade bleeding the operation could rapidly degenerate into an uncontrolled situation. Although no fatality from intraoperative hemorrhage has been reported, the risk of severe bleeding during VATS is a major concern and it is agreed that the ability to deal with such an injury and to have the necessary instruments immediately available is a prerequisite for performing this type of surgery.[28,41,42]

Tumor recurrence complicating video-assisted thoracic surgery

A recent publication of anecdotal reports from members of the Video-Assisted Thoracic Surgery Study Group reported 21 cases of tumor implants thought to be related to VATS techniques.[43] This included 14 incision recurrences, 2 staple line recurrences, 2 pleural recurrences and 3 combination recurrences. Some of the cases were mesotheliomas, which are notorious for recurring in thoracic incisions, but these reports highlight a complication that before was rarely reported in the thoracic surgical literature.

There are, however, some documented reports of tumor recurrence at VATS ports. Four recurrences followed resection of primary non-small cell lung cancers,[39,44,45] 1 followed talc insufflation for a malignant effusion,[25] and 4 followed resection of sarcoma metastases.[46]

The reports of recurrence following VATS resection of non-small cell lung cancers detail a total of 6 recurrences which were treated with chest wall resections. One chronicles the course of a patient who developed a second and fatal recurrence after a chest wall resection for the first recurrence.[44] It was generally felt that the chest wall had been seeded at the initial operation when the uncovered specimen was squeezed through one of the port sites.

The reports of sarcoma recurrence highlight several issues. The first is that VATS resection of metastatic sarcoma may greatly underestimate the extent of disease. The technique relies heavily on CT imaging and eliminates the surgeon's ability bimanually to palpate the lung and identify masses not visualized on the preoperative studies. Furthermore, it has been established that CT scans can significantly underestimate the extent of metastatic disease,[47,48] and some authors feel that it may be possible to miss up to one-half of the metastatic nodules when the VATS approach is employed.[42] In keeping with this last statement is a study in which metastatic osteosarcoma lesions were excised from 7 patients, 3 of whom had recurrent lesions within 4-6 months. It was felt that these rapid recurrences were the result of leaving small, undetected nodules at the time of the initial operation. It was the authors' conclusion that this was a failure of the VATS technique which essentially limited their resections to lesions visualized on the preoperative CT scans.[49]

Chest wall recurrences may occur as a result of pulling the specimen directly through the wound. The current recommendation is that all potentially malignant specimens be placed in a water tight specimen bag prior to removal from the chest.[39,50,51] Furthermore, some recommend that VATS resection of malignant nodules be restricted to peripheral lesions less than 2 cm.[45,52] and that open resections remain the procedure of choice for metastatic sarcoma as this offers the best chance of cure.[28,42,46,50]

Putting the issue in context, VATS is a relatively new technique and reports of complications are even more recent. Tumor seeding of thoracoscopic ports is essentially a new disease in thoracic surgery and it remains to be seen whether the current recommendations for wound protection are followed and, if so, whether they will decrease the incidence of this unacceptable complication.

CONCLUSION

There is no question that VATS has dramatically changed the practice of thoracic surgery, but as a relatively new technology, the indications and applications remain in flux. VATS is, arguably, the state of the art for diagnosis of the indeterminate pulmonary nodule. It certainly is the definitive diagnostic procedure should other modalities like transthoracic fine needle aspirates prove inconclusive. It boasts a near perfect sensitivity and specificity in the diagnosis of both benign and malignant lesions. Any lesion suspected of malignancy should be removed from the chest in a sealed specimen bag. A strong argument could be made to abandon VATS and perform an open operation to allow full palpation of the lung if the nodule is thought to be a metastatic sarcoma.

The use of VATS for treatment of non-small cell lung cancer remains controversial. The optimal treatment for early stage non-small cell lung cancers is a formal anatomic resection such as lobectomy or, at least, segmentectomy. Thus, there is only a limited role for wedge resection in the treatment of a known pulmonary malignancy, and it must be recognized that it is a compromise procedure applicable only if it is felt that the patient cannot tolerate lobectomy. This leaves the surgeon with the option of performing a lobectomy by thoracotomy or the VATS approach. Currently, the VATS approach requires a 6-10 cm utility incision for a safe dissection as well as specimen retrieval. Thus, it is more invasive than VATS procedures performed entirely through two or three small ports. The benefits of the minimally invasive approach for lobectomy and pneumonectomy have not been conclusively demonstrated, though it appears there may be some decreased discomfort in the immediate postoperative period. However, at 1 year, it does not appear that there is any significant difference between the open or the minimally invasive approach. The conservative view is that VATS may potentially compromise a patient's first and best chance at a curative cancer operation. Furthermore, there is concern regarding the ability to safely control an intraoperative catastrophy from the VATS approach. There have not been any large series of VATS lobectomies or pneumonectomies and the long-term results from those that have been reported are still pending.

The cost-effectiveness of VATS is also a matter of debate. The dramatic decrease in hospital stay achieved with laparoscopic cholecystectomy has not been conclusively demonstrated as an advantage of VATS. There does appear to be a somewhat shorter hospital stay for patients who undergo a VATS biopsy as compared to a biopsy through a thoracotomy, but VATS procedures tend to incur higher operating room costs.

Finally, there are some major complications specific to VATS. The greatest concern is bleeding, and more specifically hemorrhage in a setting where immediate digital or instrument control may not be readily applied. Most VATS dissections depend upon staplers for division and ligation of vascular structures. Staplers are highly reliable, but they do occassionally fail. A common etiology of bleeding in thoracic surgery is traction injury to the delicate pulmonary vasculature. This has also been reported with VATS procedures, necessitating expedient conversion to an open operation for definitive control of the injured vessel. To date there has been no report of a fatal hemorrhage during a VATS procedure, although there are several reports of significant bleeding from vascular injuries.

The second complication specific to VATS is that of tumor recurrence, particularly at port sites. Given the number of reports for the number of procedures performed, this is essentially a new disease entity in thoracic surgery. It appears that many of the initial resections that resulted in port site recurrences were performed without using a specimen bag to extract the specimen from the chest. Greater attention needs to be focused on protecting wounds from contact with malignant cells which could potentially lead to seeding.

Many surgeons continue to perform pulmonary VATS procedures, including lobectomies, and data will continue to accumulate. There is obviously a need for prospective randomized trials to illuminate the advantages and disadvantages of this technology. The most conservative view in thoracic surgery, however, remains that anatomic resections be performed in an open manner and that wedge biopsies for metastatic sarcomas also be resected using an open approach. A VATS procedure is a useful adjunct to mediastinoscopy in the invasive staging evaluation of some patients with lung cancer in that lymph nodes not accessible by mediastinoscopy (posterior level 7, levels 5,6) may be sampled. Also, the pleural surface may be inspected prior to proceeding with definitive resection to rule out the possibility of pleural metastases if the presence of a pleural effusion has raised this suspicion.

VIDEO-ASSISTED THORACIC SURGERY IN DIAGNOSIS AND TREATMENT OF MASSES IN THE MEDIASTINUM

There is far less experience with mediastinal VATS than has been accumulated for pulmonary disease. Most articles are case reports and no randomized studies have been published. It can be assumed, however, that most of the operative principles, benefits, complications and cost issues for pulmonary VATS apply to mediastinal VATS as well. Although this is an oncology text it is worth noting that mediastinal VATS is also being used for other procedures including: sympathetic denervation for autonomic disorders, treatment of thoracic outlet syndrome, spine surgery, diaphragmatic plication, pericardial windows for cardiac tamponade and various cardiac surgical procedures.

Procedure

The preparation for mediastinal VATS is similar to pulmonary VATS except that some authors prefer the patient in a 30-45° off-center position as opposed to the 90° standard thoracotomy position.[2,53] As with pulmonary VATS; a utility incision may be required and this is usually placed in the submammary location, especially if the patient is not in the full lateral decubitus position. Currently, only benign masses are resected with mediastinal VATS techniques. Thus, some authors have advocated morcellating a large specimen in the chest within a specimen bag in order to remove it through the intercostal spaces.[54]

Diagnostic applications

Surgical biopsies of mediastinal masses have traditionally been performed either through an open approach or mediastinoscopy. Cervical mediastinoscopy is a simple and cost effective procedure with good diagnostic yield and, in skilled hands, minimal morbidity. The instruments are widely available and most thoracic surgeons and operating room personnel are trained and comfortable with the procedure. Furthermore, it does not require single-lung ventilation.

Mediastinoscopy, however, does have its limitations. There is poor access to the posterior mediastinum and the surgeon must operate through a very restrictive port using relatively small biopsy forceps. Albeit more complicated and costly, VATS offers some advantages that may make it more desirable than mediastinoscopy in certain situations. Visualization is excellent with VATS and this is particularly true when viewing the mediastinum. VATS also allows the surgeon to examine the rest of the hemithorax at the same time. VATS enables the surgeon to take any size biopsy that is necessary. For example, this permits the surgeon to remove an enlarged lymph node intact, enhancing its diagnostic yield in certain diseases. Finally, the argument could be made that VATS is actually safer than mediastinoscopy which affords the surgeon a very limited view and a small channel through which to operate.[55]

It is cautioned, however, that the transthoracic approach employed in mediastinal VATS may prove oncologically unfavorable. Tumors such as thymomas, which have a propensity to spread by drop metastases, may contaminate the pleural space with VATS. This is unlikely to occur with traditional anterior mediastinotomy which can be performed extrapleurally.[28]

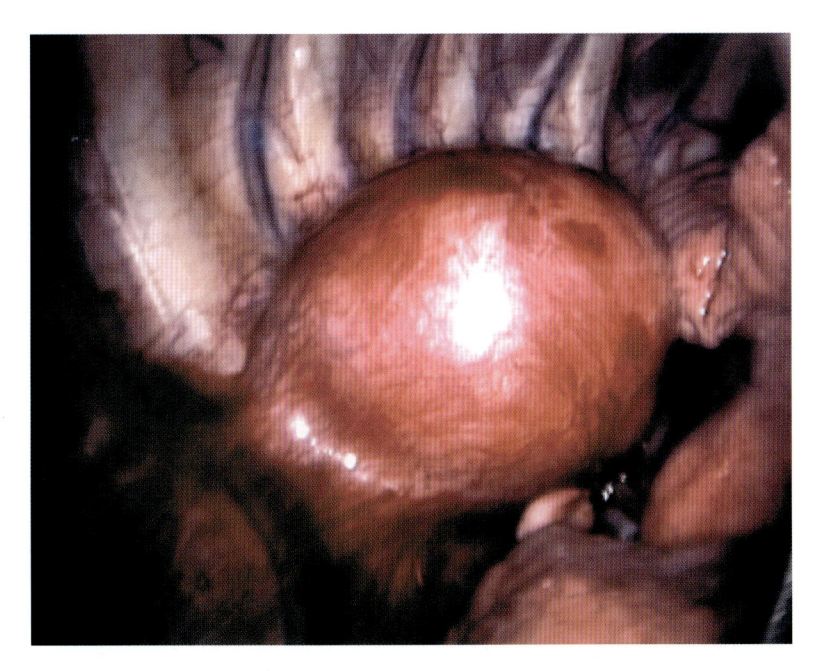

Figure 8.5 – A solid posterior mediastinal mass overlying the vertebral bodies. Lesions in this location are most likely neurogenic in origin and this proved to be a ganglioneuroma. MRI scan had demonstrated no tumor within the neural foramen and the entire lesion was resected with a video-assisted thoracoscopic approach.

Mediastinal VATS has been successfully used in the diagnosis of: lymphoma, thymoma, tuberculosis, sarcoidosis, lymph node metastases and teratoma.[56] In all reports the authors conclude that VATS is a useful and safe modality in helping to establish these diagnoses. Given the sparse literature and youth of this surgery, it is not yet possible critically to evaluate the use of mediastinal VATS for these procedures.

Therapeutic applications

Most authors agree that until further experience is gained, mediastinal VATS should be reserved for resection of benign lesions only.[2,53,55,57] Tumors which are readily accessible by the VATS approach and have been excised include: neurogenic tumors, lipomas, fibrous tumors of the mediastinum, bronchogenic cysts, pleuropericardial cysts, benign thymomas and thymic cysts (Fig. 7.5).[2,54-56,58,59] There is one report of using VATS combined with a posterior laminectomy for resection of a dumbbell-shaped cystic schwannoma.[60] The largest series reports resections in approximately 20 patients and, again, it is too early to draw any critical conclusions.

Of special interest are VATS thymectomies. In a series of 8 thymectomies for myasthenia gravis, the authors felt they accomplished complete thymic excision.[61] They claim that not only is the procedure feasible, but that it is associated with a lower postoperative analgesia requirement and a shorter hospital stay. They based this claim on a retrospective comparison to a similar group of patients resected via sternotomy.

It is our bias that combining the VATS approach with a transcervical approach facilitates complete excision of all thymic tissue.[2,57] With this approach the thymus gland is initially mobilized in the neck and branches to the innominate vein are divided. The dissection is then carried down into the mediastinum until the thymoma is encountered. The neck is then closed and the patient is positioned 30° left side up for the VATS portion. Using this approach the operation is completed and the specimen is removed through one of the chest incisions. We have used this combined approach in 15 resections for benign conditions without any mortality or significant morbidity.

It is worth noting a benchmark against which minimally invasive surgery for myasthenia gravis could be judged. Complete thymectomy for myasthenia gravis has been performed by the cervical approach with an average postoperative hospital stay of 38 hours (18-72 hours) and with resumption of normal activity between the 3rd and 7th postoperative day.[29] The only series reporting exclusively on VATS thymectomies for myasthenia gravis stated the average postoperative hospital stay for the 8 patients was 5 days (2-37 days).[61]

Complications

As with pulmonary VATS, mediastinal VATS shares the same complications as its corresponding open counterpart. However, one complication which appears specific to the VATS approach has been reported.[55] In this case, the monopolar electrocautery device was flawed with a deficient area of insulation. This area came into contact with the aorta and the authors reported, "severe bleeding requiring urgent thoracotomy and suture of aorta". The authors recommend care and inspection of all thoracoscopic instruments as well as being prepared to deal with such a complication in an expeditious manner.

Neurologic deficits have also been reported with VATS surgery and seem to be most common with mediastinal procedures. Reported complications include both temporary and permanent recurrent laryngeal nerve palsies and transient phrenic nerve palsies. One group reported neurologic complications in 4 of 49 patients in their series of mediastinal VATS procedures.[39]

CONCLUSION

The evolution of VATS for mediastinal masses is still in its early stages. There is insufficient data to render any concrete assessments of its comparative usefulness or cost effectiveness. It has been shown that diagnostic biopsies of mediastinal masses and resection of benign lesions can be performed with minimal morbidity. As with pulmonary VATS, there are complications peculiar to VATS though no operative fatalities have been reported. There appears to be a role for VATS biopsies in accessing areas of the mediastinum that are not easily reached with mediastinoscopy. Whether mediastinal VATS becomes a standard method of tumor resection, however, remains to be seen.

REFERENCES

1. Jacobaeus HC. Ueber die Moglichkeit die Zystoskopie bei untersuchung seroser hohlungen anzuwenden (Possibility of use of the cystoscope for investigation of serous cavities). *Munchen Med Wochenschr* 1910;**57**: 2090-2092.
2. Kaiser LR. Video-assisted thoracic surgery, current state of the art. *Ann Surg* 1994;**220**:720-734.
3. Kaiser LR. Diagnostic and therapeutic uses of pleuroscopy (thoracoscopy) in lung cancer. *Surg Clin North Am* 1987;**67**:1081-1086.
4. Kirby TJ, Rice TW. Thoracoscopic lobectomy. *Ann Thorac Surg* 1993;**56**:784-786.
5. Lewis RJ. Simultaneously stapled lobectomy: a safe technique for video-assisted thoracic surgery. *J Thorac Cardiovasc Surg* 1995;**109**:619-625.
6. Yim AP, Liu HP. Complications and failures of video-assisted thoracic surgery: Experience from two centers in Asia. *Ann Thorac Surg* 1996;**61**:538-541.
7. Ferson PF, Landreneau RJ, Dowling RD et al. Comparison of open versus thoracoscopic lung biopsy for diffuse infiltrative pulmonary disease. *J Thorac Cardiovasc Surg* 1993;**106**:194-191
8. Cortese DA, McDougal JC. Biopsy and brushing of peripheral lung cancer with fluoroscopic guidance. *Chest* 1982;**75**:141-145
9. Di Donna A, Bazzocchi M, Dolcet F, Springolo E. CT-guided transthoracic needle aspiration of solitary lung lesions. Personal experience in 118 cases. *Radiol Med (Torino)* 1995;**89**:287-294.
10. Milman N, Faurschou P, Grode G. Diagnostic yield of transthoracic needle aspiration biopsy following negative fiberoptic bronchoscopy in 103 patients with peripheral circumscribed pulmonary lesions. *Respiration* 1995;**62**:1-3.
11. Levine MS, Weiss JM, Harrell JH, Cameron TJ, Moser KM. Transthoracic needle aspiration biopsy following negative fiberoptic bronchoscopy in solitary pulmonary nodules. *Chest* 1988;**93**:1152-1155.
12. Klein JS, Salomon G, Stewart EA. Transthoracic needle biopsy with coaxially placed 20-gauge automated cutting needle: result in 122 patients. *Radiology* 1996;**198**715-720.
13. Landreneau RJ, Hazelrigg SR, Mack MJ et al. Thoracoscopic mediastinal lymph node sampling: useful for mediastinal lymph node stations inaccessible by cervical mediastinoscopy. *J Thorac Cardiovasc Surg* 1993;**106**:554-558.
14. Mitruka S, Landreneau RJ, Mack MJ et al. Diagnosing the indeterminate pulmonary nodule: percutaneous biopsy versus thoracoscopy. *Surgery* 1995;**118**:676-684.
15. Wain JC. Video-assisted thoracoscopy and the staging of lung cancer. *Ann Thorac Surg* 1993;**56**:776-778.
16. Roth JA, Fossella F, Komaki R, et al. A randomized trial comparing perioperative chemotherapy and surgery with surgery alone in resectable stage IIIA non-small-cell lung cancer. *J Natl Cancer Inst* 1994;**86**:673-80.
17. Rosell R, Gomez-Codina J, Camps C et al. A randomized trial comparing preoperative chemotherapy plus surgery with surgery alone in patients with non-small-cell lung cancer. *N Engl J Med* 1994; **330**:153-158.

18. Kirby TJ, Mack JM, Landreneau RJ, Rice TW. Lobectomy - Video assisted thoracic surgery versus muscle sparing thoracotomy. *J Thorac Cardiovasc Surg* 1995;**109**:997-1002.

19. Mentzer SJ, DeCamp MM, Harpole DH Jr, Sugarbaker DJ. Thoracoscopy and video-assisted thoracic surgery in the treatment of lung cancer. *Chest* 1995;**107**(Suppl):298S-301S.

20. Mack MJ, Shennib H, Landreneau RJ, Hazelrigg SR. Techniques for localization of pulmonary nodules for thoracoscopic resection. *J Thorac Cardiovasc Surg* 1993;**106**:550-553.

21. Schwarz RE, Posner MC, Plunkett MB, Ferson PF, Keenan RJ, Landreneau RJ. Needle-localized thoracoscopic resection of indeterminate pulmonary nodules: impact on management of patients with malignant disease. *Ann Surg Oncol* 1995;**2**:49-55.

22. Ohtsuka T, Furuse A, Kohno T, Nakajima J, Yagyu K, Omata S. Application of a new tactile sensor to thoracoscopic surgery: experimental and clinical study. *Ann Thorac Surg* 1995;**60**:610-613; discussion 614.

23. Ginsberg RJ, Rubinstein LV. Randomized trial of lobectomy versus limited resection for T1 N0 non-small cell lung cancer. Lung Cancer Study Group. *Ann Thorac Surg* 1995;**60**:615-622; discussion 622-623.

24. Miller JI Jr. Limited resection of bronchogenic carcinoma in the patient with impaired pulmonary function. *Ann Thorac Surg* 1993;**56**:769-771.

25. Yim AP, Ko KM, Chau WS, Ma CC, Ho JK, Kyaw K. Video-assisted thoracoscopic anatomic lung resections. The initial Hong Kong experience [see comments]. *Chest* 1996;**109**:13-17.

26. DeCamp MM, Jaklitsch MT, Mentzer SJ, Harpole DH, Sugarbaker DJ. The safety and versatility of video-thoracoscopy: a prospective analysis of 895 consecutive cases. *J Am Coll Surg* 1995;**181**:113-120.

27. Roviaro G, Varoli F, Rebuffat C et al. Videothoracoscopic staging and treatment of lung cancer. *Ann Thorac Surg* 1995;**59**:971-974.

28. Ginsberg RJ. Thoracoscopy: a cautionary note. *Ann Thorac Surg* 1993;**56**:801-803.

29. Cooper JD. Perspectives on thoracoscopy in general thoracic surgery. *Ann Thorac Surg* 1993;**56**:697-700.

30. Liu HP, Chang CH, Lin PJ, Chang JP, Hsieh MJ. Thoracoscopic-assisted lobectomy. Preliminary experience and results. *Chest* 1995;**107**:853-855.

31. Giudicelli R, Thomas P, Lonjon T et al. Video-assisted minithoracotomy versus muscle-sparing thoracotomy for performing lobectomy. *Ann Thorac Surg* 1994;**58**:712-718.

32. Landreneau RJ, Mack MJ, Hazelrigg SR, et al. Prevalence of chronic pain after pulmonary resection by thoracotomy or video-assisted thoracic surgery (see comments). *J Thorac Cardiovasc Surg* 1994;**107**:1079-1085; discussion 1085-1086.

33. Craig SR, Walker WS. Initial experience of video assisted thoracoscopic pneumonectomy. *Thorax* 1995;**50**:392-395.

34. Roviaro G, Varoli F, Rebuffat C et al. Major pulmonary resections: pneumonectomies and lobectomies. *Ann Thorac Surg* 1993;**56**:779-783.

35. Hazelrigg SR, Nunchuck SK, Landreneau RJ et al. Cost analysis for thoracoscopy: thoracoscopic wedge resection. *Ann Thorac Surg* 1993;**56**:624-629.

36. Molin LJ, Steinberg JB, Lanza LA. VATS increases costs in patients undergoing lung biopsy for interstitial lung disease. *Ann Thorac Surg* 1994;**58**:1595-1598.

37. Miller JI Jr. The present role and future considerations of video-assisted thoracoscopy in general thoracic surgery. *Ann Thorac Surg* 1993;**56**:804-806.

38. Kaiser LR, Bavaria JE. Complications of thoracoscopy. *Ann Thorac Surg* 1993;**56**:796-798.

39. Jancovici R, Lang-Lazdunski L, Pons F et al. Complications of video-assisted thoracic surgery: a five-year experience. *Ann Thorac Surg* 1996;**61**:533-537.

40. Yim AP, Ho JK. Video-assisted thoracoscopic lobectomy: a word of caution. *Aust NZ J Surg* 1995;**65**:438-441.

41. Craig SR, Walker WS. Potential complications of vascular stapling in thoracoscopic pulmonary resection. *Ann Thorac Surg* 1995;**59**:736-737; discussion 737-738.

42. Rusch VW. VATS: quo vadis? *J Am Coll Surg* 1995;**181**:165-167.

43. Downey RJ, McCormack P, LoCicero Jr. Dissemination of malignant tumors after video-assisted thoracic surgery: a report of twenty-one cases. The Video-Assisted Thoracic Surgery Study Group. *J Thorac Cardiovasc Surg* 1996;**111**:954-960.

44. Fry WA, Siddiqui A, Pensler JM, Mostafavi H. Thoracoscopic implantation of cancer with a fatal outcome. *Ann Thorac Surg* 1995;**59**:42-45.

45. Buhr J, Hurtgen M, Kelm C, Schwemmle K. Tumor dissemination after thoracoscopic resection for lung cancer. *J Thorac Cardiovasc Surg* 1995;**110**:855-856.

46. Walsh GL, Nesbitt JC. Tumor implants after thoracoscopic resection of metastatic sarcoma. *Ann Thorac Surg* 1995;**59**:215-216.

47. McCormack PM, Ginsberg KB, Bains MS et al. Accuracy of lung imaging in metastases with implications for the role of thoracoscopy. *Ann Thorac Surg* 1993;**56**:863-865; discussion 865-866.

48. Cerfolio RJ, Allen MS, Deschamps C et al. Pulmonary

resection of metastatic renal cell carcinoma. *Ann Thorac Surg* 1994;**57**:339-344.
49. Yim AP, Lin J, Chan AT, Li CK, Ho JK. Video-assisted thoracoscopic wedge resections of pulmonary metastatic osteosarcoma: should it be performed? *Aust NZ J Surg* 1995;**65**:737-739.
50. Allen MS, Pairolero PC. Inadequacy, mortality, and thoracoscopy. *Ann Thorac Surg* 1995;**59**:6.
51. Lewis RJ, Caccavale RJ, Sisler GE, Bocage JP. Does video-assisted thoracic surgery disseminate tumor? *J Thorac Cardiovasc Surg* 1996;**111**:1109-1111.
52. Buhr J. Does video-assisted thoracic surgery disseminate tumor? *J Thorac Cardiovasc Surg* 1996;**111**:1110-1111.
53. Sugarbaker DJ. Thoracoscopy in the management of anterior mediastinal masses. *Ann Thorac Surg* 1993;**56**:653-656.
54. Rieger R, Schrenk P, Woisetschlager R, Wayand W. Videothoracoscopy for the management of mediastinal mass lesions. *Surg Endosc* 1996;**10**:715-717.
55. Dmitriev EG, Sigal EI. Thoracoscopic surgery in the management of mediastinal mass. *Surg Endosc* 1996;**10**:718-720.
56. Yim AP. Video-assisted thoracoscopic management of anterior mediastinal masses. Preliminary experience and results. *Surg Endosc* 1995;**9**:1184-1188.
57. Kaiser LR. Thymoma. The use of minimally invasive resection techniques. *Chest Surg Clin N Am* 1994;**4**:185-194.
58. Naunheim KS. Video thoracoscopy for masses of the posterior mediastinum. *Ann Thorac Surg* 1993;**56**:657-658.
59. Hazelrigg SR, Landreneau RJ, Mack MJ, Acuff TE. Thoracoscopic resection of mediastinal cysts. *Ann Thorac Surg* 1993;**56**:659-660.
60. McKenna RJ Jr, Maline D, Pratt G. VATS resection of a mediastinal neurogenic dumbbell tumor. *Surg Laparosc Endosc* 1995;**5**:480-482.
61. Yim AP, Kay RL, Ho JK. Video-assisted thoracoscopic thymectomy for myasthenia gravis. *Chest* 1995;**108**:1440-1443.

8

Minimally Invasive Techniques in the Management of Esophageal Cancer

Cathal J. Kelly, David Galvin and Patrick J. Broe

Carcinoma of the esophagus accounts for 4% of all cancers in the USA, with approximately 13,000 new cases reported each year.[1] Overall survival is poor, with a 5-year survival rate of approximately 15% regardless of therapy. Over the past 10 years there has been a slight rise in incidence and a marked change in the histology of this disease. Previously, over 70% of these tumors were squamous, but since the mid 1970s there has been more than a 100% rise in the incidence of adenocarcinoma, mostly at the gastroesophageal junction.[2]

STAGING

Accurate staging of esophageal cancer is important to decide appropriate therapy, assess new treatments, and inform individual patients of prognosis. Approximately two-thirds of patients presenting with esophageal cancer will have abnormal regional lymph nodes. For disease confined to the field of resection, radical surgery is currently the best modality of treatment, although more than 50% of these patients die of metastatic disease within 2 years of resection.[3] Patients with metastatic disease outside the field of resection do not benefit from radical surgery.[4] Recent therapeutic protocols that include chemotherapy and radiation therapy, have improved survival results but are associated with increased morbidity.[5] Accurate pre-operative lymph-node staging and detection of disseminated disease identifies those patients who may benefit from neoadjuvant radiation or chemotherapy before esophagectomy and spares those who would not benefit from these therapies. Despite the lack of evidence of metastatic spread by routine non-invasive testing, the pathologic stage after resection is frequently higher due in part to the tendency of esophageal carcinoma to involve lymph nodes without obvious enlargement. Picus et al[6] demonstrated that 40 out of 43 (93%) surgically resected metastatic lymph nodes measured less than 7 mm in diameter.

Laparoscopic staging

Laparoscopy is now routinely used in many centers to stage gastrointestinal malignancies. Its role is complementary to current imaging modalities, such as ultrasonography, CT scan and MRI. Its use is justified when the information obtained changes the treatment plan. Laparoscopy may provide data that avoids unnecessary laparotomy in cancer patients, including increased morbidity and increased length of hospital stay and convalescence. These benefits of laparoscopy are of particular importance in patients with advanced malignancies whose life-span is limited.

Laparoscopic assessment for metastatic disease in patients with esophageal and esophagogastric cancer has been widely reported.[7,8] Over 50% of esophageal cancers are unresectable at the time of diagnosis. Laparoscopic staging can prevent unnecessary laparotomy or thoracotomy by detecting hepatic disease, peritoneal seeding or celiac lymph-node involvement, missed by radiological investigations.[9] Laparoscopy is accurate in assessing the resectability of gastric cancer, in addition to detecting extraluminal disease spread and hepatic metastases. It has the added advantage of allowing biopsy under direct vision. Laparoscopy facilitates visualization of the anterior gastric wall and assessment of the posterior wall, palpation of the visceral surface to determine tumor infiltration into the gastric wall and assessment of the posterior wall by probing and palpation through the anterior wall.[8] A palpating probe may also be passed through the avascular portion of the gastrocolic omentum, lifting the posterior wall of the stomach to assess mobility.

Another technique for assessing the lesser sac in gastric cancer has been described by Asenico-Arana.[10] The lesser sac is entered through the gastrocolic omentum after the stomach is raised by a transparietal suture placed throught the seromuscular layer of the corpus. In a series of 14 patients he described one false-negative and no false positives results or major complications. Studies have reported an accuracy of 89-98% for detection of metastatic spread or unresectable disease, raising resectability rates at laparotomy from 72% to 87%.[8,11,12] In a prospective study of 140 patients with adenocarcinoma of the esophagogastric junction or squamous cell carcinoma of the distal esophagus, O'Brien et al, compared combined imaging (chest X-Ray, abdominal ultrasound and CT scan of the abdomen and chest) with laparoscopy.[13] Unsuspected peritoneal metastases were detected in 17% and hepatic metastases in 10% of patients at surgery. These were detected by laparoscopy in 96% and 64% of cases, respectively, compared with 21% and 50% by combined imaging. While laparoscopy was superior to combined imaging, it was only 60% sensitive in the detection of hepatic metastases. Laparoscopic ultrasonography may further increase this detection rate.[14]

Thoracoscopic staging

Lymph-node staging in esophageal carcinoma is a significant independent prognostic indicator.[15] Akiyama et al[16] described in detail the pattern of lymph-node spread in patients with esophageal cancer; 70% had lymph node involvement to at least one of the thoracic lymph-node stations. Spread to distant lymph node stations was common. Lesions of the upper third of the esophagus may have metastasis only to lymph nodes near the diaphragm and lesions of the lower third may have metastasis only to the upper thoracic lymph nodes. Pre-operative staging of thoracic lymph node stations will reflect the actual status of lymph-node involvement provided all lymph-node stations can be assessed pre-operatively.

Lymph-node staging by non-operative means has not been particularly useful in esophageal cancer. Both CT scan and MRI have been shown to be unreliable predictors of lymph-node involvement.[17] CT scan accuracy of regional lymph node status is less than 69%. The radiologic criterion for an abnormal node is a transverse diameter of 10 mm or more. Nodes less than 10 mm infiltrated with tumor will be interpreted as normal and swollen inflammatory nodes may be interpreted as abnormal. CT scan is a very accurate tool for detecting distant metastases in the chest or abdomen. Liver metastases can be detected with 90% accuracy. No significant benefit has been shown for MRI versus CT scanning[17] with conventional T1-weighted and T2-weighted spin-echo images. Gadolinium enhancement is currently being evaluated.[18]

While endoscopic ultrasonography (EUS) is useful in determining tumor invasion pre-operatively, in one study its use in lymph-node assessment was correct in only 69% of patients.[19] It cannot distinguish between metastatic and hyperplastic lymphadenopathy.[20, 21] EUS fails in a significant number of patients because of obstruction (26-62%). In addition, hepatic and peritoneal metastases are difficult to detect by this method.[22]

Invasive or operative staging of esophageal cancer to differentiate localized from advanced esophageal cancer is not new. Murray et al,[23] reported the use of mediastinoscopy and 'mini-laparotomy' in staging 30 patients. Five patients had positive lymph nodes at mediastinoscopy and 16 had positive nodes at 'mini-laparotomy'.

Thoracoscopy allows evaluation of the mediastinum and assessment of the local spread of malignancy. Krasna et al,[24] compared non-invasive staging (CT scan, MRI and endoesophageal ultrasonography) with thoracoscopic staging in a group of 13 patients with esophageal cancer. Thoracoscopy was performed through the left chest. Using a 3-port technique and atraumatic lung retraction the aortopulmonary window was exposed and mediastinal pleura incised. Biopsies of American Thoracic Society lymph node levels 5 and 6 (aortopulmonary window and periaortic lymph nodes) were performed. All patients had correct thoracic lymph-node staging confirmed at subsequent surgical exploration. Two patients with adenocarcinoma of the distal third/gastroesophageal junction were found at laparotomy to have positive celiac lymph nodes. Two patients who had positive lymph nodes at CT scan and MRI were found to have negative lymph nodes at thoracoscopy and subsequent resection. In a further prospective multi-center trial of 49 patients, thoracoscopic lymph-node staging was achieved in 44 patients (95%).[25] In the 33 patients who underwent esophageal resection, 29 were correctly staged (88%). In this study, thoracscopy was carried out in the right chest, allowing maximal dissection of the paraesophgeal lymph nodes, avoiding the aortic arch (unless non-invasive studies indicated enlarged aortopulmonary window lymph nodes (level 5 or 6). Additional information on the depth of invasion and metastatic spread was obtained.[25] Three patients were correctly down-staged to T3 despite pre-operative non-invasive investigations suggesting T4 stage. In 2 patients thoracoscopy correctly predicted T4 invasion of the aorta and trachea, while in a further 2 thoracoscopy missed T4 lesions. One patient, who had questionable pulmonary metastasis on CT and MRI scans, was proven to have pulmonary metastasis on thoracoscopic lung biopsy.

Combined thoracoscopic/ laparoscopic staging

Krasna et al,[25] demonstrated that thoracoscopic staging can accurately assess lymph node (N) and primary tumor (T) status.[25] However, based on a 7% incidence of unsuspected celiac lymph node involvement, they prospectively evaluated the role of combined thoracoscopic/laparoscopic assessment.[25, 26] In a group of 19 patients, right-sided thoracoscopy was combined with a 4-port laparoscopic technique (1 camera port, liver retractor and 2 operating ports). During laparoscopy celiac and lesser-curve lymph nodes were routinely sampled. Six of the 19 patients in whom laparoscopic staging was used had unsuspected celiac lymph node involvement. Laparoscopic staging was accurate in staging lymph-node involvement in 16 of 17 patients (94%) who had subsequent esophagectomies. Thoracic staging was 93% accurate in detecting thoracic lymph node involvement. Three patients in this study were downstaged to N0 status after chemotherapy/radiotherapy.

This preliminary study suggests that thoracoscopic/laparoscopic staging can be used to accurately assess thoracic and abdominal lymph-node status in esophageal cancer. This may allow stratification of patients into those likely to have residual disease, those likely to benefit from neoadjuvant therapy and those benefiting from immediate curative resection. This approach also allows placement of a feeding jejunostomy tube for nutritional support and a vascular access device for administration of chemotherapy.

THORACOSCOPIC ESOPHAGECTOMY

Total esophagectomy is traditionally performed using a full thoracotomy or a blunt transhiatal approach, in addition to full gastric mobilization and cervical anastomisis. Open thoracotomy is associated with considerable morbidity. Orringer[27] first described blunt transhiatal esophagectomy, avoiding thoracotomy and reducing pulmonary complications. However, it is a blind procedure and carries a risk of hemorrhage, particularly from azygous vein or chylous leak following thoracic duct injury.[28] The risk of tumor rupture and bronchial injury are also higher.[29] Furthermore, complete lymph-node dissection is not usually achieved, and may possibly compromise patient survival.[30]

Mobilization of the esophagus using a mediastinoscope was described by Buess et al,[31] though lymph node dissection was limited and dissection of the lower esophagus was difficult. Several groups have described a right-sided thoracoscopic technique for full thoracic mobilization of the esophagus.[32, 33] This procedure is performed under general anaesthesia with a double-lumen endotracheal tube to allow collapse of the right lung during endoscopic dissection. The first part of the operation consists of the endoscopic dissection of the thoracic esophagus in the right thorax. In the second part, the stomach is mobilized through an upper midline incision while the cervical esophagus is mobilized through an incision anterior to the left sternocleidomastoid muscle in the neck. The cervical esophagus is divided and the esophagus and tumor are delivered through the abdominal wound. The stomach is then pulled through the mediastinum into the neck and anastomosed to the cervical esophagus. Four thoracoscopic ports are used. The upper two (5 and 10 mm) are placed in front and behind the lower angle of the scapula. The lower two (both 12 mm) are placed several costal interspaces below the first and just above the diaphragm. The procedure is started with the camera in the lower anterior port. Dissection of the esophagus is greatly facilitated by the use of a flexible endoscope placed within the esophagus. Dissection starts in an area of normal esophagus, leaving mobilization of the tumor until the remaining esophagus has been fully mobilized. The parietal pleura is divided above and below the azygous vein, which is mobilized and divided with an Endo GIA linear stapler. The mediastinal pleura from the thoracic inlet to the inferior pulmonary vein is then divided. An articulated dissector is used to dissect the esophagus from the adjacent tissues. Lymph nodes may be dissected *en-bloc*. A rubber sling is passed around the proximal esophagus and the middle third of the esophagus is mobilized by moving the sling in a caudal direction. Large arteries encountered can be clipped and divided under direct vision. For dissection of the lower third of the esophagus, the camera port is moved to the upper anterior porthole.

Several studies have demonstrated that thoracoscopic mobilization of the esophagus is technically feasible.[32-35] The mean time for esophageal mobilization ranges from 100 to 390 min, depending on the extent of the mediastinal dissection. The procedure has to be abandoned in patients with very bulky tumors or with extensive pleural adhesions. Pathologic assessment of dissected specimens have disclosed a number of lymph nodes ranging from 21 to 51.[32]

In addition to the three-stage esophagectomy, a modification of the Ivor-Lewis technique has been described.[36] Following the initial laparotomy to mobilize the stomach, a right thoracoscopic approach is again used to mobilize the esophagus. The head of a circular stapling gun is withdrawn through a small esophagotomy into the esophagus above the tumor after transection of the esophagus above the esophagotomy with a linear staple gun. A double-stapling technique is used to perform the intrathoracic anastomosis.

Thoracoscopic esophagectomy is, however, associated with a high incidence of respiratory complications. All patients developed some degree of right lung consolidation in one study, 3 requiring bronchoscopy, and all but 1 patient requiring ventilation for at least 72 hours.[32] Other studies have confirmed these findings.[37,38] The causes of pulmonary complications are multifactorial, including perioperative pulmonary aspiration, intraoperative pulmonary manipulation and retraction, postoperative pain, reflex diaphragmatic dysfunction and distension of the intrathoracic stomach.[39] Prolonged one-lung ventilation also may cause absorption atelectasis and transudation of fluid in the dependent lung, while alveolar overdistension may contribute to ventilator-induced pulmonary edema and acute lung injury, progressing in some patients to respiratory failure.[40,41]

In a review of 17 patients who underwent thoracoscopic-assisted Ivor-Lewis esophagectomy, thoracoscopy conferred no advantage over the open approach.[42] The incidence of respiratory complications was higher, with 76% of patients having radiologic evidence of atelectasis. There were also more technical difficulties with this operation: 4 patients required conversion to open thoracotomy because of technical failure of the anastomosis and the anastomotic leak rate was 18%. Technical problems with thoracosocpic esophagectomy and stapled anastomosis include: the untested double-stapling technique for esophageal anastomosis and the inevitable spillage of esophageal contents during withdrawal of the staple gun anvil into the esophagus; difficulty in docking the detached anvil into the circular stapling gun and difficulty in assessing the tension of the tissues during the process.[42] The postoperative stricture rate was also high because a small 25 mm staple gun was used.

ENDODISSECTION IN TRANSHIATAL ESOPHAGECTOMY

Conventional transhiatal esophagectomy with blunt dissection of the esophagus allows removal of the thoracic esophagus without thoracotomy, but does not permit mediastinal lymphadenectomy. Since this technique is performed blindly it can lead to hemorrhage and damage to associated mediastinal structures. In addition, compression of the patient's heart during dissection can lead to circulatory compromise and arrhythmias. Buess et al[31] first described the use of a mediastinoscope to dissect periesophageal tissues. Recently, specific instruments with microsurgical tools have been designed.[43] The mediastinoscope has at its tip a tissue dilator for the creation of a hollow space in the mediastinum. The dilator has several openings for the fiberoptic bundle and working, flushing and suction channels. The instrument's tip can rotate through 360° which allows circumferential esophageal dissection with the instrument's handle in a fixed position.[44]

The operation is carried out by two teams working synchronously. The endodissection is carried out via a left cervical approach and the cervical dissection is carried out as for a standard transhiatal esophagectomy. The instrument is then inserted into the upper mediastinum and dissection is continued along the mediastinum. Bumm et al.[44,45] prospectively evaluated their experience in 57 patients. Their overall clinical mortality was 5.3%, but no fatality was related to the endodissection. Only 1 patient had damage to the right main bronchus during dissection of a parabronchial lymph node and following transthoracic suture of the main bronchus this patient made an uneventful recovery. When their first 30 patients were compared with a historically matched group who underwent transhiatal esophagectomy, fewer pulmonary complications (13.3% vs 30%) and a lower rate of recurrent laryngeal nerve palsy (6.6% vs 13.3%) were seen in the endodissection group. The major benefit of this approach is that endoscopic vision allows controlled dissection of the thoracic esophagus. In addition, it can be performed simultaneously with the abdominal procedure, thereby minimizing operative delay. Periesophageal and parabronchial/tracheal nodes can be dissected for staging purposes, but a systematic lymphadenectomy cannot be performed.

Whilst Bumm et al have demonstrated that the technique is feasible, long-term clinical results are unknown. In elderly patients or patients at risk of pulmonary complications, this procedure may offer a safe alternative. A variation of this technique using a laparoscope to dissect the thoracic esophagus through the esophageal hiatus has also been described[46] but a clinical series using this technique has not yet been reported.

ENDOSCOPIC RESECTION OF MUCOSAL CANCER OF THE ESOPHAGUS

In T1 cancer of the esophagus, lymph-node metastases and vascular invasion are rare for mucosal cancer and submucosal cancer.[47] The incidence of lymph-node metastasis was 4% in mucosal cancer and 40% in submucosal cancer. Vascular invasion, involves 10% and 70%, of cases respectively. Based on this evidence, the indications for endoscopic resection in this population are: 1. Mucosal cancer without gross invasion of the muscularis mucosae; 2. A tumor of less than 2 × 2 cm in size or involving less than one third of the esophageal circumference; and 3; absence of nodal involvement. There are two procedures for mucosal resections: excision of the mucosal lesion by a grasper or suction of the lesion into the endoscope followed by snare excision. In both cases, the extent of the mucosal lesion should be marked by staining with Lugol's solution. Injection of saline into the submucosal space is helpful in excising larger mucosal specimens. Seventeen patients have been reported in whom this type of resection was carried out. No recurrences have been reported during a follow-up ranging from 8 months to 3 years. The 5-year survival rate of resected mucosal cancer is 100% and that of submucosal cancer is 62%.[48]

CONCLUSIONS

After widespread early enthusiasm for minimally invasive surgery (MIS), its place in the management of esophageal cancer is being established. MIS has a clear role in staging of esophageal cancer. While thoracoscopic esophageal resection is feasible, it does not offer substantial advantages over more conventional open procedures in terms of operating time, pulmonary complications, or duration of hospital stay. In patients in whom transhiatal esophagectomy is indicated, endodissection may offer advantages in allowing better control of hemorrhage and lymph-node sampling, but large prospective clinical trials are necessary to confirm this. In Western populations, the number of patients presenting with mucosal cancer is small; however results from centers with extensive experience suggest that endoscopic dissection is a good option in these patients.

REFERENCES

1. Boring CC, Squires TS, Tong T. Cancer statistics. *CA Cancer J Clin* 1993; **43**: 7-26.
2. Blot WJ, Devesa SS, Kneller RW, et al. Rising incidence of adenocarcinoma of the esophagus and gastric cardia. *JAMA* 1991; **265**: 1287-1289.
3. Morita M, Kuwano H, Ohno S, et al. Characteristics and sequence of the recurrent patters after curative esophagectomy for squamous cell carcinoma. *Surgery* 1994; **116**: 1-7.
4. Earlam R, Cunha-Melo JR. Esophageal squamous cell carcinoma: A critical review of surgery. *Br J Surg* 1980; **67**: 381-390.
5. Orringer MB, Forastiere AA, Perez-Tamayo C, et al. Chemotherapy and radiation therapy before transhiatal esophagectomy for esophageal carcinoma. *Ann Thorac Surg* 1990; **119**: 348-355.
6. Picus D, Balfe DM, Koehler RE, et al. Computed tomography in the staging of esophageal carcinoma. *Radiology* 1983; **146**: 433-438.
7. Dagnini G, Caldironi MW, Marin G, et al. Laparoscopy in abdominal staging of esophageal carcinoma. Report of 369 cases. *Gastrointest Endosc* 1986; **30**: 400-402.
8. Kriplani AK, Kapur BML. Laparoscopy for pre-operative staging and assessment of operability in gastric carcinoma. *Gastrointest Endosc* 1991;**37**:441-443.
9. Watt I, Stewart I, Anderson D, et al. Laparoscopy, ultrasound, and computed tomography in cancer of the oesophagus and gastric cardia: A prospective comparison for detecting intra-abdominal metastases. *Br J Surg* 1989; **76**: 1036-1039.
10. Asenico-Arana F. Laparoscopic access to the lesser sac in gastric cancer staging. *Surg Laparosc Endosc* 1994; **4**:438-440.
11. Molloy RG, McCartney JS, Anderson JR. Laparoscopy in the management of patients with cancer. *Br J Surg* 1995; **82**:352-354.
12. Possik RA, Franco EL, Pires DR, et al. Sensitivity, specificity and predictive value of laparoscopy for the staging of gastric cancer and for the detection of liver metastasis. *Cancer* 1986; **58**: 1-6.
13. O'Brien MG, Fitzgerald EF, Lee G, et al. A prospective comparison of laparoscopy and imaging in the staging of esophagogastric cancer before surgery. *Am J Gastro* 1995; **90**: 2191-3194.
14. Hunerbein M, Rau B, Schlag PM. Laparoscopy and laparoscopic ultrasound for staging of upper gastrointestinal tumors. *Eur J Surg Oncol* 1995; **21**: 50-55.
15. Ellis FH Jr, Watkins E Jr, Krasna MJ et al. Staging of carcinoma of the esophagus and cardia; a comparison of different staging criteria. *J Surg Oncol* 1993;**52**:231-235.
16. Akiyama H, Tsurumaru M, Kawamura T, Ono Y. Principles of surgical treatment for carcinoma of the esophagus. *Ann Surg* 1981; **194**: 438-446.
17. Maas R, Nicholas V, Grimm H, et al. MRI of esophageal carcinoma with ECG gating at 1.5 Tesla. In: Ferguson MN, Little AG, Skinner DB (eds) *Diseases of the esophagus*. New York: Futura Publishing, 1990, pp 145-155.
18. Templeton PA, Krasna MJ. Use of gadolinum-enhanced MRI to evaluate for airway invasion in patients with esophageal carcinoma. Radiological Society of North America 1994 (Abst).

19. Rice TW, Boyce GA, Sivall MV. Esophageal ultrasound and the pre-operative staging of carcinoma in the esophagus. *J Thorac Cardiovasc Surg* 1991; **101**: 536-543.

20. Siewert JR, Sendler A, Dittler HJ et al. Staging gastrointestinal cancer as a pre-condition for multi-modal treatment. *World J Surg* 1995; **19**: 168-177.

21. Caletti G, Ferrari A, Brocchi E et al. Accuracy of endoscopic ultrasonography in the diagnosis and staging of gastric cancer and lymphoma. *Surgery* 1993; 113: 14-27.

22. Greenberg J, Durkin M, Van Drunen M et al. Computed tomography or endoscopic ultrasonography in pre-operative staging gastric and esophageal tumours. *Surgery* 1994; **116**: 696-702.

23. Murray GF, Wilcox BR, Stared PIK. The assessment of operability of esophageal carcinoma. *Ann Thorac Surg* 1977; **23**: 393.

24. Krasna MJ, McLaughlin JS. Thoracoscopic lymph node staging for esophageal cancer. *Ann Thorac Surg* 1993; **56**: 671-674.

25. Krasna MJ, Reed CE, Jaklitsch MT et al. Thoracoscopic staging of esophageal cancer: A prospective, multi-institutional trial. *Ann Thorac Surg* 1995; **60**: 1337-1340.

26. Krasna MJ, Flowers JL, Attar S, McLaughlin J. Combined thoracoscopic/laparoscopic staging of esophageal cancer. *J Thorac Cardiovasc Surg* 1996; **111**: 800-807.

27. Orringer MB. Transthoracic versus transhiatal esophagectomy; what difference does it make? *Ann Thorac Surg* 1987; **44**:116-118.

28. Fok M, Siu KF, Wong J. A comparison of transhiatal and transthoracic resection for carcinoma of the thoracic esophagus. *Am J Surg* 1989; **158**: 414-419.

29. Bolger G, Walsh TN, Tanner WA et al. Chylothorax after oesophagectomy. *Br J Surg* 1991; **78**: 587-589.

30. Khoury GA. Oesophageal surgery under Akiyama. *Lancet* 1989; **1**: 91-92.

31. Buess G, Becker MD, Memtges R et al. Die Endoskopisch - mikrochirurgische Dissection der Speiserohre. *Chirugie* 1990; **61**: 308-311.

32. McAnena OJ, Rogers J, Williams NS. Right thoracoscopically-assisted oesophagectomy for cancer. *Br J Surg* 1994; **81**: 236-238.

33. Darzi A, Monosn JRT. Minimally invasive esophageal surgery. Throacoscopic esophagectomy-minimally invasive direct vision esophageal mobilization for cancer. *Dis Esophag* 1994; **7**: 27-31.

34. Collard JM, Lengele B, Otte JB, Kestens PJ. En Bloc and standard esophagectomies by thoracoscopy. *Ann Thorac Surg* 1993; **56**: 675-679.

35. Gossat D, Fourquier p, Celerier M. Thoracoscopic esophagectomy: Technique and initial results. *Ann Thorac Surg* 1993; **56**:667-670.

36. Lloyd DM, Vipond M, Robertson GSM et al. Thoracoscopic oesophagogastrectomy–a new technique for intra-thoracic stapling. *Endo Surg Allied Technol* 1994; **2**: 26-31.

37. Chui PT, Mainland P, Chung SCS, Chung DC. Anaesthesia for three stage thoracoscopic oesophagectomy: An initial experience. *Anaesth Intensive Care* 1994; **22**: 593-596.

38. Robertson GSM, Lloyd DM, Wicks ACB, Veitch PS. No obvious advantages for thoracoscopic two stage oesophagectomy. *Br J Surg* 1996; **83**: 675-678.

39. Bonser RS, Goldstraw P. Management of complications of intra-thoracic resection. In: Hurt RL (ed) *Management of Oesophageal Carcinoma*. London: Springer-Verlag 1989; pp 267-291.

40. Barker SJ, Clarke C, Trivedi N, Hyatt J et al. Anaesthesia for thoracoscopic laser ablation of bullous emphysema. *Anaesthesiology* 1993; **78**: 44-50.

41. Hickling KG, Henderson SJ, Jackson R. Low mortality associated with low volume pressure limited ventilation with permissive hypercapnia in severe adult respiratory distress syndrome. *Intensive Care Med* 1990; **16**: 372-377.

42. Robertson GSM, Lloyd DM, Wicks ACB, Veitch PS. No obvious advantages for thoracoscopic two-stage oesophagectomy. *Br J Surg* 1996; **83**: 675-678.

43. Bumm G, Holscher AH, Feussner H et al. Endodissection of the thoracic esophagus: Technique and clinical results in transhiatal esophagectomy. *Ann Surg* 1993; **218**: 97-104.

44. Bumm R, Siwert JR. Endodissection in trashiatal esophagectomy: technical aspects and clinical results. *Dis Esophag* 1994; **7**: 32-35.

45. Bumm R, Holscher AH, Feussner H et al. Endodissection of the thoracic esophagus: Techniques and clinical results in transhiatal esophagectomy. *Ann Surg* 1993; **218**: 97-104.

46. Sadanaga N, Kuwano H, Watanabe M et al. Laparoscopy-assisted surgery: A new technique for transhiatal esophageal dissection. *Am J Surg* 1994; **168**: 355-357.

47. Endo M Takeshita K, Kawano T, Inoue H. Endoscopic resection of mucosal cancer of the esophagus. *Dis Esophag* 1994; **7**: 24-26.

48. Endo M, Ide H, Yoshino K, Yoshida M. Diagnosis and treatment of early esophageal cancer. In: Siewert J, Holscher AH (eds) *Diseases of the Esophagus*. Berlin: Springer-Verlag, 1986; pp 375-380.

9

Laparoscopy and Other Minimally Invasive Techniques in Patients with Advanced Intraperitoneal Malignant Disease

David M. Thompson, Cihat Tetik and Maurice E. Arregui

With improved technology and advanced skills, cure and palliation of gastrointestinal tumors has entered the domain of laparoscopy. This approach provides a more humane means of palliation. Laparoscopic techniques are the latest of the minimally invasive procedures that must be compared with well established endoscopic, percutaneous radiologic and ultrasound-guided approaches and with open surgery. This chapter discusses the indications, risks and benefits associated with various minimally invasive approaches (laparoscopic, endoscopic and percutaneous) as they apply to advanced malignancies causing obstruction of the upper gastrointestinal tract, biliary tree and small and large bowel. Laparoscopic approaches to enteral feeding tube placement, implantation of drug-delivery catheters and cryosurgery for liver metastasis are also reviewed.

MINIMALLY INVASIVE GASTRIC BYPASS

Gastric bypass is most commonly performed in patients with duodenal obstruction from pancreatic cancer. The prognosis is poor and 90% die within 1 year of diagnosis. Up to 50% of patients develop duodenal obstruction at some point in their disease process.[1] The necessity for gastric bypass is obvious when the patient has nausea and vomiting caused by duodenal compression or distortion. The need for prophylactic gastrojejunostomy, however, is less clear. Gastrojejunostomy can provoke delayed gastric emptying and prolonged hospitalization. The 30-day mortality rates are 40% and 70% after traditional gastrojejunostomy for patients without duodenal obstruction and for those with duodenal impingement, respectively.[2] However, the patients in this study with established gastric outlet obstruction causing nausea and vomiting were not followed-up to determine if their bypasses were patent. Nineteen of 21 had a poor outcome as defined by death within 30 days of operation or discharge from hospital. Mortality resulted from progression of the disease. The other 2 were able to tolerate a diet.

Other malignancies which may require gastric bypass include gastric, duodenal and ampullary cancers or any extraluminal malignancy obstructing the gastroduodenal passage. Only 30% of patients with gastric cancer are suitable for curative therapy.[3] Pyloric obstruction caused by a tumor may be effectively palliated by resection or by gastrojejunostomy. Obstruction of the cardia is relieved by resection or stenting. Acute hemorrhage and ulcer-like pain is treated preferably by resection when possible.

Excellent palliation of malignant gastric outlet obstruction can be achieved by laparoscopic and endoscopic bypass procedures. Gastric resections, gastrojejunostomies, truncal vagotomies and chemical destructions of celiac ganglia can also be performed laparoscopically. In *laparoscopic-assisted gastric bypass*, the gastric ligaments that restrain the stomach are freed laparoscopically and the stomach is brought out through a small incision. The gastric anastomosis is then performed using a traditional open technique. In a *totally laparoscopic approach*, the surgeon should choose an anastomotic technique consistent with his or her laparoscopic skills and the condition of the patient. Anastomotic techniques, such as single-layer, double-layer, interrupted, continuous suturing or mechanical stapling techniques can be used for laparoscopic gastrojejunal anastomoses. Rhodes et al[4] looked at 16 patients with unresectable carcinoma of the pancreas who underwent laparoscopic palliation for biliary obstruction, gastric outlet obstruction or both. A total of 8 laparoscopic gastrojejunostomies were performed and normal gastric emptying was present within 1 week in 7 (88%). Median operating room time for the entire group was 75 min and median hospital stay 4 days. Fourteen of the 16 patients were discharged within 7 days of surgery and they returned to normal activity within 2 weeks. La Ferla & Murray[5] looked at a group of 14 patients who underwent open biliary diversion and gastrojejunostomy. The mean hospital stay for this group was 20 days and the mortality was 20%. These enteric bypasses were done prophylactically. In both studies[4,5] the patients were diagnosed at the initial laparotomy and were determined to be unresectable. Four of the 8 patients in the first study who underwent laparoscopic gastrojejunostomy had duodenal obstruction while none of the patients in the second study presented in this way. There are no retrospective or prospective studies comparing open to laparoscopic bypass in patients with pancreatic cancer. The best that can be done is to compare studies with similar groups of patients.

More than 65% of patients with pancreatic cancer who are suitable for palliative bypass surgery have moderate to severe pain.[1] The chemical destruction of the celiac ganglia with injection of 95% alcohol is an effective and easy technique to perform laparoscopically in patients with intractable pancreatic pain. The morbidity for this is low.

Endoscopic dilation and placement of an endoprosthesis can be considered if gastric obstruction is the result of an extraluminal tumor. Endoscopic stent placement at a narrowed gastrojejunostomy may also be helpful if gastric stasis occurs after gastric bypass.[6,7] Balloon- or self-expandable endoprostheses have been applied to malignant stenoses of the esophagus and cardia because of the suitability of a straight lumen. If an endoprosthesis is placed in a curved intestinal lumen, there is a greater risk of perforation. Tumor ingrowth into the lumen through the struts or overgrowth around the ends of the stent can occur as late complications. Occlusion of the endoprosthesis can also be caused by vegetable fiber clogging the lumen. Inadequate deployment of the stent may result in an inadequate passage. This sometimes results from the balloon- and self-expandable endoprostheses shortening during placement. These endoprosthesis can only be removed surgically. There are only case reports of the use of expandable metallic stents in gastric outlet obstruction and no long-term data is available to compare it with laparoscopic bypass.

Although gastrojejunostomy may improve obstruction of the gastroduodenal passage, it may be ineffective for bleeding caused by the malignancy and for the pain caused by extragastric extension of tumor. Radiation may be helpful if hemorrhage is not acute. Endoscopic cautery can be used to stop the hemorrhage. When resection is not feasible, one study[8] has shown that the neodymium(Nd): YAG laser is safe and effective when applied to intraluminal tumors. However, only 3 of the 22 obstructing lesions in this study were gastric in origin. These patients achieved palliation with an average of two treatments and had a mean survival of 10.6 months. In a second, retrospective study by Laukka & Wang[9], 20 patients with malignant duodenal tumors underwent Nd:YAG laser treatment for either gastrointestinal hemorrhage (95%) and/or obstructive symptoms (45%). This group required an average of three treatments and all showed improvement in their obstructive symptoms. The complication rate was 5% and no mortalities related to the treatments occured. The overall survival was poor, similar to the previous study. No studies have compared Nd:YAG laser treatment with open, laparoscopic or endoscopic palliation of malignant obstructions.

In some cases, simple gastrostomy may be carried out in patients with gastric obstruction who require intermittent gastric suction. This can be done laparoscopically if there is any contraindication to endoscopic gastrostomy.

It is too early to compare laparoscopic or endoscopic approaches to traditional open approaches in gastric bypass surgery. There are no prospective studies comparing operative time, length of hospitalization and return to full activity in open versus laparoscopic or endoscopic techniques for palliative gastrointestinal bypass, although studies in small groups of patients suggest the less invasive techniques offer the patient less morbidity and earlier return to full activity.[4,5]

ENDOSCOPIC/ LAPAROSCOPIC BILIARY BYPASS

Biliary obstruction may result from primary cancers of the pancreas, ampulla and bile ducts or metastatic cancers to the liver or perihilar lymph nodes. Prolonged obstruction may result in malabsorbtion, malnutrition, coagulopathy, pruritus, liver insufficiency, renal failure and cholangitis. The mean survival time after diagnosis of unresectable malignant disease causing biliary obstruction is low. Therefore, an optimal form of biliary drainage should not only be effective, but be associated to a low morbidity and capable of minimizing hospitalization and the recovery period.

Malignant biliary obstruction can be managed by several methods. Traditional techniques include open surgical methods, such as cholecystojejunostomy, choledochojejunostomy, hepaticogastrostomy, hepaticojejunostomy or pancreaticoduodenectomy. Today, these operations can be done laparoscopically. An alternative approach is percutaneous stent placement with or without external drainage. The most commonly used method is internalized stent placement by either endoscopic or combined percutaneous-endoscopic techniques. The Nd-YAG laser has been used for recanalization of bile-duct cancers but simple stenting is generally more successful and safer. The methods of minimal access biliary bypasses are listed in Table 9.1.

Nasobiliary catheter placement has not been used for long term bypass of distal bile duct obstruction in malignant disease because of patient discomfort, the necessity for flushing and dressing the catheter, the possibility of bile leakage, and infection and pain at the catheter entry site. Nasobiliary catheters have been placed for short term use in some patients with advanced malignancies. There is very little role for

Table 9.1 - Minimal access biliary bypasses in patients with malignant obstructive jaundice.

Endoscopic sphincterotomy
Nasobiliary catheter
Percutaneous transhepatic stent (PTS)
Endoscopic plastic stent (EPS)
Endoscopic metal stent (EMS)

Nd:YAG Laser recanalization

Laparoscopic cholecystojejunostomy (LCCJ)
Laparoscopic choledochojejunostomy (LCDJ)
Laparoscopic hepaticojejunostomy
Laparoscopic hepaticogastrostomy

---

nasobiliary catheters. Unresectable tumors in the region of the pancreatic head or involving the porta hepatis may be managed by the placement of a endoscopic or percutaneous prosthesis. These minimally invasive approaches to restore bile duct patency are preferable to open surgical alternatives in patients without other indications for operative therapy. The ideal endoprosthesis should be easily insertable with minimal complications, should remain in place, and should stay open until death. Plastic and metal stents have been used for biliary drainage. The big disadvantage of plastic biliary stents is the need for frequent stent changes. These stents occlude within 3 to 6 months.

Expandable metal stents have been developed to reduce the polyethylene stent complications such as occlusion and migration. Their placement is more successful in patients with small, flexible ducts. Additionally, they increase the luminal diameter and decrease the occlusion rate. Despite their large internal diameter (8-10 mm), tumor ingrowth or overgrowth can occur. Tumor ingrowth between the struts of the stent causes occlusion. Tumor ingrowths are observed in 6.5% of metal endoprostheses with a narrow woven mesh whereas prostheses with large distances between the struts have ingrowths rates of 19% to 50%.[10] In some cases, the insertion of metal stents may be more difficult technically, and more expensive (5 to 10 times more than that of polyethylene stents). However, metal endoprostheses may be more cost effective because of the need for fewer admissions for stent complications and stent changes. Metal stents can cause hemobilia and erosion through the wall of the biliary tree. Additionally, their inability to be removed nonsurgically limits their application. Recanalization of occluded metallic stents requires a second metallic or polyethylene endoprosthesis through the existing lumen of the occluded stent. More complicated methods such as thermal and laser probes to open the lumen are associated with higher complication rates.

All forms of biliary stent placements may result in complications such as cholangitis, acute cholecystitis, stent fracture, occlusion, migration, bleeding, bile leaks and hyperamylasemia. Life-threatening cholangitis is the most common complication. The incidence of this complication is approximately 10% to 20% after the stent placement.[11,12] Pancreaticobiliary sepsis is a major cause of death after Endoscopic Retrograde Colangiopancratography (ERCP)[13] and patients with obstructive bile duct disease should receive antibiotic prophylaxis before undergoing this procedure.[14] Drainage of obstructed ductal segments is essential if cholangitis does develop and this may require a percutaneous transhepatic approach if the endoscopic approach is not possible. The early cholangitis rate is 2-3% in patients with distal common bile-duct strictures and occurs principally in those endoscopic failures in which contrast is injected into an obstructed biliary tree which is unsuccessfully stented.[14,15] Stent placement may narrow the lumen of the cystic duct, leading to acute cholecystitis. This infrequent complication may be related to the mechanical obstruction of the cystic duct by prosthesis, tumor or inflammation and edema caused by the stent.[16]

Endoscopic stent placement is currently the preferred alternative to traditional operative biliary-digestive bypass in the palliative treatment of patients with unresectable malignant biliary obstruction because of the comfort of a completely indwelling endoprosthesis. Endoscopic stent placement has better patient acceptance, and lower morbidity and mortality rates than percutaneous stent insertion.[12] Duodenal perforation is a complication of the endoscopic approach, adding to the other complications of stent placement. The frequency of duodenal perforation in biliary endoprostheses placement is low. In patients with silent retroperitoneal perforations and malignant disease, these perforating stents may be left in place because they continue to drain the biliary tree. Intraoperative and postoperative 30-day mortality after endoscopic stent placement is 10-18% and after traditional bypass surgery is 15-30%.[5]

The difference in mortality seems to be due to patient selection and natural progression of the disease and not to the procedure. Endoscopically placed internal plastic stents become occluded over time requiring periodic stent changes. The major cause of occlusion is adherence of bacteria and encrustation of bile.[10] One approach to preventing stent occlusion and the subsequent complications of biliary sepsis is prophylactic replacement at scheduled intervals. However, premature stent replacement causes additional patient discomfort and increases procedure related expenses. The time interval for stent replacement can be extended to 6 months, resulting in decreased patient discomfort and cost. After 6 months, there is a significant increase in the rate of stent occlusion. Distal stent migration out of the common bile duct is seen at a rate of up to 6%[10,17] and proximal stent migration at approximately 5%.[17] Bleeding and bile leaks may result from injury to the bile ducts or liver and may increase mortality.[12] Serum amylase may rise transiently after biliary stent placement, but pancreatitis is infrequent and usually mild. Although pancreatitis may also result from the introduction of an infected stent, it is more likely to occur after excessive and repeated injections of contrast substances. Endoscopy-related mortality is <2% and the technical success rate is 90%.[10,18]

Percutaneous transhepatic biliary drainage is most commonly used for palliation in patients with unresectable malignant hilar obstruction in whom an endoscopic attempt has failed or is not feasible. Percutaneous transhepatic stent (PTS) placement is performed with local anesthesia and fluoroscopic guidance and is usually successful for bilateral drainage via one percutaneous tract.[19] Percutaneous biliary drainage resolves pruritus and metabolic derangements in more than 80% of patients with extrahepatic biliary obstruction.[20] Major complications occur in up to 25% of these patients and include bleeding, bacteremia and liver abscess.[21] Most can be managed with antibiotics, transfusions or catheter manipulation and they rarely require surgical intervention. Catheter-related complications include unintentional removal, leakage around the catheter, fractured guidewire and fractured catheter. Although the fluid leaking around the catheter is usually bile, ascitic leaks can also develop and PTS is not advised in patients with ascites. Bile leak and pneumothorax are other possible complications.

The 30-day mortality rate of the external-internal biliary drainage is 10-27%.[11,20,22] Morbidity and mortality rates are higher when PTS is placed for palliation of patients with end-stage malignancies[20] but, the underlying disease process may be the most important factor in determining the outcome of PTS.

Although the placement of biliary endoprostheses is the preferred approach to unresectable malignant biliary obstruction, readmission rates of up to 40% have been reported.[23] Surgical biliary bypasses such as cholecystojejunostomy, choledochojejunostomy, hepaticojejunostomy and hepaticogastrostomy are being reconsidered for palliation of malignant bile duct obstruction because of long term patency, absence of endoprosthesis-related complications and the ability to use a minimally invasive technique.

Laparoscopic biliary bypass procedures have not been prospectively compared to open techniques but would intuitively seem to offer real benefits such as reduction of postoperative stay in hospital, minimal wound complications, less postoperative pain, early return to full activity and work and lower cost of treatment. Additionally, laparoscopy allows accurate staging of the malignancy and the possibility of performing concomitant gastroenterostomy if indicated. Laparoscopic biliary bypass operations do not require more personnel or devices than laparoscopic cholecystectomy.

Careful selection of the type of biliary bypass is necessary to ensure long-term function. Intraoperative cholangiography and laparoscopic ultrasound help the surgeon select the appropriate site for bypass. *Laparoscopic cholecystojejunostomy* is indicated when the gallbladder and the cystic duct-common hepatic duct junction are intact and the tumor is unlikely to obstruct them in the patient's lifetime. The majority of patients are not suitable for cholecystojejunostomy because of prior biliary surgery (29%), hilar obstruction (17%) or a closed hepatocystic junction.[24] If the surgeon chooses open anastomosis, cholecystojejunostomy can be achieved by a laparoscopic-assisted approach. To perform a totally laparoscopic cholecystojejunostomy, laparoscopic surgical experience is the most important requirement. If cholecystojejunostomy is contraindicated, alternatives such as choledochojejunostomy, hepaticojejunostomy or hepaticogastrostomy should be considered.

Laparoscopic choledochojejunostomy is a feasible alternative to laparoscopic cholecystojejunostomy if a 2-3 cm section of normal common bile duct is clearly visible between the hepatic parenchyma and the upper limit of the tumor. This is a more technically demanding procedure than a laparoscopic cholecystojejunostomy. No randomized studies have compared laparoscopic cholecystojejunostomy to laparoscopic choledochojejunostomy but if the open surgical data comparing these two procedures is extrapolated, the latter procedure results in fewer postoperative complications and significantly fewer long-term failures in regards to recurrent jaundice.[25] Since anastomosis between common bile duct and jejunum cannot be performed out of the peritoneal space a totally laparoscopic technique must be used.

Recently, *hepaticogastrostomy* under fluoroscopic, endoscopic and laparoscopic guidance has been reported with a success rate of 100% in 7 patients with advanced carcinoma.[26] Unlike other laparoscopic approaches, this procedure requires more devices and equipment. It is carried out in two parts: the first in a radiological intervention room and the second in the operating room. This requires a team approach from a radiologist, endoscopist and laparoscopic surgeon. This procedure has also been performed without laparoscopic guidance. Patients undergoing this procedure experience significant discomfort because of the necessity of internal-external drainage for a 15-day period to avoid the potential complication of bile leak. Subcapsular hematoma and cholangitis are additional complications. The complication rate is approximately 30%. Bile leak, bile gastritis and symptomatic reflux are potential complications although they have not yet been reported. Hepatico-gastrostomy is performed away from the tumor site and therefore obstruction of the biliary bypass by tumor invasion is avoided. In Soulez et al's. study,[26] 3 of the 7 patients died; 3, 6 and 9 months postoperatively. None had recurrence of jaundice. The remaining four patients are alive without jaundice. This procedure avoids multiple interventions to treat stent complications and is very useful for palliation of patients with slow-growing tumors such as cholangiocarcinomas.

The debate about surgical versus endoscopic/percutaneous palliation of obstructive jaundice rages on. Several prospective, randomized trials have compared these two interventional modalities.[27-30] The overall conclusion from these studies is that the two methods are equally effective in the short-term relief of jaundice. Endoscopic stenting seems to be associated with a lower procedure related complication rate and a shorter hospital stay. The 30-day mortality is also lower than in the surgical group, although this does not reach statistical significance probably because of the small study group sizes. The combined data from the four studies shows a 30-day mortality rate of 11% for the non-operatively-stented group and 18% for the surgically bypassed group.[31] In one of the studies, 33 of the patients randomized to endoscopic stent placement underwent 54 stent placements and the number of endoscopic procedures ranged from 1 to 5 per patient.[28] No similar studies have compared

Table 9.2 – Minimal access procedures carried out in 29 patients with obstructive jaundice caused by unresectable malignancy within the last 5 years.

Procedure (number)	Success rate (number)	Operative complications (number)	Additional procedures (number)
Percutaneous transhepatic stent (10)	100 %	Bile leak from the gallbladder (1)	Endoscopic stent placement (3) Laparoscopic gastrojejunostomy (1)
Endoscopic plastic stent (34)	82 %	False tract with extravasation of dye at the hilum (1)	Endoscopic sphincterotomy (8) Stent change (7) Percutaneous transhepatic stent placement (2)
Endoscopic cholecystojejunostomy (14)	100%	None	Endoscopic sphincterotomy (3) Percutaneous transhepatic stent removal (4)
Laparoscopic cholecystojejunostomy (2)	100%	None	Ablation of liver metastasis and injection of pancreatic mass (1)
Laparoscopic choledochojejunostomy (4)	100%	None	Laparoscopic gastrojejunostomy (1)

Table 9.3 – Diagnosis for and minimal access procedures carried out in 29 patients with obstructive jaundice caused by unresectable malignancy (over the past 5 year period).

Diagnosis (No of Patients)	PTS (Prs/Pts)	EPS (Prs/Pts)	EMS (Prs/Pts)	LCCJ (Prs/Pts)	LCDJ (Prs/Pts)	OCCJ (Prs/Pts)	OCDJ (Prs/Pts)	Total (Prs/Pts)
Pancreatic cancer (15)	3/1	10/7	7/7	2/2	3/3	0/0	0/0	25/15
Cholangiocarcinoma (7)	6/4	17/7	3/3	0/0	0/0	0/0	0/0	26/7
Metastatic colon cancer (4)	1/1	6/4	3/3	0/0	0/0	0/0	0/0	10/4
Gall bladder cancer (1)	0/0	0/0	1/1	0/0	0/0	0/0	0/0	1/1
Metastatic esophageal cancer (1)	0/0	1/1	0/0	0/0	0/0	0/0	0/0	1/1
Metastatic breast cancer (1)	0/0	0/0	0/0	0/0	1/1	0/0	0/0	1/1
Total (29)	10/6	34/19	14/14	2/2	4/4	0/0	0/0	64/29

PTS= Percutaneous transhepatic stent; EPS= endoscopic plastic stent; EMS= endoscopic metal stent; LCCJ= laparoscopic hepaticojejunostomy. LCDJ= laparoscopic choledochojejunostomy; OCCJ= open cholecystojejunostomy; OCDJ= open choledochojejunostomy; Prs= number of procedures; Pts= number of patients.

laparoscopic bypass with endoscopic palliation. Cholecystoduodenostomy and choledochoduodenostomy should not be used as palliative procedures for periampullary malignancies because of the high incidence of recurrent biliary obstruction. The procedures we have performed to palliate malignant bile duct obstructions are shown in table 9.2 and the patient diagnoses are described in table 9.3. Our data supports both endoscopic/percutaneous and surgical bypass procedures. The average length of stay in hopital for the surgical bypass group was 4 days. The endoscopic bypass group required multiple stent changes for occlusion, a drawback of endoscopic palliation also identified in larger studies.

ENDOSCOPIC/ LAPAROSCOPIC PLACEMENT OF FEEDING TUBES: GASTROSTOMY AND JEJUNOSTOMY

Enteral feeding is superior to parenteral feeding because it is safer, cheaper, easier to administer, physiologic and avoids septic complications. Nasogastric or nasojejunal feeding tubes are rarely suitable in patients with advanced malignant disease because they are uncomfortable and can lead to pulmonary aspiration. Gastrostomies and jejunostomies are currently being performed endoscopically. Gastrostomy is chosen for the majority of patients because the stomach is an excellent reservoir for bolus feedings and the incidence of osmotic diarrhea with gastrostomy feeding is less than with jejunostomy feeding. In oncology, gastrostomy tubes for long-term feeding are usually placed in patients with obstruction caused by tumors of the head and neck, esophagus and proximal stomach. They have also been used as a conduit for the replacement of bile if internal drainage cannot be established. They can also provide gastrointestinal decompression in patients with bowel obstruction.

Percutaneous endoscopic and non-endoscopic gastrostomy and percutaneous endoscopic jejunostomy (PEJ) were first described in 1980 and 1982, respectively. They have now replaced surgical gastrostomies because of decreased morbidity, mortality and cost. Percutaneous endoscopic gastrostomy (PEG) and PEJ are carried out in the endoscopy suite or at the patient's bedside. The former is performed using a flexible fiberoptic gastroscope and a PEG kit. To carry out the PEJ, the gastrostomy tube is placed first. The PEJ tube is inserted through the lumen of the gastrostomy tube and carried from the stomach into the duodenum with the gastroscope and grasping forceps. Percutaneous non-endoscopic gastrostomy must be carried out in the radiology department under local anesthesia and with the assistance of fluoroscopy.

Percutaneous endoscopic placement of feeding tubes is significantly quicker and less expensive than the open surgical approach. However, surgical placement can be carried out by one operator with basic surgical instruments while percutaneous techniques can require two operators and endoscopy or fluoroscopy. Surgical techniques also offer the advantage of intraabdominal inspection and lower risk of injury to surrounding structures. Surgical placement of feeding tubes is obligatory when the gastrointestinal wall cannot be apposed to the abdominal wall or the endoscope cannot be introduced into the stomach because of oropharyngeal or esophageal pathology. *Laparoscopic gastrostomy* or *laparoscopic jejunostomy* should be considered for patients in whom none of the percutaneous methods is technically feasible. If there is a technical problem associated with the percutaneous technique, laparoscopic assisted gastrostomy can be carried out.

Laparoscopic placement of jejunal feeding tubes has been achieved by several methods such as using T-fasteners as retractors and anchors or simply by bringing the intestinal loop out of the peritoneal cavity through a trocar site.[32-34]

Contraindications to the placement of feeding tubes include peritonitis, massive ascites, low serum protein, coagulopathy and pathology of the gastrointestinal wall.

Complications of the open procedures (at a rate of 56%) are infection, abscess, poor drainage, inflammatory or gastrointestinal fluid drainage around the tube, dermatitis, bleeding, separation of the gastrointestinal tract and abdominal walls, intraperitoneal leakage, peritonitis, ileus, prolapse around the feeding tube and injury to the posterior gastrointestinal wall or adjacent organs.[35,36] Retrospective data suggest that non-surgical gastrostomies are associated with a lower incidence of complications.[37] Complications of laparoscopic techniques may occur at the laparoscopic stoma. Infection is the commonest complication after percutaneous endoscopic techniques, followed by aspiration which probably relates to the underlying disease of the patient. Although PEJ, a modification of PEG involving transpyloric passage of a small bore feeding tube, was advocated for use in patients with aspiration, this complication is more common in patients with PEJs than in those with PEGs.[38] Aspiration results from tube migration back into the stomach or esophagus and anatomical displacement of the stomach. PEJ is not recommended routinely in patients requiring tube feedings because of the increased incidence of tube dysfunction and the failure to prevent aspiration in predisposed patients. Additionally, some tube-related complications, such as peritube leakage, plugging, fracture and migration, are more common after PEJ than PEG.[38] Jejunal tube placement with the assistance of the laparoscope has been advised because of the ability to prevent aspiration, kinking and coiling.[34] Separation of the gastrointestinal tract and abdominal wall, pneumoperitoneum, poor drainage, intraperitoneal leakage and peritonitis, extraperitoneal leakage and gastrointestinal bleeding are other complications of percutaneous endoscopic techniques. Furthermore, catheter-site metastasis may occur in patients with head and neck tumors who undergo PEG or PEJ placement.[39] Complication rates after PEG have been reported at a rate of up to 20%.[40,41]

The 30-day mortality rates with open gastrostomy tube placement range from 6 to 37%, while those reported with laparoscopic gastrostomy tube placement have been as high as 35%. It must be remembered that the procedure itself is rarely the cause of death. Typically, the underlying disease is the cause that leads to the patient's demise. The 30-day mortality for PEGs is 0 to 16%, and only 8% after percutaneous non-endoscopic gastrostomy.[37,40]

PEG is the prefered approach when feasible because of the simplicity and relatively lower complication rate. When not feasible, a laparoscopic approach is a reasonable alternative to open gastrostomy, although there are no studies demonstrating any advantage. When a gastrostomy tube is contraindicated because of the risk of aspiration, a surgical jejunostomy becomes the preferred approach. The laparoscopic approach may provide better patient comfort and perhaps a lower morbidity, but again there are no studies to demonstrate advantage with the laparoscope.

DIVERTING COLOSTOMY

In patients with advanced malignancies, fecal diversion is commonly carried out to relieve obstruction, incontinence, complicated fistula-in-ano, rectovaginal or rectourinary tract fistulas and severe perianal sepsis. These conditions may result from advanced malignancies such as tumor of the colon, anus, ovary or prostate.[42]

Laparoscopic fecal diversion does not require as large an abdominal incision as laparotomy and does not limit intraabdominal exploration as trephine stoma formation does. Laparoscopic colostomy is technically simple and requires minimal equipment. Some authors have advocated laparoscopic fecal diversion procedures for surgeons with limited experience in laparoscopic intestinal surgery because of its relative simplicity.[42] Additionally, it allows the patient to recover without laparotomy pain and related complications. Laparoscopic colostomy decreases the common complications of open colostomy such as wound infection, evisceration and incisional hernia. Bowel function returns more quickly after laparoscopy than laparotomy and the smaller abdominal incision means less narcotics because of less pain. Laparoscopic colostomy theoretically has the additional advantage of reduced adhesion formation. It is also safe as laparoscopic colostomy allows the surgeon to identify and mobilize the bowel segment more accurately and easily than trephine stoma formation. However, in some cases, such as in patients with dilated colon or small bowel, visualization may not be enough to allow the surgeon to accomplish sufficient intestinal mobilization safely, and conversion to an open procedure is necessary.

No studies have compared open and laparoscopic colostomy to confirm the theoretical advantages of the latter.

LAPAROSCOPIC IMPLANTATION OF DRUG-DELIVERY CATHETERS

Implantation of drug-delivery catheters is necessary in some patients with advanced malignant disease who require peritoneal infusion for regional chemotherapy.

Bacteriologically safe devices such as Tenckhoff catheters have been used for this purpose since 1968. In patients undergoing peritoneal dialysis, complications after implantation of Tenckhoff catheters has been reported in up to 70% of cases, and 39% of these ultimately require catheter removal. The most frequent complication is peritonitis and in the majority of the cases, this can be treated on an outpatient basis with intraperitoneal antibiotics.[43,44] The commonest mechanical problem is outflow obstruction, which may be associated with omental and peritoneal adhesions to the catheter, fibrin or blood-clot formation, extraperitoneal placement or catheter migration. Other complications are catheter-site infections, genital edema, abdominal wall hernias, dialysate leakage out of the abdomen, bleeding, cuff extrusion, respiratory compromise and back, abdominal, scrotal or rectal pain.[43,44-46] The majority of these complications are not due to surgical technique but associated with peritoneal dialysis. Complications of intraperitoneal chemotherapy do not include the full list of the complications of peritoneal dialysis. Bleeding is associated with difficult insertion of the catheter and is usually seen in patients with abdominal adhesions. This complication may be avoided by laparoscopic assistance.

The placement or repositioning of Tenckhoff catheters has been performed laparoscopically.[47] Laparoscopic placement or manipulation allows the surgeon to explore the abdomen, to see the exact cause of catheter malfunction, to accurately place the catheter without bleeding and to carry out the lysis of adhesions and subtotal resection of the omentum if the adhesions and the omentum are the causes of outflow obstruction. These advantages have encouraged the use of laparoscopic techniques, particularly in patients with previous extensive abdominal operations or multiple prior catheter insertions. The laparoscopic technique allows early resumption of peritoneal drug-delivery after surgery and rapid recovery of social and professional activities with less pain and fewer pulmonary complications.

Complications associated with the laparoscopic technique of placement of drug-delivery catheters are similar to those of other laparoscopic procedures. Prospective studies documenting the morbidity and mortality are necessary to ascertain the best approach for the placement of drug-delivery catheters.

LAPAROSCOPIC CRYOSURGERY

Cryosurgery is the *in situ* destruction of tissue by freezing with cooled liquid nitrogen. In surgical oncology, cryosurgery has been mainly applied to hepatic malignancies that are surgically unresectable by traditional criteria. Chemotherapy and radiation therapy have not increased the survival of patients with hepatic malignancies. Cryosurgery is a focal treatment and extends the benefit of surgical excision of liver tumors by saving larger amounts of normal liver surrounding the tumor. Tumors located near the inferior vena cava or major portal branches have been treated without injury to these structures. Therefore, cryosurgery has increased the chance of cure in patients with unresectable liver malignancies.

Cryotherapy and intraoperative ultrasonographic (IOUS) imaging of liver tumors allows the surgeon two modalities that are repeatable and may offer the patient with hepatic malignancies long-term survival. IOUS allows delineation of the extent and margins of hepatic malignancies. Additionally, IOUS enhances the detection of small intrahepatic masses and guides the biopsy of liver tumors. It is an essential part of the evaluation for resection of liver tumors. During cryosurgery, IOUS may be used to guide needles or probes precisely into the tumor and to measure the freezing process in real time, demonstrating how much of the tumor and how much of the normal tissue has been frozen. The development of laparoscopic ultrasonography has allowed the surgeon to carry out laparoscopic cryosurgery.

Complications of cryosurgery include thrombocytopenia and coagulopathies, superficial liver capsule tear, bleeding at the probe site, gas embolism and right-sided pleural effusion. The liver tears are probably related to thermal gradients. If there is troublesome bleeding resulting from the tears, suturing the hepatic parenchyma can stop it. Bleeding at the probe site is a common complication and can be avoided by selecting the safest path to the tumor using IOUS guidance. Nitrogen embolus is a rare complication seen in patients undergoing cryosurgery with an open probe system.[48] In the older system liquid nitrogen comes into direct contact with the liver parencyhema, while nitrogen flow in newer systems is through a closed probe tip. Pleural effusion is associated with posteriorly located large tumors.[49]

Two large series with fairly long term follow-up have been reported in the literature. Ravikumar et al.[50] reported their 5-year experience in 32 patients. The majority (75%) had metastatic colon cancer. The median hospital stay for the group was 6 days. There were two significant complications: a right subphrenic abscess, which was treated by CT-guided drainage and a wound dehiscence. There were no operative mortalities. After a median follow-up of 24 months with Carcino-embryonic antigen (CEA) levels and CT scans, 28% remained disease free, 34% were alive with disease and 38% had died.

The majority of failures were in patients with liver and extrahepatic disease and only 9% of failures occurred at the treatment site. Those patients who had residual tumor after treatment faired considerably worse than those with no residual tumor. In those with no residual tumor after treatment, there was a 78% survival rate and a 39% disease-free survival rate over a median follow-up of 24 months.

Zhou et al[51] reported 5-year follow-up results from 60 patients in whom cryosurgery alone was utilized (45% of cases) or combined with resection. No perioperative morbidity or mortality was reported and the overall 1- and 5-year survival rates were 51.7% and 11.4%, respectively. In the subset of patients who had cryosurgery alone, the 1- and 5-year survival rates were 33.3% and 4.3%. Those with smaller tumors faired better overall.

The only report of laparoscopic cryosurgery is from Cuschieri et al[49] in which cryosurgery was performed on 18 patients, and in 6 this was done laparoscopically. They used prototype laparoscopic cryoprobes. The operative complications were few and consisted of bleeding and parenchymal tears which were easily controlled. There was a slight survival benefit in 3 of the patients with follow-up of 18 months or longer. No randomized studies have compared laparoscopic with open cryosurgery.

Laparoscopic cryosurgery adds potential complications that are not seen with laparoscopy alone. Although there are currently no reports of carbon dioxide embolism, it is a potential complication of laparoscopic cryosurgery because of parenchymal tears communicating with hepatic veins. It also adds potential benefits such as shorter hospital stay and quicker return to preoperative activity. Our experience with cryosurgery of the liver includes a group of 9 patients, 5 of whom underwent laparoscopic and 4 open cryosurgery (Table 9.4). The median hospital stay in those who underwent laparoscopic cryosurgery was 4 days, while the median length of stay for the open group was 7.5 days. There was one patient in the laparoscopic group who required an extended postoperative stay for cardiac problems unrelated to the cryosurgery. The complications were all minor and all in the laparoscopic group. They included minor intraoperative bleeding requiring transfusion, a biloma requiring percutaneous drainage and frost bite of the skin at a probe insertion site requiring no further treatment.

Table 9.4 – Cryosurgery carried out in our patients with primary or metastatic carcinoma of the liver.

Patient number	Diagnosis	Technique	Indication	Additional procedure	Posoperative hospital stay (days)	Complications
1	Colon cancer	Laparoscopic	Multiple lesions in both lobes and cirrhosis	None	4	None
2	Colon cancer	Laparoscopic	High risk patient	None	13	Frost bite of skin at cryo probe site
3	Colon cancer	Open	Multiple lesions in both lobes	Right hepatic lobectomy, partial resection of diaphragm	7	None
4	Colon cancer	Open	Multiple bilateral lesions	Biopsy of right adrenal gland	8	None
5	Liver cancer (Hepatoma)	Laparoscopic	Lesion in left lobe, cirrhosis, ascites	None	5	Minor bleeding
6	Esophageal cancer	Laparoscopic	Single large lesion at the dome of the liver. For palliation	Laparoscopic cholecystectomy	2	Biloma
7	Lung cancer	Laparoscopic	One lesion in liver. For palliation	None	2	None
8	Ovarian cancer	Open	One lesion in liver. Debulking surgery	None	10	None
9	Leiomyosarcoma of the groin	Open	Several metastases to the liver. For palliation	None	7	None

CONCLUSION

The indications as well as the risks and benefits of various minimally invasive approaches to advanced malignancies causing obstruction of the upper gastrointestinal tract, biliary tree and small and large bowel have been discussed. Additionally, minimal access approaches to enteral feeding-tube placement, implantation of drug-delivery catheters and the use of cryosurgery for non-resectable liver lesions have been reviewed. It is too early to determine which of the newer laparoscopic approaches will replace open surgical and other established minimally invasive approaches in patients with advanced unresectable malignancies.

REFERENCES

1. Singh SM, Reber HA. Surgical palliation for pancreatic cancer. *Surg Clin North Am* 1989;**69**: 599-611.
2. Weaver DW, Wiencek RG, Bouwman DL, Walt AJ. Gastrojejunostomy: Is it helpful for patients with pancreatic cancer? *Surgery* 1987;**102**: 608-613.
3. Smith JW, Brennan MF. Surgical treatment of gastric cancer. *Surg Clin North Am* 1992;**72**: 381-399.
4. Rhodes M, Nathanson L, Fielding G. Laparoscopic biliary and gastric bypass: a useful adjunct in the treatment of carcinoma of the pancreas. *Gut* 1995;**36**: 778-780.
5. La Ferla G, Murray WR. Carcinoma of the head of the pancreas: bypass surgery in unresectable disease. *Br J Surg* 1987; **74**:212-213.

6. Solt J, Papp Z. Strecker stent implantation in malignant gastric outlet stenosis. *Gastrointest Endosc* 1993;**39**: 442-444.

7. Topazian M, Ring E, Grendell J. Palliation of obstructing gastric cancer with steel mesh, self-expanding endoprostheses. *Gastrointest Endosc* 1992;**38**: 58-60.

8. Eckhauser ML. The neodymium-YAG laser and gastrointestinal malignancy. *Arch Surg* 1990;**125**: 1152-1154.

9. Laukka MA, Wang KK. Endoscopic Nd:YAG laser palliation of malignant duodenal tumors. *Gastrointest Endosc* 1995;**41**: 225-229.

10. Lammer J. Biliary endoprostheses: plastic vs. metal stents. *Radiol Clin North Am* 1990;**28**: 1211-1222.

11. Stoker J, Laméris JS, Blankenstein M. Percutaneous metallic self-expandable endoprostheses in malignant hilar obstruction. *Gastrointest Endosc* 1993;**39**: 43-49.

12. Speer AG, Cotton PB, Russell RCG, et al. Randomised trial of endoscopic versus percutaneous stent insertion in malignant obstructive jaundice. *Lancet* 1987;**2**: 57-62.

13. Bilbao MK, Dotter CT, Lee TG, Katon RM. Complications of endoscopic retrograde cholangiopancreatography (ERCP). *Gastroenterology* 1976;**70**: 314-320.

14. Niederau C, Pohlmann U, Lübke H, Thomas L. Prophylactic antibiotic treatment in therapeutic or complicated diagnostic ERCP: Results of a randomized controlled clinical study. *Gastrointest Endosc* 1994;**40**: 533-537.

15. Lichtenstein DR, Carr-Locke DL. Endoscopic palliation for unresectable pancreatic carcinoma. *Surg Clin North Am* 1995;**75**: 969-988.

16. Lillemoe KD, Pitt HA, Kaufman SL, Cameron JL. Acute cholecystitis occurring as a complication of percutaneous transhepatic drainage. *Surg Gynecol Obstet* 1989;**168**: 348-352.

17. Johanson JF, Schmalz MJ, Geenen JE. Incidence and risk factors for biliary and pancreatic stent migration. *Gastrointest Endosc* 1992;**38**: 341-346.

18. Siegel JH, Snady H. The significance of endoscopically placed prostheses in the management of biliary obstruction due to carcinoma of the pancreas: results of nonoperative decompression in 277 patients. *Am J Gastroenterol* 1986; **81**: 634-641.

19. Kubota Y, Seki T, Yamaguchi T, et al. Bilateral drainage of biliary hilar malignancy via a single percutaneous track: role of percutaneous transhepatic cholangioscopy. *Endoscopy* 1992;**24**: 194-198.

20. Stambuk EC, Pitt HA, Pais OS, et al. Percutaneous transhepatic drainage: risks and benefits. *Arch Surg* 1983;**118**: 1388-1394.

21. Lois JF, Gomes AS, Grace PA, et al. Risks of percutaneous transhepatic drainage in patients with cholangitis. *AJR* 1987;**148**: 367-371.

22. Mueller PR, vanSonnenberg E, Ferrucci JT Jr. Percutaneous biliary drainage: Technical and catheter related problems in 200 procedures. *AJR* 1982;**138**: 17-23.

23. Cotton PB. Nonsurgical palliation of jaundice in pancreatic cancer. *Surg Clin North Am* 1989;**69**: 613-627.

24. Tarnasky PR, England RE, Lail LM. et al. Cystic duct patency in malignant obstructive jaundice. An ERCP-based study relevant to the role of laparoscopic cholecystojejunostomy. *Ann Surg* 1995;**221**: 265-271.

25. Sarfeh IJ, Rypins EB, Jakowatz JG et al. A prospective, randomized clinical investigation of cholecystoenterostomy and choledochoenterostomy. *Am J Surg* 1988;**155**: 411-414.

26. Soulez G, Gagner M, Therasse E, et al. Malignant biliary obstruction: preliminary results of palliative treatment with hepaticogastrostomy under fluoroscopic, endoscopic, and laparoscopic guidance. *Radiology* 1994;**192**: 241-246.

27. Andersen JR, Sorenson SM, Kruse A, et al. Randomized trial of endoscopic endoprothesis versus operative bypass in malignant obstructive jaundice. *Gut* 1989;**30**: 1132-1135.

28. Bornman PC, Harries-Jones EP, Tobias R, et al. Prospective controlled trial of trans hepatic biliary endoprothesis versus biliary surgery for incurable carcinoma of head of pancreas. *Lancet* 1986;**1**: 69-71.

29. Dowsett JF, Rusell RCG, Hatfield ARW, et al. Malignant obstructive jaundice: A prospective randomized trial of bypass surgery versus endoscopic stenting. *Gastroenterology* 1989;**96**: 128A.

30. Shepard HA, Royle G, Ross APR, et al. Endoscopic biliary endoprothesis in the palliation of malignant obstruction of the distal common bile duct. *Br J Surg* 1988;**75**: 1166-1168.

31. Lillemoe KD, Barnes SA. Surgical palliation of unresectable pancreatic carcinoma. *Surg Clin North Am* 1995;**75**: 953-968.

32. Morris JB, Mullen JL, Yu JC, Rosato EF. Laparoscopic-guided jejunostomy. *Surgery* 1992;**112**: 96-99.

33. Duh Q-Y, Way LW. Laparoscopic jejunostomy using T-fasteners as retractors and anchors. *Arch Surg* 1993;**128**: 105-108.

34. Eltringham WK, Roe AM, Galloway SW, et al. A laparoscopic technique for full thickness intestinal biopsy and feeding jejunostomy. *Gut* 1993;**34**: 122-124.

35. Gauderer MW, Stellato TA. Gastrostomies: evolution, techniques and complication. *Curr Probl Surg* 1986;**23**: 658-719.
36. Wasijev BK, Ujiki GT, Beal JM. Feeding gastrostomy: complications and mortality. *Am J Surg* 1982;**143**: 194-195.
37. Rogers DA, Bowden TA. Gastrostomy: Operative or nonoperative. *Surg Clin North Am* 1992;**72**: 515-524.
38. Wolfsen HC, Kozarek RA, Ball TJ. Tube dysfunction following percutaneous endoscopic gastrostomy and jejunostomy. *Gastrointest Endosc* 1990;**36**: 261-263.
39. Strodel WE, Kenady DE, Zweng TN. Avoiding stoma seeding in head and neck cancer patients. *Surg Endosc* 1995;**9**: 1142-1143.
40. Zera RT, Nava HR, Fischer JI. Percutaneous endoscopic gastrostomy (PEG) in cancer patients. *Surg Endosc* 1993;**7**: 304-307.
41. Ponsky JL. Percutaneous endoscopic stomas. *Surg Clin North Am* 1989;**69**: 1227-1236.
42. Hashizume M, Haraguchi Y, Ikeda Y, et al. Laparoscopy-assisted colostomy. *Surg Laparosc Endosc* 1994;**4**: 70-72.
43. Fleisher AG, Kimmelstiel FM, Lattes CG, Miller RE. Surgical complications of peritoneal dialysis catheters. *Am J Surg* 1985;**149**: 726-729.
44. Olcott C, Feldman CA, Coplon NS, et al. Continuous ambulatory peritoneal dialysis. Technique of catheter insertion and management of associated surgical complications. *Am J Surg* 1983;**146**: 98-102.
45. Kopecky RT, Funk MM, Kreitzer PR. Localized genital edema in patients undergoing continuous ambulatory peritoneal dialysis. *J Urol* 1985;**134**: 880-884.
46. Cronen PW, Moss JP, Simpson T, et al. Tenckhoff catheter placement: surgical aspects. *Am Surg* 1985;**51**: 627-629.
47. Kittur DS, Gazaway PM, Abidin MR. Laparoscopic repositioning of malfunctioning peritoneal dialysis catheters. *Surg Laparosc Endosc* 1991;**1**: 179-182.
48. Schlinkert RT, Chapman TP. Nitrogen embolus as a complication of hepatic cryosurgery. *Arch Surg* 1990;**125**: 1214.
49. Cuschieri A, Crosthwaite G, Shimi S, et al. Hepatic cryotherapy for liver tumors. Development and clinical evaluation of a high-efficiency insulated multineedle probe system for open and laparoscopic use. *Surg Endosc* 1995;**9**: 483-489.
50. Ravikumar TS, Kane R, Cady B, et al. A 5-year study of cryosurgery in the treatment of liver tumors. *Arch Surg* 1991;**126**: 1520-1524.
51. Zhou XD, Tang ZY, Yu YQ, et al. Clinical evaluation of cryosurgery in the treatment of primary liver cancer: report of 60 cases. *Cancer* 1988;**61**: 1889-1892.

10

Operative Laparoscopy in Gynecologic Oncology

Joel M. Childers and Earl A. Surwit

Modern operative laparoscopy entered the world of gynecologic oncology with the introduction of laparoscopic pelvic lymphadenectomy. This procedure, originated in France by Daniell Dargent, was initially performed on patients with early cervical cancer using a retroperitoneal approach.[1,2] Laparoscopic transperitoneal pelvic lymphadenectomies were reported shortly thereafter by Querleu et al.,[3] again for staging of patients with early cervical carcinoma.

It was the development of laparoscopic para-aortic lymphadenectomy that attracted widespread attention to the use of endoscopy in gynecologic oncology. The technique was developed simultaneously in France and the United States. Initial case reports included patients with non-Hodgkin's lymphoma, cervical cancer, endometrial cancer and ovarian cancer.[4-7] Reports of small series of patients undergoing laparoscopic para-aortic lymphadenectomy soon followed and suggested that the procedure was both adequate and safe.[8-12]

While operative laparoscopy in gynecologic oncology is still in its infancy, there appear to be several clinical situations in which it could be used routinely. This chapter reviews the history and current use of this surgical approach in patients with gynecologic malignancies.

CANCER OF THE CERVIX

Laparoscopic lymphadenectomy in candidates for radical hysterectomy

In 1987 Daniell Dargent described his experience combining laparoscopic retroperitoneal pelvic lymphadenectomy with radical hysterectomy in patients with early cervical cancer.[13] Subsequently, Denis Querleu pioneered a transperitoneal approach to the sampling of pelvic lymph nodes.[3] He demonstrated that, with this surgical technique, open radical hysterectomy could be avoided in patients with early cervical carcinoma if positive lymph nodes were found. Like his predecessor Dargent, Querleu detected no lymph nodes containing metastatic disease in those patients who underwent radical abdominal hysterectomy following laparoscopic lymphadenectomy.

The first American series in which laparoscopic lymphadenectomy was used in the management of cervical cancer was reported by Childers et al.[8] Unlike their European colleagues, these authors incorporated both pelvic and para-aortic lymphadenectomy in their patients with early and advanced cervical carcinoma (Fig 10.1). They confirmed the feasibility of both

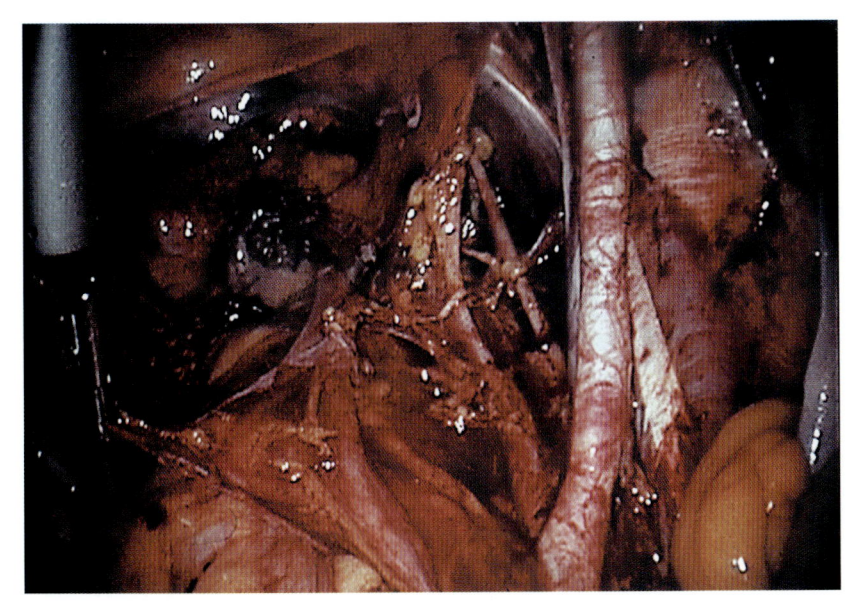

Figure 10.1 - View from the umbilical port after a laparoscopic pelvic lymphadenectomy. The right external iliac artery can be seen lying on the psoas muscle and its tendon. The bifurcation of the right common iliac is at the bottom of the picture, illustrating the origin of the internal iliac artery and its continuation as the superior vesicle artery and the obliterated umbilical artery. The obturator nerve can be seen between the external iliac artery and the obliterated umbilical artery in the obturator space.

pelvic and para-aortic lymphadenectomy and the advantage of precluding the need for laparotomy in patients with metastatic disease. These authors also discovered that obesity can be a limiting factor in the adequacy of laparoscopic lymphadenectomy. In their patients who underwent laparotomy following laparoscopic lymphadenectomy, 91% of the lymph nodes normally taken at the time of a radical hysterectomy had been removed, but this percentage varied according to the weight of the patient.

In addition to obesity, experience plays a role in the adequacy of laparoscopic lymphadenectomy. Fowler et al.[14] reported 12 patients with stage Ib cervical carcinoma who underwent laparoscopic transperitoneal lymphadenectomy followed immediately by laparotomy. The yield of lymph nodes obtained laparoscopically was 75%; 282 nodes were obtained at laparoscopy and 95 at laparotomy. A clear improvement in yield was evident as the operators gained experience in the technique. The percentage of lymph nodes removed through the laparoscope increased from 63% in the first 6 patients to 85% in the last 6. It must be noted, however, that after only 12 lymphadenectomies the surgeon is still in the early learning phase. As in all previous publications, these authors discovered no undetected nodal metastases when laparotomy was performed.

These early reports confirmed the feasibility of pelvic and para-aortic laparoscopic lymphadenectomy in patients with cancer of the cervix. Few complications were reported, the estimated blood loss was remarkably low (<100 ml), operative times were acceptable and hospital stays were short (1-2 days). Node counts and visual inspection of dissection sites were comparable to laparotomy, particularly in non-obese patients and as operator experience increased.

Radical hysterectomy

(Table 10.1)

As operative experience in the retroperitoneal space improved, several investigators were tantalized by the concept of avoiding laparotomy in patients who required radical hysterectomy. This has now been accomplished both laparoscopically and vaginally.[6,15-22] A complete laparoscopic radical hysterectomy was first described by Canis et al.[15] and Nezhat et al.[16] Their patients benefited from short hospitalizations; however, the operative times were long (4-8 hours).

Table 10.1 – Uses of operative laparoscopy in cervical cancer

I. Radical hyserectomy without laparotomy
- Laparoscopic assisted radical vaginal hysterectomy
- Laparoscopic radical hysterectomy
- Radical vaginal hysterectomy after laparoscopic lymphadenectomy

II. Avoid laparotomy in node patients
- Laparoscopic lymphadenectomy with frozen section

III. Define radiation fields in patients recieving radiotherapy
- Laparoscopic lymphadenectomy with frozen section

IV. Ovarian function preservation in patients recieving radiotherapy
- Oophoropexy

V. Assist in placement of transperitoneal interstitial implants in advanced disease.

VI. Determine eligibility for pelvic exenteration

The second alternative offered by laparoscopy is its use in radical vaginal hysterectomy (Schauta procedure). The primary advantage is utilization of a proven 'radical' hysterectomy technique and this has been successfully utilized by Dargent in Lyon. His experience in performing more than 200 Schauta operations makes him the ideal surgeon to combine laparoscopic lymphadenectomy with the Schauta procedure. Unfortunately, most physicians who practise gynecologic oncology have not been trained in this technique.

The third alternative to laparotomy is provided by the combination of both laparoscopic and vaginal approaches to hysterectomy. Laparoscopically assisted vaginal hysterectomy has been reported by several authors and has many variations. Querleu[17] described these variations and how the operation can be tailored to the specific needs of individual patients. We prefer a combined laparoscopic and vaginal approach. Our experience suggests that the vaginal margins are best obtained vaginally, and in most cases it is quicker, easier and safer to transect the uterosacral ligaments vaginally, as is closure of the vaginal cuff. Laparoscopically, the uterine vessels and cardinal ligaments are transected and the ureter is dissected down to the bladder. This anterior laparoscopic/posterior vaginal approach can usually be accomplished in 2-4 hours.

While many factors are important when comparing new cancer management options, none is as important as overall patient survival. Unfortunately, with operative laparoscopy in the oncologic setting still in its infancy, traditional 5-year survival rates are not available. However, Querleu and LeBlanc[23] reported an 83% 4-year survival rate for their first 106 patients with early cervical carcinoma managed with laparoscopic transperitoneal lymphadenectomy. This is similar to the survival rate of an historical group matched for age, stage and therapy. There were only 3 pelvic sidewall recurrences in the 84 node-negative patients. This 4% sidewall recurrence rate is similar to the 2-5% rate reported after laparotomy.[24,25]

Laparoscopy has changed our approach to patients with early cervical cancers who are candidates for radical hysterectomy. First, laparoscopic pelvic node dissection is performed using the transperitoneal approach. Patients with negative nodes are then managed with a laparoscopically assisted radical vaginal hysterectomy, as described above. When pelvic node metastases are discovered, the radical hysterectomy is abandoned and a para-aortic node dissection is performed to select patients who might benefit from extended-field radiation therapy.

Surgical staging and other procedures for advanced cervical cancer

A handful of publications have documented several other uses for operative laparoscopy in patients with advanced carcinoma. Laparoscopic removal of para-aortic lymph nodes to determine whether extended-field radiotherapy should be included in the treatment plan has been reported.[8,26] While this individual tailoring of radiotherapy fields makes sense, the potential morbidity of extended-field radiotherapy in patients who have undergone laparoscopic transperitoneal para-aortic lymphadenectomy is an obvious concern. Vasilev et al.[27] have pioneered the use of an extraperitoneal laparoscopic para-aortic lymph node dissection to avoid adhesion-related complications. While only 4 cases have been reported, this certainly represents an attractive option for patients with advanced cervical cancer. When compared to extraperitoneal para-aortic lymphadenectomy, studies have clearly shown a higher incidence of radiotherapy complications in patients undergoing transperitoneal para-aortic lymphadenectomy via laparotomy and subsequently receiving extended-field radiotherapy.[27] Whether transperitoneal laparoscopic para-aortic lymphadenectomy will confer the same risk is unknown.

Another novel use for operative laparoscopy in patients with advanced carcinoma is the creation of a colostomy. Boike and Lurain[28] reported good results in 3 such patients. Laparoscopy can also be utilized in patients with cervical cancer for the placement of transperitoneal interstitial implants.[26] Needle depth and localization can be visualized and altered as necessary, and the intraperitoneal cavity can be assessed for disease outside the radiation field. Lymph-node assessment would include a low bilateral para-aortic lymph node dissection. An omental carpet can be created for protection from bowel injuries. In an attempt to emulate the 'open' procedure pioneered by DiSaia et al.,[29] we have reported 1 case in whom all these procedures were performed laparoscopically.[26]

CANCER OF THE ENDOMETRIUM

Surgical staging of endometrial cancer includes intraperitoneal exploration, cytologic washings and pelvic and para-aortic lymph-node sampling. The hysterectomy specimen is evaluated pathologically for depth of invastion and spread to the adnexa or cervix for staging. Most oncologists base recommendations for adjuvant chemotherapy or radiotherapy on the information gleaned from surgical staging.[30] This information becomes extremely important for individualizing treatment of this disease. All of this staging information can be obtained without laparotomy - by the use of laparoscopic and vaginal surgery, making laparoscopy an attractive alternative not only for the patient whose uterus has not yet been removed, but also for those patients who have been referred to the oncologist for recommendations after hysterectomy but who have not undergone surgical staging. While scientific publications on the role of laparoscopy in endometrial carcinoma are few, its use in patients both with and without uteri has been described. Table 10.2 outlines the uses of laparoscopy in patients with early endometrial cancer.

Childers et al.[9] reported 59 patients with clinical stage I endometrial carcinoma who underwent

Table 10.2 – Uses of operative laparoscopy in endometrial cancer

I. Avoidance of laparotomy for hysterectomy
- Laparoscopically assisted vaginal hysterectomy
- Laparoscopic hysterectomy

II. Avoidance of laparotomy for staging
- Patients with uterus in place
- Unstaged patients already having hysterectomy
  - Remove ovaries
  - Sample lymph nodes
  - Inspect upper abdomen
  - Obtain washing for cytology

laparoscopically assisted surgical staging (LASS) and laparoscopically assisted vaginal hysterectomy (LAVH). Fig. 10.2 outlines the schema used in this study. Frozen sections were used to determine the risk of lymph-node metastasis. Low-risk patients (grade 1, less than one-half myometrial invasion) did not undergo laparoscopic lymphadenectomy.

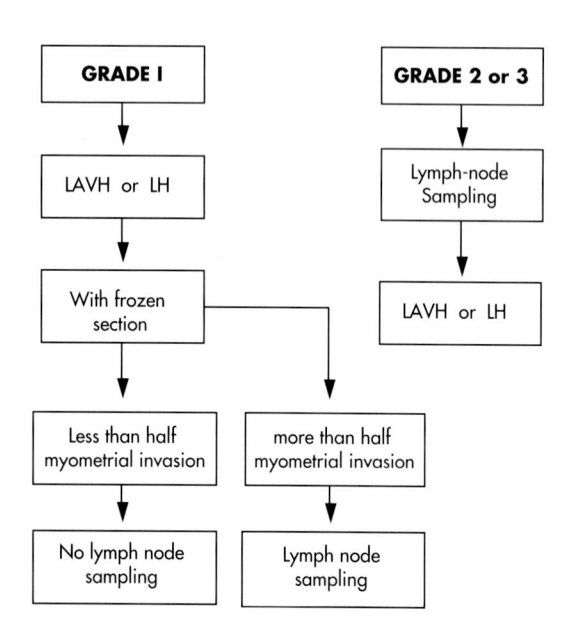

Figure 10.2 - Laparoscopically assisted surgical staging (LASS) schema for clinical stage I endometrial carcinoma. LAVH = laparoscopically assisted vaginal hysterectomy; LH = laparoscopic hysterectomy.

Intermediate- and high-risk patients (grade 1 with outer-half myometrial invasion and grade 2 and 3 carcinomas) underwent pelvic and para-aortic lymph node sampling.

This series clearly demonstrates that metastatic disease can be discovered at the same rate one would expect if laparotomy were used. When all grades were considered, metastatic disease was discovered in 14% of patients, and in 36% (9 of 25) of grade 2 and 3 patients. Metastatic disease was discovered on the peritoneum of the pelvis and upper abdomen, on the ovary, omentum, right diaphragm and in the pelvic and para-aortic nodes.

The procedure is safe, with only 5% (5 of 29) of the initial patients requiring laparotomy. The estimated blood loss in all cases was <200 ml, and the average hospital stay was 2.9 days, including those patients with complications. Obesity, again, was the most signficant limitation in this setting and the authors were unable to perform laparoscopic lymphadenectomy in 6% (2 of 32) of the patients who should have had sampling according to this schema.

Investigators from Northwestern University[31] presented the results of a nonrandomized retrospective review comparing laparotomy and laparoscopy in managing stage I endometrial carcinoma. Thirty-seven patients were managed using both methods. Four laparoscopic procedures could not be completed endoscopically. The number of lymph nodes removed from the pelvis and para-aortic areas was identical in both groups. While laparoscopic management required 23 additional minutes to complete compared to laparotomy, these women were discharged from hospital 2.6 days sooner (2.4 days versus 5.0, statistically significant). Obesity precluded para-aortic lymphadenectomy in some of the 10 patients who underwent pelvic lymph-adenectomy only, and 2 obese patients required laparotomy.

There were 3 significant complications in the laparoscopy group: 2 patients required reoperation for small-bowel herniation through 12-mm lateral port sites (diagnosed on days 5 and 10 postoperatively) and 1 developed a high left ureteral leak from delayed thermal injury (3 weeks postoperatively).

To evaluate the learning-curve experience of laparoscopic staging of endometrial cancer, we looked retrospectively at our first 125 patients with clinical stage I endometrial carcinoma.[32] Their ages ranged from 29-89 years, with a mean of 68.6, and their weights from 44 to 149 kg. On final pathology 66 patients had grade 1 lesions, 34 grade 2 and 25 grade 3. No extrauterine disease was discovered in any of the patients with well-differentiated lesions. However, metastatic disease was discovered in 18% of patients with grade 2 lesions and in 44% of patients with poorly differentiated lesions. This rate of detection of metastasis is equal to or better than that described in existing reports on surgical staging using laparotomy. Futhermore, there was no difference in the rate of detection of metastatic disease throughout the study, indicating that the ability to detect extrauterine disease laparoscopically does not relate to operator experience.

In contrast, operative times for patients staged without lymphadenectomy decreased significantly throughout the experience, from a mean of 163 min to 99 min (p<0.0001) (Fig. 10.3). Operative times for staging of patients with lymphadenectomy also decreased significantly, from a mean of 196 min to 128 min (p<0.0002) (Fig. 10.4). The most significant improvement with experience was hospital stay which decreased from a mean of 3.2 days in the first 25 patients to 1.8 days in the last 25 (p<0.0001) (Fig. 10.5).

The overall major complication rate did appear to relate to experience. The rate of 4% appears somewhat high but includes 2 enterotomies, which occurred during adhesiolysis and were both recognized and repaired at the time of surgery, as well as two small cystectomies, again both of which were recognized and repaired at the time of the primary surgical procedure. The 1 truly major complication was a transected left ureter that occurred in the first 25 procedures, when an endoscopic stapling device was used to transect the left uterine artery. This was an error in technique resulting from our inexperience with laparoscopic hysterectomies at that time. In

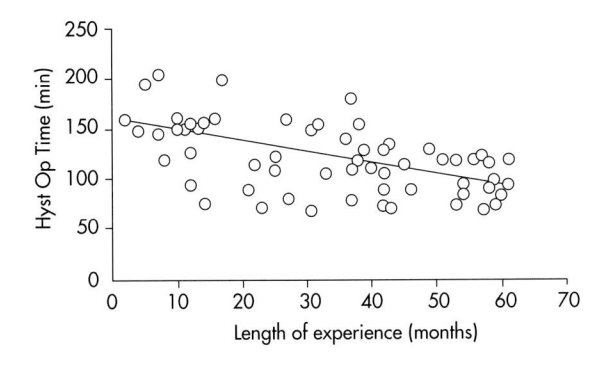

Figure 10.3 - Linear regression curve demonstrating the statistically significant drop in hysterectomy time when compared to length of operator experience (p<0.0001).

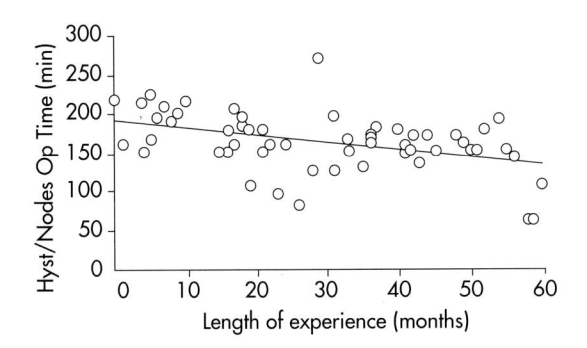

Figure 10.4 - Linear regression curve demonstrating the statistically significant drop in operative time for hysterectomy and lymphadenectomy for surgical staging of endometrial cancer (p<0.0002).

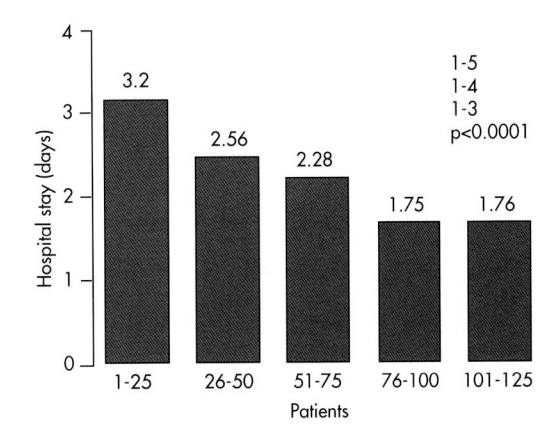

Figure 10.5 - Decrease in hospital stay for patients undergoing laparoscopic surgical staging for endometrial carcinoma. The patients have been ordered chronologically and grouped in blocks of 25.

contrast to the complication rate, the rate of conversion to laparotomy dropped significantly as our laparoscopic skills improved, from 8% (2 of 25) in the first 25 patients to 0 (0 of 100) in the later patients. There were no complications related to the lymphadenectomy.

Laparoscopic staging of patients with endometrial cancer can also be utilized for patients who are referred to oncologic surgeons after hysterectomy and incomplete surgical staging. Laparoscopic staging includes inspection of the intraperitoneal cavity, procurement of pelvic washings, removal of remaining ovaries and pelvic and/or para-aortic lymphadenetomy.

Our initial experience (and currently the only published report) with these unstaged patients included 13 women, whose ages ranged from 36 to 74 years (mean 64) and weights from 60 to 91 kg (mean 67 kg).[33] The intervals between hysterectomy and laparoscopic staging ranged from 14 to 63 days (mean 47 days). Extrauterine disease was discovered in 23% (3 of 13). One patient had positive washings and 2 had microscopically involved pelvic lymph nodes. There were no intraoperative complications. Estimated blood loss averaged <50 ml and the mean hospital stay was 1.5 days. Nine of 11 intermediate-risk patients were spared external radiation.

Our overall experience confirms that LASS is a safe, feasible and adequate procedure that offers remarkably short hospital stay and recovery times for patients with endometrial cancer. There are, however, several disadvantages to incorporating LASS into oncologic practice. First, in performing these sophisticated, advanced surgical procedures, an experienced assistant is necessary. The assistant should have experience in operative laparoscopic techniques as well as sound knowledge of the retroperitoneal space. Even with an experienced assistant, a new surgical learning curve is begun, which lengthens operative time. Futhermore, because of the difficulty in accomplishing para-aortic lymphadenectomies by this method, the surgeon must individualize and perform lymphadenectomy only on intermediate- to high-risk patients. This requires reliance on frozen section, which does not afford 100% accuracy. However, this individualization of surgical management works well for the patient with endometrial carcinoma because of the well-known association between increased patient weight and well-differentiated carcinoma.[34-36] Because most obese patients will have well-differentiated lesions, many will not require lymphadenectomy.

Table 10.3 – Uses of operative laparoscopy in endometrial cancer

I. **Second-look laparoscopy**
II. **Staging early ovarian cancer**
• At time of removal of malignant mass
• Unstaged patient after mass is removed

However, if one's surgical philosophy is to perform pelvic and para-arotic lymphadenectomy on all patients with endometrial carcinoma, regardless of their risk for metastatic disease, obesity will be a significant limiting factor.

CANCER OF THE OVARY

Ovarian cancer is also a surgically staged malignancy. Staging includes a systematic inspection of the intraperitoneal cavity, including infracolic omentectomy, sampling of the pelvic and para-aortic lymph nodes, multiple biopsies of the pelvic, abdominal, visceral and parietal peritoneum and peritoneal cytology specimens. Random diaphragmatic biopsies or scrapings for cytology are also recommended. Table 11.3 outlines the uses of operative laparoscopy in ovarian cancer if these surgical dictums are followed.

We began to assess our ability to evaluate both the intraperitoneal cavity and the retroperitoneal lymph nodes to detect metastatic ovarian carcinoma in candidates who where eligible for second-look ovarian cancer operations.[36] Our initial experience consisted of 40 women with advanced (stage II-IV) disease who had completed surgical debulking that was 'optimal' in 39 of the patients, and had received platinum-based chemotherapy. Examinations and serum CA-125s were negative in all patients. A total of 44 laparoscopic procedures were performed (4 patients had positive second-look laparoscopic procedures followed by third-look laparoscopies after treatment with intraperitoneal monoclonal-tagged yttrium). The mean age of these patients was 61 years and their weights ranged from 48 to 84 kg, with a mean of 61 kg. Twenty-four of the 44 second-look laparoscopic procedures (56%) were positive for persistent disease. Microscopic disease only was discovered in 5 (21%), located in the omentum, para-aortic nodes (2 patients), pelvic peritoneum and peritoneal washings (Figs 10.6 and 10.7).

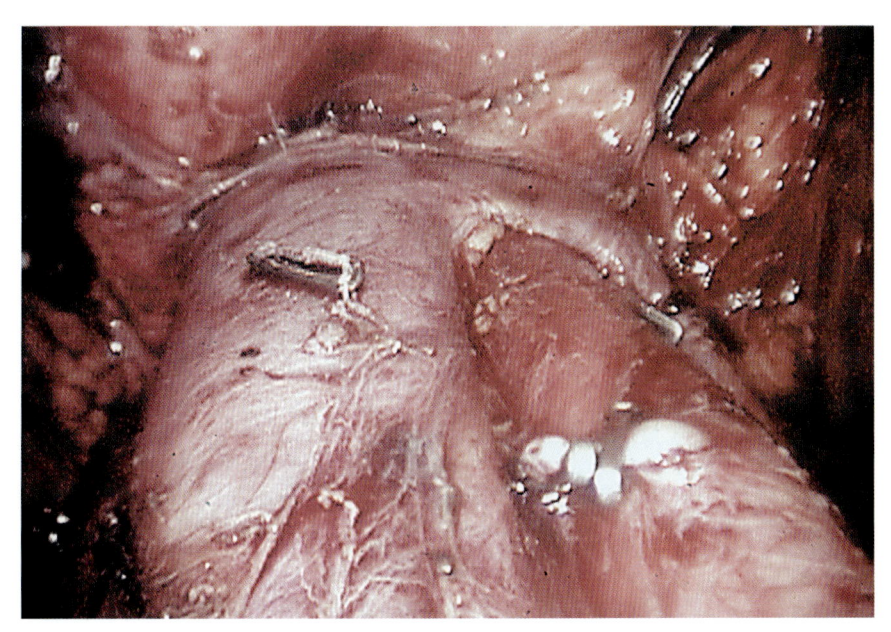

Figure 10.6 - View from the umbilical port looking in the cephalad direction after high para-aortic lymph node sampling. The vena cava is on the left and the aorta on the right. Note the left renal vein crossing the aorta to empty into the vena cava. Clips have been placed on the surface of the vena cava and the aorta.

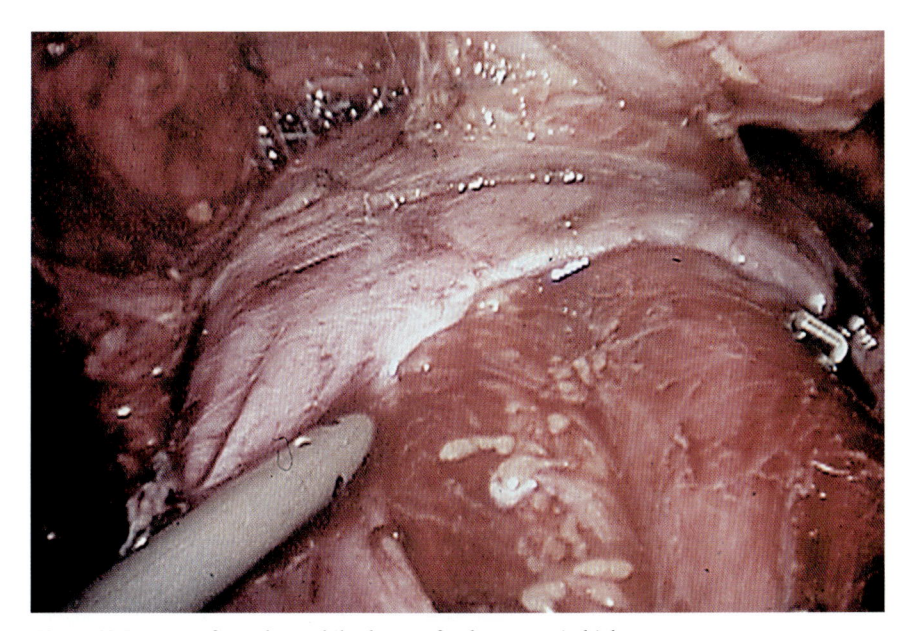

Figure 10.7 - View from the umbilical port after laparoscopic high para-aortic lymph node sampling. The irrigation instrument separates the vena cava on the left from the aorta on the right to demonstrate that most of the lymph nodes between these two structures can be well sampled. The left renal vein is seen crossing the aorta to empty into the vena cava in the background.

Twenty of the 44 patients (44%) had negative restaging procedures. However, 5 of these were deemed inadequate at the time of surgery because of extensive intraperitoneal adhesions that prevented successful evaluation of the intraperitoneal and/or retroperitoneal space. Disease recurred in all 5 of these patients, compared to a 20% recurrence rate in the remaining 15 patients.

The significant complication rate was comparable to that of open second-look procedures. Significant complications occurred in 6 (14%) of the 44 procedures and in 3 of these the patients required laparotomy, 1 for repair of a hole in the vena cava, 1 to repair a trocar injury to the transverse colon, and 1 to repair a small-bowel enterotomy.

The hospital stay, however, was dramatically reduced compared to open second-look operations. Excluding the 6 patients with significant complications, hospital stay for the remaining 39 patients ranged from 0 to 3 days with a mean of 1.1 days.

Casey et al.[38] compared 57 second-look laparoscopies and 69 second-look laparotomies for ovarian cancer and there were no significant differences between the two groups with respect to patient age, tumor histology, degree of primary cytoreduction and tumor stage or grade. The ability to detect disease was similar in the two groups, 52.6% and 53.6% respectively, despite 50% fewer biopsies being obtained during the laparoscopic procedures.

Significant differences between laparoscopy and laparotomy were found when the following variables were evaluated: estimated blood loss, operative time (81 min vs 130 min), hospital stay (0.3 days vs 6.8 days) and cost (50% lower).

Armed with the knowledge that modern operative laparoscopy is as useful as laparotomy in detecting both gross and microscopic disease in the second-look setting, we began to offer laparoscopic surgical staging to patients with presumed stage I ovarian carcinoma. Our experience with second-look procedures confirmed that the areas most likely to have early metastatic disease from ovarian carcinoma (washings, pelvic peritoneum, paracolic gutters, omentum, hemidiaphragm, and pelvic and para-arotic lymph nodes) can be more than adequately evaluated by laparoscopic inspection.

Our initial experience consisted of 14 women with presumed ovarian carcinoma whose ages ranged from 17 to 75 years (mean 64.5 years) and weight from 50 to 91 kg (mean 73 kg).[38] Five were referred unstaged after their malignant masses had been removed. These patients underwent laparoscopic staging as their second procedure. The remaining 9 had malignant ovarian tumors discovered during the laparoscopic management of their adnexal masses and underwent laparoscopic staging at the time of their primary procedures (Fig. 10.8). Twelve of the 14 patients had epithelial ovarian tumors (5 well-differentiated, 3 grade 2 and 4 grade 3 tumors). The remaining 2

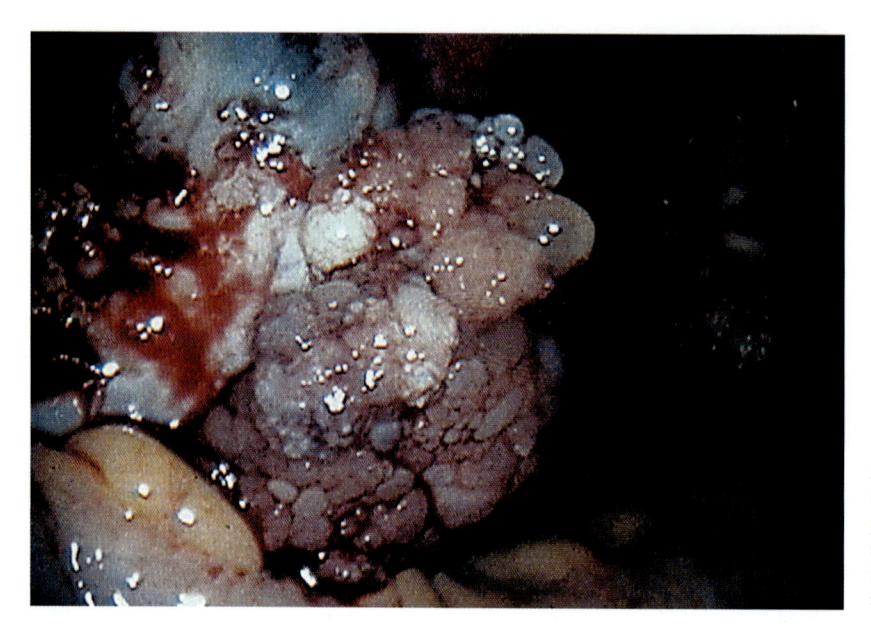

Figure 10.8 - Laparoscopic view of a left ovarian carcinoma. This patient underwent laparoscopic surgery for a suspicious adnexal mass and subsequently underwent surgical staging.

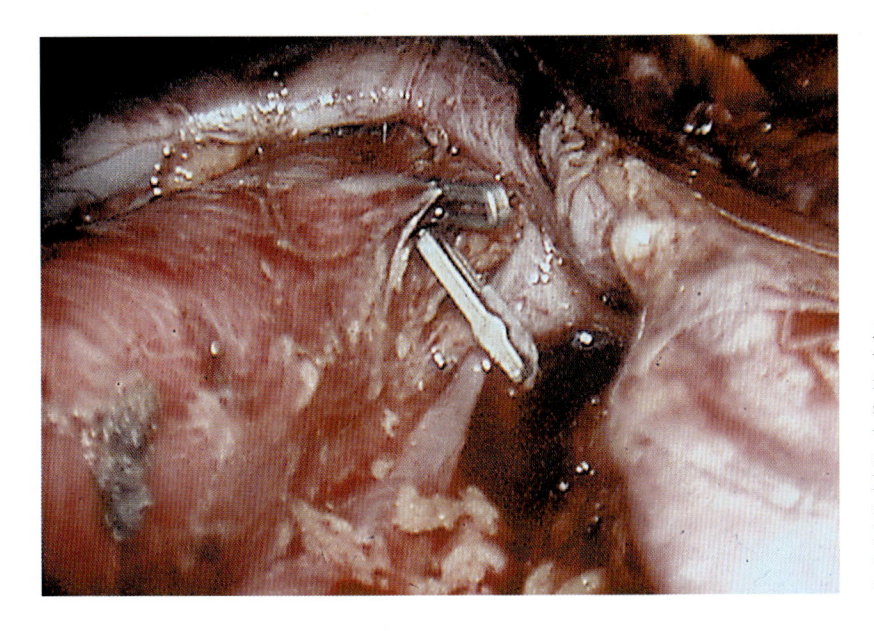

Figure 10.9 - View of the lumbar vein from the umbilical port looking in a cephalad direction. The aorta is seen on the left and the left ovarian vein on the right, heading in a cephalad direction to empty into the left renal vein, which crosses the aorta at the top of the picture. A clip has been applied to a lumbar vein coming from beneath the aorta to empty into the left ovarian vein.

patients had a Sertoli-Leydig cell tumor and a dysgerminoma respectively.

Metastatic disease was discovered in 8 (57%) of the 14 patients. Two were upstaged to stage IC based on washings that contained adenocarcinoma; 3 were upstaged to stage II for positive pelvic biopsies; 3 were upstaged to stage IIIC, based on metastatic disease to para-aortic lymph nodes. Two patients also had microscopic omental metastases. Hospital stay ranged from 0 to 3 days, with a mean of 1.6 days.

Use of laparoscopy in ovarian cancer patients was successful in detecting microscopic disease in high-risk areas: washings, pelvic peritoneum, omentum and pelvic and para-arotic lymph nodes, at a rate similar to that reported in the current literature. Laparoscopy offers an excellent opportunity to inspect peritoneal surfaces and especially the diaphragm. Visualization is enhanced because of the magnification offered by endoscopic techniques.

The main advantage of laparoscopic staging relates to the avoidance of a large abdominal incision, i.e. hospitalization and recovery times are significantly shorter. We believe better inspection of the pelvic peritoneum and of a majority of the diaphragm can be obtained because of the superbly illuminated and magnified view that laparoscopy offers. However, the entire diaphragmatic surface cannot be fully visualized or palpated. Futher disadvantages include the difficulties inherent in acquiring the laparoscopic skills to accomplish this difficult surgical procedure, particularly the left infrarenal lymphadenectomy. Exposure can be difficult to obtain and lumbar veins can be difficult to visualize, dissect around and control if injured (Fig. 10.9). Surgical assistants need to be skilled in endoscopic procedures and familiar with retroperitoneal anatomy.

CONCLUSION

Operative laparoscopy is being used by many gynecologic oncologists in the management of patients with cervical, endometrial and ovarian carcinoma. Patients with cervical cancer who are candidates for radical hysterectomy can undergo laparoscopic lymphadenectomy and avoid laparotomy if nodes are positive. Furthermore, with appropriate skills the surgeon can preclude laparotomy in node-negative patients by performing laparoscopic radical hysterectomy, laparoscopically assisted radical vaginal hysterectomy or radical vaginal hysterectomy.

Patients with clinical stage I endometrial carcinoma are being managed by LASS. Obesity is not a significant limitation for these patients if lymphadenectomy is not performed on patients with well-differentiated lesions with less than one-half myometrial invasion. Patients referred after hysterectomy who are at intermediate or high risk for metastasis can be offered laparoscopic staging with minimal morbidity, allowing adjuvant therapy recommendations to be based on full staging information.

Table 10.4 – Disadvantages of operative laparoscopy in gynecologic oncology

- Longer operative times initially
- Lack of direct tactile palpation
- Inability to visualise behind liver
- Requires skilled assistant for certain procedures
- Lack of long-term survival data
- Lack of data regarding cost effectiveness
- Dependability of laparoscopic equipment

Patients with presumed stage I carcinoma of the ovary who are unstaged at the time of their original surgery can undergo laparoscopic surgical staging rather than empiric chemotherapy. The laparoscopic management of patients with suspicious adnexal masses will also identify some patients with presumed stage I ovarian cancer who can be staged at the same time that the mass is being managed laparoscopically.

The advantages and disadvantages of laparoscopy in gynecologic oncology have yet to be fully delineated. Most importantly, it appears that metastatic disease can be detected in cervical, endometrial and ovarian malignancies at a rate similar to that when laparotomy is employed. Futhermore, its use appears safe, and indeed the morbidity may be lower than when laparotomy is utilized. Hospital stay and recovery time are clearly shorter than following laparotomy, and evaluation of certain intraperitoneal areas may be better as well. When all things are considered, potentially the socioeconomic costs of laparoscopy may also be an important advantage of this surgical technique.

The disadvantages are numerous as well (Table 10.4). First, the oncologic surgeon has new surgical skills to learn. The aquisition of these skills requires a serious time commitment, and most assuredly during the learning process operative times will be much longer than those of laparotomy. The oncologic surgeon who can perform sophisticated cancer operations with a relatively untrained assistant will discover that the advanced operative laparoscopist requires the assistance of a skilled surgeon, a luxury that many gynecologic oncologists are not afforded. In addition, there are some areas, such as the hemidiaphragm deep behind the liver, that cannot be fully visualized laparoscopically.

Perhaps of most importance is the lack of long-term follow-up of patients whose malignancies have been managed laparoscopically. Future studies will need to address overall survival, radiotherapy complications, costs and the applicability of these advanced techniques on a broader scale. Certainly, operative laparoscopy is not a passing fad but its exact role is yet to be defined.

REFERENCES

1. Wurtz, Mazman E, Gosselin B *et al*. Vilan anatomique des adenopathies retroperitoneales par endoscopie chirurgicale. *Ann Chirug* 1987;**41**:258-263.

2. Dargent D, Salvat J. *Envahissenent Ganglionnaire Pelvien: Place de la Pelviscopie Retroperitoneale*. Paris: Medsi, 1989.

3. Querleu D, LeBlanc, Castelain B. Laparoscopic lymphadenectomy in the staging of early carcinoma of the cervix. *Am J Obstet Gynecol* 1991;**164**:579-581.

4. Childers JM, Surwit EA. Combined laparoscopic and vaginal surgery for the management of two cases of stage I endometrial carcinoma. *Gynecol Oncol* 1992;**45**: 46-51.

5. Childers JM, Surwit EA. Laparoscopic para-aortic lymph node biopsy for diagnosis of a non-Hodgkin's lymphoma. *Surg Laparosc Endosc* 1992;**2**:139-142.

6. Nezhat C, Burrell M, Nezhat F. Laparoscopic radical hysterectomy with para-aortic and pelvic node dissection. *Am J Obstet Gynecol* 1992;**166**:864-865.

7. Querleu D. Laparoscopic para-arotic lymph node sampling in gynaecologic oncology: A preliminary experience. *Gynecol Oncol* 1993;**49**:24-29.

8. Childers JM, Surwit EA, Hatch KD. The role of laparoscopy in the management of cervical carcinoma. *Gynecol Oncol* 1992;**47**:38-43.

9. Childers JM, Brzechffa PR, Hatch KD, Surwit EA. Laparoscopically assisted surgical staging (LASS) of endometrial cancer. *Gynecol Oncol* 1993;**51**:33-38.

10. Childers JM, Hatch KD, Tran AN, Surwit EA. Laparoscopic para-arotic lymphadenectomy in gynecologic malignancies. *Gynecol Oncol* 1993;**82**: 741-747.

11. Nezhat CR, Nezhat FR, Burrell MO *et al*. Laparoscopic radical hysterectomy and laparoscopic-assisted vaginal radical hysterectomy with pelvic and para-aortic lymph node dissection. *J Gynecol Surg* 1993;**9**:105-120.

12. Querleu D, LeBlanc E. Laparoscopic infrarenal para-aortic node dissection for restaging of carcinoma of the ovary or fallopian tube. *Cancer* 1994;**73**: 1467-1471.

13. Dargent D. A new future for Schauta's operation through a pre-surgical retroperitoneal pelviscopy. *Eur J Gynaecol Oncol* 1987;**8**:292-296.
14. Fowler J, Carter J, Carlson J *et al*. Lymph node yield from laparoscopic lymphadenectomy in cervical cancer: A comparative study. *Gynecol Oncol* 1993;**51**: 187-192.
15. Canis M, Mage G, Wattiez A *et al*. Vaginally assisted laparoscopic radical hysterectomy. *J Gynecol Surg* 1992;**8**:103-105.
16. Nezhat C, Nezhat FR, Burrell MO. Laparoscopic radical hysterectomy and laparoscopic-assisted vaginal radical hysterectomy with pelvic and para-aortic lymph node dissection. *J Gynecol Surg* 1993;**9**:105-120.
17. Querleu D. Laparoscopically assisted radical vaginal hysterectomy. *Gynecol Oncol* 1992;**51**:248-254.
18. Dargent D. Laparoscopic surgery in gynecologic cancer. *Curr Opin Obstet Gynecol* 1993;**2**:135-142.
19. Kadar N, Riech H. Laparoscopic-assisted radical Schauta hysterectomy and bilateral pelvic lymphadenectomy for the treatment of bulky stage Ib carcinoma of the cervix. *Gynaecol Endosc* 1993;**2**: 135-142.
20. Jobling T, Wood C. Laparoscopic modified radical hysterectomy and lymphadenectomy simulating open operation for stage 1a2 cervical carcinoma. *Aust NZ J Obstet Gynaecol* 1993;**33**:400-403.
21. Kadar N. Laparoscopic vaginal radical hysterectomy: An operative technique and its evolution. *Gynaecol Endosc* 1994;**3**:109-122.
22. Dargent D, Matevet P. Hysterectomie elargie laparoscopico-vaginale. *J Gynecol Obstet Biol Reprod* 1993;**21**:709-710.
23. Querleu D, LeBlanc E. Neoplasia. In: Gomel V, Taylor P (eds) *Diagnostic and Operative Gynecologic Laparoscopy*. St Louis: Mosby, 1995, pp.143.
24. Ng H, Kan Y, Chao K, Yuan C, Shyu S. The outcome of the patients with recurrent cervical carcinoma in terms of lymph node metastases and treatment. *Gynecol Oncol* 1987;**26**:355-363.
25. Webb M, Symmonds R. Site of recurrence of cervical cancer after radical hysterectomy. *Am J Obstet Gynecol* 1980;**138**:813-817.
26. Childers JM, Brainard P, Rogoff EE, Surwit EA. Laparoscopically assisted transperineal interstitial irradiation and surgical staging for advanced cervical carcinoma: A case report. *Endocurietherapy/Hyperthermia Oncol* 1994;**10**:83-86.
27. Vasilev SA, McGonigle KF. Extraperitoneal laparoscopic para-aortic lymph node dissection. *Gynecol Oncol* 1996;**61**:315-320.
28. Boike GM, Lurain JR. Laparoscopic descending colostomy in three patients with cervical cancer. *Gynecol Oncol* 1994;**54**:381-384.
29. DiSaia PJ, Syed N, Puthawala A. Malignant neoplasm of the upper vagina. *Endocurietherapy/Hyperthermia Oncol* 1990;**6**:251-256.
30. Gretz HF, Economos K, Husain A *et al*. The practice of surgical staging and its impact on adjuvant treatment recommendations in patients with stage I endometrial carcinoma. *Gynecol Oncol* 1996;**61**:409-415.
31. Boike GM, Lurain JR, Burke JJ. A comparison of laparoscopic management of endometrial cancer with traditional laparotomy. *Gynecol Oncol* 1994;**52**: 105(Abstract).
32. Melendez T, Childers J, Harrigill K, Surwitt EA. Laparoscopic staging of endometrial cancer: The learning experience. 1997 (in press).
33. Childers JM, Spirtos NM, Brainard P, Surwit EA. Laparoscopic staging of the patient with incompletely staged early adenocarcionma of the endometrium. *Obstet Gynecol* 1994;**83**:597-600.
34. Cauppila A, Gronroos M, Nieminen U. Clinical outcome in endometrial cancer. *Obstet Gynecol* 1982;**60**: 473-480.
35. Bokhman JV. Two pathogenic types of endometrial carcinoma. *Gynecol Oncol* 1983;**15**:10-17.
36. Larson DM, Johnson K, Olson KA. Pelvic and para-aortic lymphadenectomy for surgical staging of endometrial cancer: Morbidity and mortality. *Obstet Gynecol* 1992;**79**:998-1001.
37. Childers JM, Lang J, Surwit EA, Hatch KD. Laparoscopic surgical staging of ovarian cancer. *Gynecol Oncol* 1995;**59**:25-33.
38. Casey AC, Farias-Eisner R, Pisani AL *et al*. What is the role of reassessment laparoscopy in the management of gynecologic cancers in 1995? *Gynecol Oncol* 1996;**60**: 454-461.

11

Application of Minimal Access Surgery in the Management of Diverse Malignancies

H. Stephan Stoldt, Riccardo A. Audisio, Amy L. Halverson and Jonathan M. Sackier

*M*ost organs and tumor types are the subject of ongoing studies examining the feasibility and relevance of a minimalist approach to surgery. Issues such as ease of access and size of tumor, amongst others, have dictated the pace of advance in the use of minimally invasive surgery. This book devotes chapters to several of these tumor types where the evidence is sufficient to debate the issues involved. In several other organs such as the pancreas, liver and kidney, the literature consists predominantly of case reports or small series. This chapter outlines the role of minimally invasive surgery for tumors of the spleen and adrenal gland as representatives of this mixed group of tumors. The theme of the section on the spleen is disease-oriented whilst that on the adrenal gland is more technique-oriented.

MINIMAL ACCESS SURGERY OF MALIGNANCIES INVOLVING THE SPLEEN

The diagnostic and therapeutic roles of splenectomy in the management of neoplastic involvement of the spleen remain undefined. Unlike other hematologic disorders, such as idiopathic thrombocytopenic pupura (ITP), in which benefits from splenectomy are quite evident, the usefulness of splenectomy in the management of hematologic malignancies appears limited. Over the past two decades, improvement in non-invasive diagnostic techniques, the development of new, non-operative biopsy procedures and increased utilization of systemic therapy for earlier-stage disease, has led to a reduced role for splenectomy in the management of various hematologic disorders. Despite the limited indications for splenectomy, the minimally invasive approach to splenectomy has rapidly expanded in recent years. With the accumulation of experience in minimal access surgery, consideration must be given to the advantages and limitations of the laparoscopic approach to the spleen.

Historical perspective

From the 16th through the 18th century, splenectomy was reported mainly for trauma, although the first therapeutic splenectomy for an enlarged spleen was performed by Leonard Fiorvanti in 1549.[1] Splenectomy for hereditary spherocytosis was first carried out in 1887 and Bryand & Billroth are credited with performing the first splenectomy for treatment of leukemia and lymphoma.[2]

In the 1960s and 70s, splenectomy was routinely used for staging and treatment of various neoplastic diseases. The introduction of computed axial tomography (CAT) and lymphangiography, as well as the addition of percutaneous biopsy of the liver and spleen, greatly reduced the need for splenectomy as a staging modality. In addition, the earlier and wider use of adjuvant chemotherapy in malignancies involving the spleen has decreased the need for extensive staging procedures. Current indications for splenectomy in the treatment of neoplastic diseases, including Hodgkin's disease, non-Hodgkin's lymphoma, leukemias and myeloid metaplasia, place greater importance on symptom palliation than diagnosis or therapy.

INDICATIONS FOR SPLENECTOMY

Hodgkin's disease

Staging is important to determine the extent of therapy necessary for the treatment of Hodgkin's disease (Table 11.1). Early stages of Hodgkin's disease, i.e. I, II and possibly IIIA, may best be treated by localized or extended area radiation. More advanced stages, i.e. IIIB and IV, respond best either to combination treatment with radiation and chemotherapy or chemotherapy alone.[3] Splenectomy, in addition to paraaortic lymph node and liver biopsies, forms part of the staging process during exploratory laparotomy for Hodgkin's disease. Percutaneous biopsy techniques, however, may replace formal laparotomy staging in many patients. Cavanna *et al*[4] reported a series of patients in which ultrasound-guided percutaneous tissue core biopsy of the spleen was used as a diagnostic and staging procedure. An adequate specimen was obtained in 45 of 46 patients. Splenic disease was found in 12 and normal tissue in 33 patients. Negative biopsy results were confirmed by splenectomy. The necessary conditions for obtaining a biopsy include a normal prothrombin (PT) and partial thromboplastin (PTT) time and a platelet count > 70 000/mm.[3] No complications were reported.

With the development of new and better adjuvant therapies, chemotherapy is being used more often for

Table 11.1 – Ann Arbor staging classification for Hodgkin's disease.

Stage	Characteristics
I	Involvement of a single lymph node region (1) in a single organ or site (IE)
II	Involvement of two or more lymph node regions on the same side of the diaphragm (II) or localized involvement of an extralymphatic organ or site (IIE)
III	Involvement of lymph nodes on both sides of the diaphragm (III) or localized involvement of an extralymphatic organ or site (IIIE) or spleen (IIIS) or both (IIISE)
IV	Diffuse or disseminated involvement of one or more extralymphatic organs with or without associated lymph node involvement. The organ(s) involved should be identified by a symbol: A, asymptomatic; B, fever, sweats, weight loss > 10% of body weight.

stage II disease in addition to stages III and IV. Studies have shown a high incidence of occult metastases in stage II disease and improved survival in stages II–IV with chemotherapy.[3] Staging laparotomy is useful only when it helps to determine whether adjuvant therapy should be added to the treatment course. For stages I and II, laparotomy is justified to rule out intraabdominal disease which may have eluded detection by other modalities.[5] In one series, 25-50 % of patients with stage I-IIIA disease were reclassified based on findings at celiotomy.[6] Following a course of radiation and/or chemotherapy, a staging laparotomy may be indicated for Hodgkin's disease to confirm remission of disease, to detect a suspected recurrence, or at the time of recurrence in a peripheral node, to document coexistent abdominal disease.[1]

Splenectomy alone has not been shown to alter B-cell function or increase the ability to administer radiation or chemotherapy.[3,5] Splenectomy may be therapeutic in the rare instances when ITP associated with Hodgkin's disease occurs. In this setting, ITP is more severe and resistant to treatment.[3]

Overall, children with Hodgkin's disease have a better outcome than adults. Although 20% of all clinical stage I patients have occult infradiaphragmatic disease, laparotomy and splenectomy are discouraged due to the risk of postsplenectomy sepsis which may occur in up to 10% of patients.[7] The risk of postsplenectomy sepsis increases as children's age decreases below 10 years. The use of chemotherapy and extended field, low-dose irradiation in all children without the use of staging laparotomy results in an 85% survival. Relapse-free survival in clinical stages I, II and III has been reported to be as high as 90%.[7]

Non-Hodgkin's lymphoma

As in Hodgkin's lymphoma, there is a diminishing role for laparotomy and splenectomy in patients with non-Hodgkin's lymphoma. Initial diagnostic work-up of a patient with lymphocytic lymphoma should include a blood count, serum chemistry, chest X-ray, abdominal CT, ultrasound and lymphangiogram. Correlation between abnormal blood counts and bone marrow infiltration is poor. One study found an abnormal blood count in only 37% of patients with bone marrow infiltration.[8] Serum chemistry may reveal an elevated creatinine with renal insufficiency, elevated uric acid, lactate dehydrogenase and liver enzymes. Chest X-ray may show hilar lymphadenopathy, pleural effusion or parenchymal involvement. Lymphangiogram is an accurate predictor of intraabdominal lymphoma. In one study, 80% of patients with positive lymphangiograms had disease in the liver or lymph nodes outside the paraaortic region at laparotomy. Eighteen to 50% of negative lymphangiograms had similar findings. Ten percent of patients with negative lymphangiograms showed disease on follow-up abdominal CT scan.[8] The extent of disease may be predicted by associated risk factors and histology with males and patients with mixed cellular or lymphocyte-depleted histology having a higher incidence of subdiaphragmatic disease.[9]

Chebner et al[10] evaluated the utility of percutaneous and peritoneoscopy-directed liver biopsy in addition to lymphography and bone marrow biopsy in staging non-Hodgkin's lymphoma. Staging is necessary to differentiate patients with local disease (stage I or II), which may be treated with radiotherapy alone, from those with disseminated disease requiring systemic therapy. Of 170 consecutive patients with the diagnosis of histiocytic, mixed lymphocytic–histiocytic, or lymphocytic lymphoma, adequate staging without laparotomy was achieved in 98 (58%) patients. Forty-four patients who were stage I to III after non-operative staging procedures underwent staging laparotomy with splenectomy, wedge liver biopsy and biopsy of paraaortic, mesenteric and porta hepatis lymph nodes and positive findings were found in 25 (57%). With regard to histology, only 5 of 81 (6.3%) patients with nodular lymphoma and 12 of 40 (30%) with histiocytic lymphoma remained with a stage I or II disease classification after non-operative staging.

Most upgrading occurs from stage III to stage IV, which has little impact on therapy.[8] Patients with lymphocytic lymphoma tend to be older than those with Hodgkin's lymphoma and may be more prone to postoperative complications. Laparotomy has been used as a diagnostic tool to rule out residual disease in patients who have undergone treatment. Other diagnostic modalities, such as CT scans, lymphangiograms and gallium scans, may overpredict residual disease. A study conducted at the National Cancer Institute of re-exploration of residual abdominal disease that had been stable for at least 2 cycles of chemotherapy, concluded that posttreatment re-exploration was unnecessary.[8] The primary indications for splenectomy in non-Hodgkin's lymphoma remain symptomatic splenomegaly, pain from splenic infarction and cytopenia from hypersplenism.

Metaplasia

Myeloid metaplasia is characterized by splenomegaly, immature granulocytes, distorted erythrocytes and erythroblasts in the peripheral blood and associated portal hypertension. The two forms of this disease are called agnogenic (AMM) and postpolycythemic (PPMM). PPMM develops in 10% of patients with previous polycythemia vera and is characterized by a worse prognosis (2 year median survival compared to 60% 5-year survival in AMM). The use of splenectomy in either form of the disease remains controversial. Reported indications for AMM include painful splenomegaly, refractory hemolytic anemia, marked thrombocytopenia, high-output cardiac failure due to shunting through the spleen and associated portal hypertension.[11] Thrombocytosis, DIC and elevated alkaline phosphatase are relative contraindications to splenectomy for AMM.[12] The high risk and uncertain benefits support a conservative approach to splenectomy.

Leukemia

The role of splenectomy in the treatment of various leukemias is similar to that described for lymphomas and metaplasia. In chronic myelogenous leukemia (CML), controlled studies have not substantiated any advantage of splenectomy on the onset of blastic phase or survival.[13,14] In both CML and chronic lymphocytic leukemia (CLL), massive splenomegaly causing abdominal pain from mass effect or intermittent infarction may develop. When patients are symptomatic, splenectomy is warranted. Historically, splenectomy was the standard approach to therapy for hairy cell leukemia (HCL) with reported complete and partial response rates of 40% and 58% respectively. Currently, splenectomy is being replaced with chemotherapy with INF-alpha and 2 deoxycofomycin and a 60-90% complete response rate is reportd with this chemotherapy.[9] Splenectomy is reserved for the correction of severe cytopenia in patients unresponsive to chemotherapy. Patients with HCL respond to splenectomy with improvement in hematologic parameters in up to 98%.[9]

Splenic tumors

Primary tumors of the spleen are uncommon. Cavernous hemangioma is the most common benign neoplasm and others include lipomas, hamartomas and fibromas. Primary malignant tumors of the spleen are mainly hemangiosarcomas. Rarely, breast, lung, skin and colon tumors may metastasize to the spleen. In hepatocellular carcinoma, splenomegaly occurs commonly secondary to portal hypertension. The treatment of these neoplasms should be dictated by the extent of the disease and the patient's overall condition.

Technical considerations

Preoperative evaluation includes assessment of the patient's overall physiologic status, which may be compromised by the underlying disease. Medical optimization may include preoperative administration of gamma globulin to raise platelet count prior to surgery.[15] All patients should receive a polyvalent pneumococcal vaccine. Determination of extent of disease via non-operative staging techniques is essential. Prior to surgery, two important points must be considered. The first is the need to rule out an accessory spleen. This may be done by preoperative scintillation scan. Accessory spleens are found most commonly in the ligaments attaching the spleen and in the perihilar space but also in remote areas of the abdomen and pelvis. Preoperative evaluation is especially important, since accessory spleens may not be easily visible with laparoscopic surgery. For most neoplastic disorders requiring splenectomy, removal of all splenic tissue is important.

A second consideration is whether preoperative splenic artery embolism is indicated. This has been advocated in high-risk patients to shorten operative time or in obese patients where dissection may be technically difficult.[16,17] Others argue that preoperative splenic artery embolization is an additional procedure with its own risks and expense without certain benefit. A worrying risk of this procedure is embolization of the tail of the pancreas with possible pancreatitis or pancreatic necrosis. Other reported complications are groin hematoma and abdominal pain.[18,19]

The position of the patient is either supine with right lateral flexion, spinal extension and a bolster behind the left chest – our favored technique – or a right lateral position. Trocar position is subject to individual variation. Generally a 10–11 mm trocar is placed through the umbilicus to accommodate the laparoscope, a 5 or 10 mm trocar in the subxyphoid area and a 10–11 mm trocar half-way between these two. A 10–11 mm trocar is placed in the left axillary line half-way between the costal margin and the iliac crest and a 12 mm trocar half-way between the umbilicus and the lateral trocar (Fig. 11.1).

The precise sequence of the procedure varies from surgeon to surgeon. Essential elements include the division of the splenic attachments, division of the short gastric vessels and division of the hilar vessels. Unger & Rosenbaum[2] recommend ligating the splenic vessels with more than one tie, because of the risk of arteriovenous fistula formation. The spleen may be removed by morselating it in a plastic bag and bringing it out through a widened trocar incision. If an intact spleen is necessary for pathologic evaluation, such as in staging Hodgkin's disease, then it may be removed through a separate, left lower quadrant incision.

Outcome

New technology does not necessarily bring improved outcome and since the popularization of laparoscopy, surgeons have evaluated its advantages and limitations carefully. Data compiled from different series shows an average operation time of 135 min for splenectomy and an average postoperative stay of 4.6 days. The average conversion rate into an open procedure is 11%. Conversion is most often due to hemorrhage or technical difficulties with splenomegaly.[2,15-18] In studies comparing laparoscopic to open splenectomy, there is no significant difference in operative time and laparoscopic surgery is associated with a significantly shorter postoperative length of stay.[16,17] Compared to the open technique, laparoscopy results in decreased complications such as atelectasis, ileus, pancreatitis and wound infection.[2] Drawbacks include the physiologic stress of a CO_2 pneumoperitoneum and limitations in removing enlarged spleens and identifying ectopic spleens.

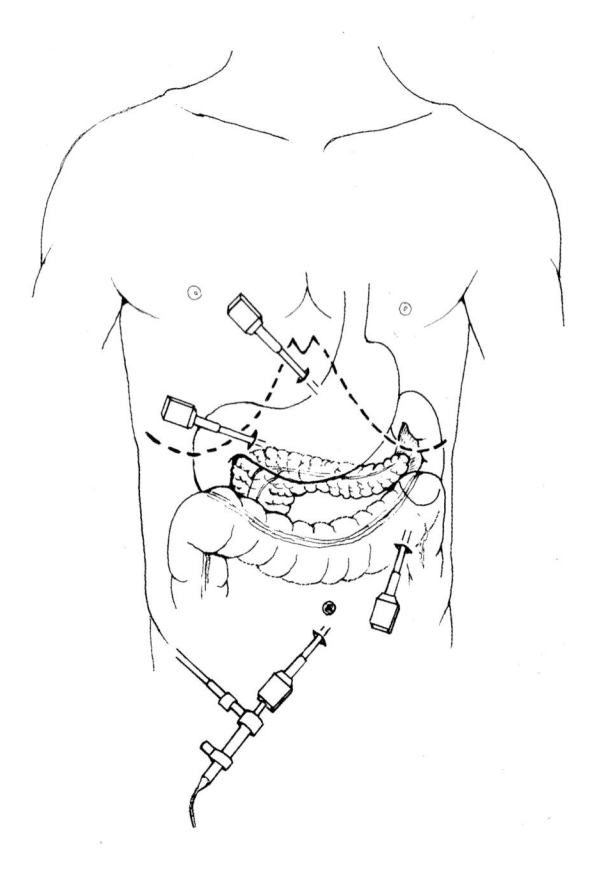

Figure 11.1 - Trocar placement for laparoscopic splenectomy.

Common complications following splenectomy include wound infection, subphrenic abscess, pulmonary embolus, stress ulcer, gastrointestinal bleed, pulmonary infection and wound dehiscence. The most worrying complication is postsplenectomy sepsis. In a recent study, 73% of postoperative deaths following splenectomy were due to septic complications.[5] Organisms that have been implicated in postsplenectomy sepsis include *Staphylococcus aureus*, *Streptococcus pneumoniae*, *Escherichia coli*, *Hemophylis influenzae*, *Enterobacter* and *Pseudomonas sp*. Neither immunization with the Pneumovax vaccine nor prophylactic antibiotics can guarantee prevention of sepsis.[3]

Morbidity and mortality following splenectomy are mainly related to the underlying disorders. Horowitz et al[5] found that patients with Hodgkin's disease and HCL have a complication rate of <20%. Mortality for conventional staging of Hodgkin's lymphoma has been reported to be 0.1%.[3] In comparison, patients with non-Hodgkin's lymphoma, CLL and CML had a complication rate of >70%.[5] In another study, the morbidity and mortality in AMM was increased compared to other hematologic disorders.[13] The chance of overwhelming postsplenectomy sepsis is 15-20 times greater in patients who have splenectomy for a hematologic disorder compared with those who have splenectomy for trauma.[20] This difference in complication rates is most likely due to associated immunologic deficiencies in patients with hypersplenism from hematologic disorders, since the only reported preoperative parameter predictive of an increased complication rate has been a large spleen (>200 g).[5]

A less commonly reported complication following splenectomy in patients with hematologic malignancies is fibrinolysis. Furthermore, splenectomy has also been implicated in the development of secondary cancers. There may be an increased risk of late development of acute leukemia following splenectomy and chemotherapy for Hodgkin's disease and these patients may also have an increased risk of secondary solid tumors.[5, 21-23]

SUMMARY

The role of splenectomy in neoplastic disorders has markedly changed over the past decade. Current indications in hematologic malignancies include staging laparotomy as a final diagnostic tool following other non-operative staging techniques. The therapeutic uses for splenectomy are primarily palliation of symptoms secondary to splenomegaly and improvement of anemia and thrombocytopenia associated with hypersplenism. The related complications following splenectomy for neoplastic disorders need to balance the risks and benefits of the procedure carefully and select each patient adequately. Laparoscopic splenectomy is a safe alternative to the open technique and it gives greater postoperative patient satisfaction.

MINIMAL ACCESS SURGERY OF MALIGNANCIES INVOLVING THE ADRENAL GLANDS

The operative exposure of the adrenal glands, which are deeply located within the retroperitoneum, has challenged surgeons for generations.[24] Conventional surgical approaches have used a variety of operative incisions including anterior transperitoneal incisions, flank and posterior (lumbar) retroperitoneal approaches with excision of the 11th or 12th rib and thoracoabdominal incisions. These differing operative exposures have their own unique advantages and disadvantages. Historically, the transabdominal approach has been used for larger unilateral or bilateral adrenal gland tumors with suspected malignancy. Its advantage is the ability to explore the entire peritoneal cavity for associated disease and to inspect and remove both adrenal glands when needed. The lateral or transthoracic approach provides the most direct and widest exposure, while the extraperitoneal approach provides direct but limited access to a single adrenal gland. Common to all open surgical approaches, however, is a large incision which confers a considerable amount of postoperative pain, significant morbidity and the need for prolonged convalescence.

Advances in laparoscopic instrumentation and increasing skill and experience in laparoscopic surgery provided surgeons with new minimal invasive techniques to explore and remove the adrenal glands. In 1992, Gagner et al[25] reported the first 3 patients who had successfully undergone laparoscopic adrenalectomy through a lateral transperitoneal approach. Like other minimally invasive procedures, laparoscopic adrenalectomy was quickly adopted and increasing numbers of these procedures are being reported.[26-29]

Three important questions are raised with respect to the adoption of minimal access surgery of the adrenal glands: Firstly, is laparoscopic adrenalectomy comparable to the conventional open methods, and can the morbidity from large incisions be improved by this method? Secondly, which approach is the more advantageous? and thirdly, should minimal access adrenalectomy be performed in the case of suspected or even proven malignancy?

Despite the lack of prospective randomized trials comparing open versus laparoscopic adrenalectomy, all retrospective reports favor the minimal invasive procedure. Although associated with longer operative times, laparoscopic adrenalectomy is associated with significantly decreased intraoperative blood loss, reduced postoperative pain and a shorter hospital stay.[30-34] These benefits have now been reproduced in many centers and in larger number of patients and this approach is clearly becoming the preferred method for removing many adrenal tumors.[35]

The routes for minimally invasive procedures on the adrenal glands parallel those of open procedures and different advantages and disadvantages can be identified for each. The anatomy of the transperitoneal approach, anterior or lateral, is more familiar to surgeons and is better suited for larger lesions, i.e. those with a higher likelihood of harboring a malignancy.[36] The retroperitoneal approach uses balloon dilatation to open up an operative field in the retroperitoneum.[31,32,37] Unlike the lateral transperitoneal approach, this technique does not require repositioning of the patient who requires bilateral adrenalectomy and it is not hindered by adhesions from previous intraabdominal disease or surgery. Nevertheless, it provides only a limited working space and does not afford the best exposure of the vena cava for right-sided lesions. It is likely that the different approaches will be used to deal with particular problems posed by individual patients.

Although clearly preferred for benign tumors, whether or not a minimally invasive approach should be considered for adrenal tumors of potential malignancy, i.e. incidentalomas larger than 6 cm in size, or for proven malignant lesions remains unclear. Absolute contraindications to laparoscopic adrenalectomy have not yet been established and the only established relative contraindication to the laparoscopic approach of adrenal tumors is a lesion that exceeds 10 cm in diameter, not only because of the increased difficulty in manipulating and removing large solid masses with available endoscopic instrumentation, but also because of the increased malignant potential of very large adrenal masses.[34]

A concern with laparoscopic adrenalectomy for malignancy is that there may be a greater likelihood of fracturing and spilling tumor cells during the procedure, which could result in local or port-site recurrences, as has been reported with laparoscopic excision of gallbladder and colon.[38,39] The principles of laparoscopic dissection that must be followed strictly to avoid this complication include extracapsular dissection of the adrenal gland, gentle manipulation of the adrenal gland and avoidance of direct and sharp grasping of the adrenal tumor, as well as careful hemostasis to maintain a clear field of dissection and to avoid further spillage.

The removal of primary adrenal malignancies, adrenal metastases or adrenal lesions indeterminate for malignancy and that do not exhibit radiographic evidence of invasion of adjacent soft tissues is reasonable if the above considerations are taken into account. However, any adrenal malignancy that shows significant invasion into surrounding tissues and organs should contraindicate a minimally invasive approach.

CONCLUSION

New and improved technology will allow most tumors to be accessed using a minimally invasive approach. This chapter demonstrates this point in two uncommon tumors. New advances in this field can be expected in the near future but it should be stated that technical advance must always be matched by an oncologically acceptable alternative to established methods.

REFERENCES

1. Fersoco SJ, Modlin. .Splenic surgery. In: Ballantyne GH, Leahy AF, Modlin IM (eds) *Laparoscopic Surgery*. WB Sanders, Philadelphia, 1994.

2. Unger SW, Rosenbaum GJ. Laparoscopic splenectomy. In: Arregui ME, Fitzgibbon RJ, Katkhouda N, Mckernan JB, Reich H (eds) *Principles of Laparoscopic Surgery*. Springer-Verlag, New York, 1995, pp356-365.

3. Devita VT, Hellman S, Jaffe ES. Hodgkins Disease. In: DeVita VT, Hellman S, Rosenberg SA (eds) *Cancer: Principles and Practice of Oncology*, 4th edn. JB Lippincott Co, Philadelphia, 1993, pp1829-1858.

4. Cavanna L, Civardi G, Fornari F et al. Ultrasonically guided percutaneous splenic tissue core biopsy in patients with malignant lymphomas. Cancer 1992;**69**:2932-2936.

5. Horowitz J, Smith JL, Weber TK, Rodriguez-Bigas MA, Petrelli NJ. Postoperative complications after splenectomy for hematologic malignancies. Ann Surg 1996;**223**:290-296.

6. Taylor MA, Kaplan HS, Nelson TS. Staging laparotomy with splenectomy for Hodgkin's disease: the Stanford experience. World J Surg 1985;**9**:449-455.

7. Poplack DG, Kin LE, Magrath IT, Pizzo PA. Leukemia and lymphoma in childhood. In:. DeVita VT, Hellman S, Rosenberg SA (eds) Cancer: Principles and Practice of Oncology, 4th edn. JB Lippincott Co, Philadelphia, 1993, pp1792-1818.

8. Longo DL, DeVita VT, Jaffe ES, Mauch P, Urbe WJ. Lymphocytic lymphomas. In: DeVita VT, Hellman S, Rosenberg SA (eds) Cancer: Principles and Practice of Oncology, 4th edn. JB Lippincott Co, Philadelphia, 1993, pp 1859-1927.

9. Saven A, Piro LD. Treatment of hairy cell leukemia. Blood 1992;**79**:111-1120.

10. Chebner BA, Johnson RE, Young RC et al. Sequential nonsurgical and surgical staging of non-Hodgkin's lymphoma. Ann Int Med 1976;**85**:149-154

11. Zenilman ME. Splenectomy for hematologic disorders .In: Cameron JL (ed) Current Surgical Therapy.1995 Mosby YearBook, Inc, St Louis, Missouri.

12. Benbassat J, Gilon D, Penchas S. The choice between splenectomy and medical treatment in patients with advanced agnogenic myeloid metaplasia. Am J Hematol 1990;**33**:128-135.

13. Medical Research Council Working Party for Therapeutic Trials in Leukemia. Randomized trials of splenectomy in Ph1 positive chronic granulocytic leukaemia, including an analysis of prognostic factors. Br J Haematol 1983;**54**:415-430

14. The Italian Cooperative Study Group on Chronic Myeloid Leukemia. Results of a prospective randomized trial of early splenectomy in chronic myeloid leukemia. Cancer 1984;**54**:333-338.

15. Gigot JF, Legrand M, Cadiere GB et al. Is laparoscopic splenectomy a justified approach in hematologic disorders? Preliminary results of a prospective multicenter study. Int Surg 1995;**80**:299-303

16. Phillips EH, Carroll BJ, Fallas MJ. Laparoscopic splenectomy. Surg Endosc 1994;**8**:931-933.

17. Friedman RL, Fallas MJ, Carroll BJ, Hiatt JR, Phillips EH. Laparoscopic splenectomy for ITP. Surg Endosc 1996;**10**:991-995.

18. Poulin EC, Thibault C, Mamazza J. Laparoscopic splenectomy. Surg Endosc 1995; **9**:172-177.

19. Haitt JR, Gomes AS, Machleder HI. Massive splenomegaly. Arch Surg 1990; **125**:1363-1367.

20. Francke EL, Neu HC. Postsplenectomy infection. Surg Clin North Am 1981;**61**:135-155.

21. van Leeuwen FE, Klokman WJ, Hagenbeek A et al. Second cancer risk following Hodgkin's disease: a 20 year follow-up study. J Clin Oncol 1994;**12**:312-325.

22. Swerdlow AJ, Douglas AJ, Vaughan Hudson G, Vaughan Hudson B, MacLennan KA. Risk of second primary cancer after Hodgkin's disease in patients in the British National Lymphoma Investigation: relationships to host factors, histology and stage of Hodgkin's disease and splenectomy. Br J Cancer 1993;**68**:1006-1011.

23. Dietrich PY, Henry-Amar M, Cossel JM, Bodis S, Bosq J, Hayat M. Secondary primary cancers in patients continuously disease-free from Hodgkin's disease: a prospective role for the spleen? Blood 1994;**84**:1209-1215.

24. Pertsemlidis D. Minimal-access versus open adrenalectomy. Surg Endosc 1995;**9**:384-386

25. Gagner M, Lacroix A, Bolte E. Laparoscopic adrenalectomy in Cushing's syndrome and pheochromocytoma. N Engl J Med 1992;**327**:103

26. Deans GT, Kappadia R, Wedgewood CM et al. Laparoscopic adrenalectomy. Br J Surg 1995;**82**: 994-995

27. Marescaux J, Mutter D, Wheeler MH. Laparoscopic right and left adrenalectomies. Surg Endosc 1996;**10**:912-915.

28. Stuart RC, Chung SCS, Lau JYW et al. Laparoscopic adrenalectomy. Br J Surg 1995; **82**:1498-1499

29. Stoker ME, Patwardhan N, Maini BS. Laparoscopic adrenal surgery. Surg Endosc 1995;**9**:387-391.

30. Brunt LM, Doherty GM, Norton JA et al. Laparoscopic adrenalectomy compared to open adrenalectomy for benign adrenal neoplasms. J Am Coll Surg 1996;**183**:1-10.

31. Heintz A, Junginger T, Bottger T. Retroperitoneal endoscopic adrenalectomy. Br J Surg 1995; **82**:215.

32. Heintz A, Walgenbach S, Junginger T. Results of endoscopic retroperitoneal adrenalectomy. Surg Endosc 1996;**10**:633-635.

33. MacGillivray DC, Shichman SJ, Ferrer FA et al. A comparison of open vs laparoscopic adrenalectomy. Surg Endosc 1996;**10**:987-990.

34. Prinz RA. A comparison of laparoscopic and open adrenalectomies. Arch Surg 1995; **130**:489-494.

35. Fernandez-Cruz L. Laparoscopic adrenal surgery. *Br J Surg* 1996; **83**:721-723.

36. Duh QY, Siperstein AE, Clark OH *et al.* Laparoscopic adrenalectomy - Comparison of the lateral and posterior approaches. *Arch Surg* 1996;**131**:870-876.

37. Mercan S, Seven R, Ozarmagan S *et al.* Endoscopic retroperitoneal adrenalectomy. *Surgery* 1995;**118**:1071-1076.

38. Copher JC, Rogers JJ, Dalton ML. Trocar-site metastasis following laparoscopic cholecystectomy for unsuspected carcinoma of the gallbladder. *Surg Endosc* 1995;**9**: 348-350.

39. Jacquet P, Averbach AM, Jacquet N. Abdominal wall metastasis and peritoneal carcinomatosis after laparoscopic-assisted colectomy for colon cancer. *Eur J Surg Oncol* 1995;**21**:568-570.

12

Minimal Access Surgery in the Evaluation of Lymph Nodes: Lessons from Breast Cancer

Theodore N. Tsangaris

Surgery for cancer consists of removal of the primary lesion and, in many cases, removal of the draining lymph nodes as well. The latter is performed both for diagnostic and therapeutic reasons. Lymphadenectomy is associated with complications such as seroma formation and lymphoedema amongst others. Given these complications, and the dubious therapeutic benefit of lymphadenectomy in many tumor types, attention has recently focused on ways of avoiding lymphadenectomy or performing minimally invasive procedures on lymphatic basins. Such innovation has of course raised questions concerning the oncologic benefit of new minimally invasive procedures. Does a laparoscopic colectomy allow as complete a lymphadenectomy as its gold standard counterpart?

This chapter addresses these issues but does not attempt to examine the concept of minimal invasion for lymph node resection in all tumor types. Instead it examines breast cancer specifically and uses this model as a platform for discussion of other tumor types.

Over the last 25 years there have been tremendous changes in our understanding of the biology of breast cancer, as well as diagnostic and some therapeutic advances in breast cancer. First, the incidence has risen worldwide; in the United States over 184 000 women are diagnosed with the disease annually[1] and over 44 000 die every year from the disease. It is the commonest cancer in women and the second leading cause of cancer deaths in women in the US. One in 8 women runs the risk of the disease, a ratio which until recently was increasing. However, women now present with earlier breast cancers; this is directly attributable to several factors including public awareness and more diligent self-breast examinations and clinical examinations by the physician. The most significant factor, however, is the expanded use of breast imaging, specifically mammography.[2-6] The number of early invasive breast cancers and non-invasive breast cancers has therefore risen dramatically. Early diagnosis along with the use of adjuvant chemotherapy and/or hormonal therapies have shown modest improvements in disease-free and overall survival for breast cancer patients.[7-10] Clinical trials have clearly shown that breast conservation therapy with radiation provides equivalent results in terms of survival when compared to modified radical mastectomy.[11-14] The treatment for breast cancer is truly becoming a multidisciplinary approach.

This chapter outlines the current controversy surrounding axillary dissection and the arguments for and against maintaining current practice. Finally, some less invasive alternatives to the standard level I and II dissection are discussed.

LYMPHADENECTOMY IN BREAST CANCER: TOWARDS A MINIMALIST APPROACH

In 1971, the National Surgical Adjuvant Breast and Bowel Project (NSABP) began a randomized trial (B-04) to compare alternative local and regional treatments in breast cancer.[15] After being stratified to clinically negative or positive axillary lymph nodes, 1665 patients were randomized to five treatment arms (Table 12.1). The most significant finding from this study was the failure to show a survival advantage of more radical surgery, specifically axillary dissection. Overall survival and disease-free survival were equivalent among treatment arms for both node-negative and node-positive groups. The other interesting finding was that 40% of the clinically node-negative group, who had modified radical mastectomy, went on to have pathologically positive lymph nodes. However, only 18% of the clinically node-negative patients who were treated with total mastectomy, required a delayed axillary dissection.

In the clinically node-positive group, regional recurrence was lower following axillary dissection (1.0%) compared with radiation to the axilla (11.9%). Again, no difference in overall or disease-free survival was noted. The B-04 study led on to a study compar-

Table 12.1 – Five treatment arms of NSABP B-04 trial

B-04[2]
Node (−)
1. Modified radical mastectomy
2. Total mastectomy with radiation treatment
3. Total mastectomy with delayed axillary dissection.
Node (+)
1. Modified radical mastectomy
2. Total mastectomy with radiation treatment

ing breast conservation vs mastectomy (B-06) and eventually adjuvant trials, and the Halstedian hypothesis of breast cancer was subsequently changed; breast cancer was now seen as a potentially systemic disease from the beginning. Surgical treatment became part of a multidisciplinary approach affecting local regional disease and the axillary lymph nodes were viewed as indicators rather than instigators of distant disease. Therefore, axillary dissection should be viewed as a prognostic or staging procedure and therapeutic only in that it may decrease local regional recurrence.

Currently, the National Cancer Institute (NCI) consensus on invasive breast cancer is that a level I and II dissection should be performed.[16] Level III nodes, interpectoral nodes (Rotters) and internal mammary lymph node dissections are rarely performed; morbidity far outweighs any prognostic or therapeutic benefit these dissections might offer.[17,18] However, morbidity for level I and II dissections is not insignificant. Although major complications such as injury to the long thoracic or thoracodorsal nerves or axillary vein are infrequent, minor complications like seroma formation and loss of intercostobrachial nerve sensation are more common. Relatively infrequent, but significant morbidities such as arm or breast edema are well documented and can reach upward of 20% in some series.[19-22] The risks for arm edema are life long. If the extent of the dissection could be altered, it would not only decrease cost and inconvenience to the patient, but also morbidity. As mentioned above, several important developments have worked together to fuel the current debate regarding limiting the extent of axillary dissection. First, screening has encouraged the increased detection of non-invasive breast cancers and smaller invasive cancers. Second, the indications for adjuvant therapy have broadened to include many node-negative patients and most premenopausal patients. Finally, an improved and expanded list of tumor prognostic markers have added to the medical oncologist's arsenal of factors that predict relapse in addition to lymph node status.

With physical examination being notoriously unreliable, tumor size remains the most important indicator of lymph node status. Haagensen[23] reviewed 935 patients between 1935 and 1972. Approximately 40% had axillary node metastasis and 28% had positive lymph nodes, even when their tumors measured between 1 and 9 mm.

Silverstein et al.[24] looked at 1128 node dissections between 1979 and 1992. All patients with T3 or smaller lesions were included in the study. Table 12.2 shows the number of node dissections per T category and the percent of positive axillary dissections. There were no positive dissections in the T_1s (ductal carcinoma in situ, DCIS) category and only 3% were positive in the T_1a (less than or equal to 0.5 cm) category. A subgroup of 43 of the 96 patients with T_1a qualified as having DCIS with microinvasion. There was no statistical difference in survival between the DCIS and T_1a patients.

In tumors between 0.6 and 1.0 cm in diameter, the incidence of positive axillary dissections was 17%, and this percentage increased in proportion to the tumor size. The authors recommended that tumors of 0.6 cm (T_1b) and larger should undergo routine axillary dissection and tumors classified as DCIS should not. This policy is supported by other studies.[25-28] Invasive tumors in category T_1a (up to 0.5 cm) may be selectively chosen for axillary dissection. Prognostic factors such as ploidy, S-phase, nuclear grade and receptor status (ER/PR) with presence of lymphatic or vascular invasion might be used in this setting to help decide who should receive axillary dissection.[24-28] Larger T_1a tumors with multiple poor prognostic signs might benefit from axillary dissections. In an expanded series, Silverstein et al.[29] suggested that the clinical presentation of the tumor (palpable versus non-palpable) along with tumor size could be used for lesions up to T_3 in determining the possibility of having a positive axillary dissection. Similar thoughts were expressed by the University Hospital of South Manchester.[30] In their series, multiple logistic regression analysis revealed that women with a screen-detected breast cancer <1 cm, or <3 cm of

Table 12.2 – Axillary lymph node involvement in relation to the size of tumor (*adapted from Silverstein et al.*[29])

T (size)	Number of patients	Node + dissection (%)
T_1s (DCIS)	189	0 (0)
T_1a (≤5 mm)	96	3 (3)
T_1b (6-10 mm)	156	27 (17)
T_1c (11-20 mm)	357	115 (32)
T_2 (21-50 mm)	330	145 (44)
T_3 (≥51 mm)	92	55 (60)

DCIS = ductal carcinoma in situ

histologic grade 1, could be spared axillary dissections. However, a retrospective review from three large urban hospitals in Tulsa, Oklahoma found a 12.0% incidence of positive axillary dissections for T1a lesions.[31]

Increasingly, patient selection based on clinical presentation, tumor histoprognostic and immunoprognostic factors may diminish the role of dissection in the determination of adjuvant therapy. In 1993, Lin et al.[22] retrospectively studied 283 breast cancer patients, 15% of whom had clinically positive lymph nodes but 86% of whom were pathologically positive. In 31% of the study group who had favorable tumor prognostic factors, and clinically negative axillary nodes, axillary lymph node dissection alone determined the indication for adjuvant therapy. Thirteen percent of this group ultimately had positive nodes. For the 54% of patients who had node-negative disease but poor tumor prognostic factors, lymph node dissection played no role in the decision-making regarding adjuvant therapy.

Between 1982 and 1989, The New England Medical Center[32] performed a prospective study of 73 women, aged 65 years or older, who were clinically node-negative. These patients received lumpectomy and radiation to the breast and axilla (without dissection). Sixty-six of the 73 who were ER positive or who had a tumor >2 cm in diameter also received tamoxifen. At a median follow-up of 54 months, 8-year rates of local and regional lymph node control were 92.5% and 100%, respectively, with a breast cancer specific survival of 93.8%. A retrospective review of women 70 years and older suggested similar results,[33] as did results from Rush Presbyterian in Chicago[34] where 492 patients with clinically negative lymph nodes were studied. Crude rates of local and distant failure were similar for patients both with and without axillary dissection. The Yale group[35] treated 327 clinically stage I and II patients with lumpectomy alone without axillary dissection followed by radiation therapy to the breast and axilla. There was a 71% overall 10-year survival rate and a nodal control rate of 97%. A prospective randomized study from France,[36] however, resulted in a different conclusion. Patients with axillary dissection and radiation had a significant advantage in terms of survival compared to those with radiation alone to the axillary lymph node basin, although radiation treatment was given to both groups. However, in this study, only the pathologically confirmed positive lymph nodes (i.e. axillary dissection group) were given adjuvant therapy, and this probably accounts for the survival benefit in this group. Thus, it would appear that the less invasive approach to the axilla would be to do nothing or else to radiate the axilla. For selected patients, this may be the correct management.

Some surgeons are more comfortable with a limited axillary dissection or axillary sampling. However, the technique up to this point is random and has been criticized. Most surgeons advocate an all-or-none approach to axillary dissection. A randomized trial from Oestersund Hospital, Sweden addressed this issue.[37] Two hundred women over a 6-year period were randomized to axillary dissection or biopsy (lower half of axillary fat and suspicious lymph nodes) of the axilla and the results suggested that the two approaches gave similar results in terms of breast cancer staging. A Japanese study[38] in 95 patients showed that intraoperative, histologic examination of frozen sections of axillary lymph nodes was significantly more effective than clinical examination. Suspicious lymph nodes (large or hard) were sampled from the axillary fat pad harvested from a complete axillary dissection. Histologic examination using frozen section was performed during surgery and the remaining axillary nodes were examined after surgery by permanent section. A diagnostic accuracy of 97%, a sensitivity of 77% and a specificity of 100% were achieved by frozen section. The authors concluded that axillary sampling of this type may be used to determine the extent of subsequent axillary dissection. Although the costs of this procedure are mentioned in the report, the time needed intraoperatively to accomplish sampling is not.

In both studies,[37,38] significant numbers of lymph nodes were removed and whether this should be considered true sampling or incomplete axillary dissection is the subject of some debate. Improvement in long-term morbidity is not known for these patients.

Lessons from melanoma

The management of lymph node basins in melanoma has pioneered novel approaches in the field of lymphadenectomy in general in oncology. There are many controversies regarding the role of lymphadenectomy in patients with melanoma. In many respects, there are similarities when comparing lymph node assessment for melanoma and for breast cancer. Differences also exist such as the fact that melanoma may occur in any region of the body and thus pertinent lymph node basins are more numerous and diverse. Secondly, the purpose of lymph node dissection in melanoma is not only prognostic but is also therapeutic. Treatment of clinically positive regional lymph nodes requires complete resection to achieve local control and to increase survival figures.

Management of clinically negative nodal basins presents a significant problem and has generated controversy as to the best approach. Neither retrospective or prospective studies regarding elective node dissection provide a definitive answer. Several studies have explored less invasive yet reliable prognostic techniques for determining the status of lymph node basins.[39-43]

MINIMALLY INVASIVE TECHNIQUES IN LYMPHADENECTOMY

Sentinel node biopsy

Minimally invasive techniques in the form of sentinel node lymphadenectomy were employed much earlier for melanoma than breast cancer. Borrowing technology initially developed and used for melanoma patients, Giuliano *et al*.[44] adopted the technique of lymphatic mapping and sentinel lymphadenectomy for breast cancer. In this method, a vital dye (isosulfan blue), is injected at and around the tumor site. After 5-10 min, the axilla is entered and blunt dissection performed until a lymphatic tract or blue-stained node is identified. This dye-filled tract is dissected until the first blue lymph node (Fig. 12.1.). The tract is followed proximally to the tail of the breast to ensure the identified lymph node is the most proximal, i.e. the sentinel node. The node and a rim of surrounding tissue are excised and submitted separately. Completion of the axillary dissection is then performed. Between 1991 and 1994, 174 lymphatic mapping and sentinel lymphadenectomies were performed in this way. Sentinel nodes were identified in 114 of 174 (65.5%) procedures and were accurate in predicting nodal status in 109 of the 114 (95.6%). As with any technique, there is a learning curve. All false negative sentinel nodes occurred in the early part of this study, while later experience demonstrated successful mappings in up to 85% of cases. In 38% of clinically negative and pathologically positive axilla, the sentinel node was the only lymph node with tumor. In 10 of the last 54 procedures, the sentinel node was located in level II and might have been missed by random sampling or low (level I) axillary dissection. When sentinel lymphadenectomy was compared 'head to head' with axillary dissection, there were some interesting findings.[45,46] Using both H&E staining and immunohistochemical techniques with antibodies to cytokeratin, the incidence of axillary nodal metastasis and micrometastasis in sentinel lymphadenectomy and axillary dissection were compared prospectively. The number of patients with axillary metastasis was 29.1% in the axillary dissected group and 42% in the sentinel node group. Of these, 10.3% and 38.2% respectively had micrometastasis ($\leq$ 2 mm). This was statistically significant.

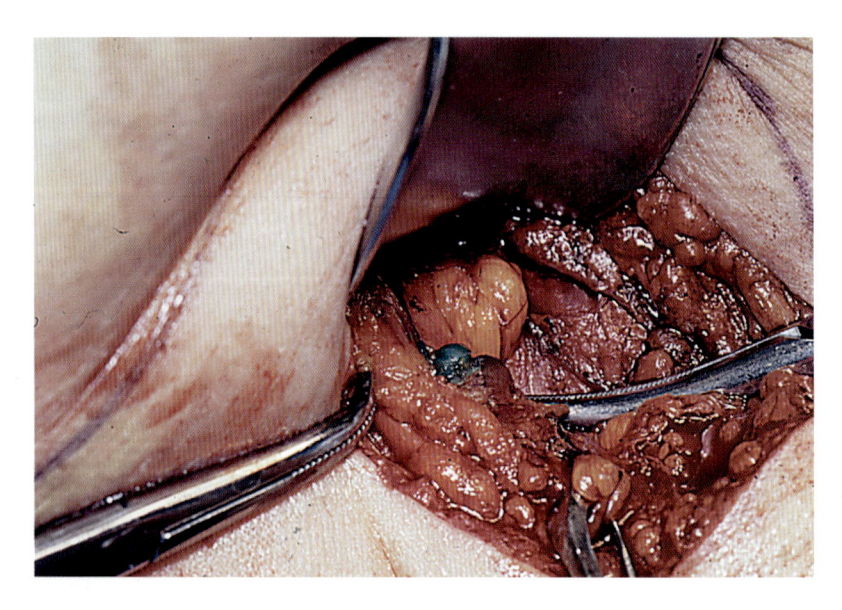

Figure 12.1 - Identification of the sentinel lymph node after injection of isosulfan blue at the primary tumor site - open technique.

With a little familiarity, the technique can be very reliable and extremely accurate when a sentinel node is identified. The first hurdle is the ability to recognize a small dye-filled lymphatic or blue-tinged lymph node; the interval between dye injection and its appearance in the axilla is variable and this can be frustrating. Medial and lower (away from the axilla) lesions might need a longer transit time, particularly if the breast is large. Some medial lesions never show dye in the axilla and are presumed to drain toward the internal mammary lymph nodes. In tumors already excised, the presence of fibrous tissue may make the dye unavailable for recruitment by the lymphatics. In our experience, 1 of 2 false negatives occurred because of mechanical obstructions to the dye, presumably due to scar tissue. The blue node was negative, but two nodes immediately adjacent were positive for tumor. Therefore, it is our practice to take the blue node with any immediately surrounding lymph nodes in patients who have had previous surgery. A potential complication is tattooing of the skin and care should be taken when injecting around the tumor site to avoid this problem.

At the same time as vital blue dye techniques were being evaluated, radiolymphoscintigraphy or gamma probe guided mapping and sentinel lymph node biopsy were also being developed. This was done in an attempt to decrease the number of unsuccessful mappings using the vital dye techniques. Initially developed for melanoma,[39-43] it has been applied to breast cancer patients. Krag et al.[47] reported encouraging initial results using a hand-held gamma probe to follow the technetium sulfur colloid from the breast to the lymph node. Recently, Albertini et al.[48] suggested in a prospective trial that lymphatic mapping using the combination of a vital blue dye and a filtered technetium-labeled sulfur colloid may enhance the ability to identify the sentinel node and, as a result, the accuracy of the procedure.

It has been questioned whether sentinel node lymphadenectomy philosophically is a throw-back to the Halstedian view of metastatic spread. In fact, the sentinel node does nothing to undermine the new paradigm of breast disease. It simply attempts to identify the first node involved should the axilla be a site of metastatic disease. The exact procedure has yet to be agreed on, but this minimally invasive approach is worthy of future study and may provide advantages over standard axillary dissection, while at the same time delivering accurate prognostic information.

Endoscopic lymphadenectomy

Considering the strong trend toward minimally invasive approaches in surgery, and the desire to be more selective in axillary dissection, we have applied endoscopic technology to the axilla. Initially, the technique was evaluated in the Endosurgical Education and Research Center at The George Washington University Medical Center using porcine and cadaver models. These initial experiments showed that a space could be developed, key anatomic structures identified and the axillary contents manipulated. We then proceeded to study and evaluate the technique in human subjects.

Endoscopic axillary exploration (EAE) was performed in 23 patients with invasive breast cancer.[49] After induction of general anesthesia, the patient is placed in a supine position with the ipsilateral arm abducted to 90°. The breast, chest wall and axilla are prepared and draped in the usual sterile fashion. The lateral aspect of the pectoralis major muscle and the anterior border of the latissimus dorsi muscle are delineated with a marking pencil. A 1 cm skin incision is made at the superior aspect of the axilla and dissection carried down bluntly to the lateral border of the pectoralis major muscle. The clavipectoral fascia is incised at this level and a tract is created into the axilla using blunt finger dissection. A balloon distension device is inserted into the tract and carefully inflated under endoscopic vision to create a working space (Fig. 12.2). The balloon is removed and replaced by a blunt-tipped cannula. Insufflation with CO_2 is initiated to a pressure of 8-12 mmHg. A 30° laparoscope with attached video camera is introduced for visualization of the axillary contents.

Under direct visualization, a 5 mm trocar is introduced at the inferior aspect of the dissected axillary space (Fig. 12.3). Use of monopolar electrosurgery is avoided throughout the procedure. After adequate exposure within the axilla has been achieved, exploration of the axilla along with the sentinel lymph node technique is initiated. The latter technique is performed as described above (Fig. 12.4).

Dissection of the axilla with the balloon distension device and insufflation allowed identification of the following anatomic landmarks: rib cage, pectoralis major muscle, serratus anterior muscle, latissimus dorsi muscle and intercostal brachial nerves. After identification of these structures, only minimal instrument dissection is required to identify the axillary vein, long thoracic and thoracodorsal nerves in their usual

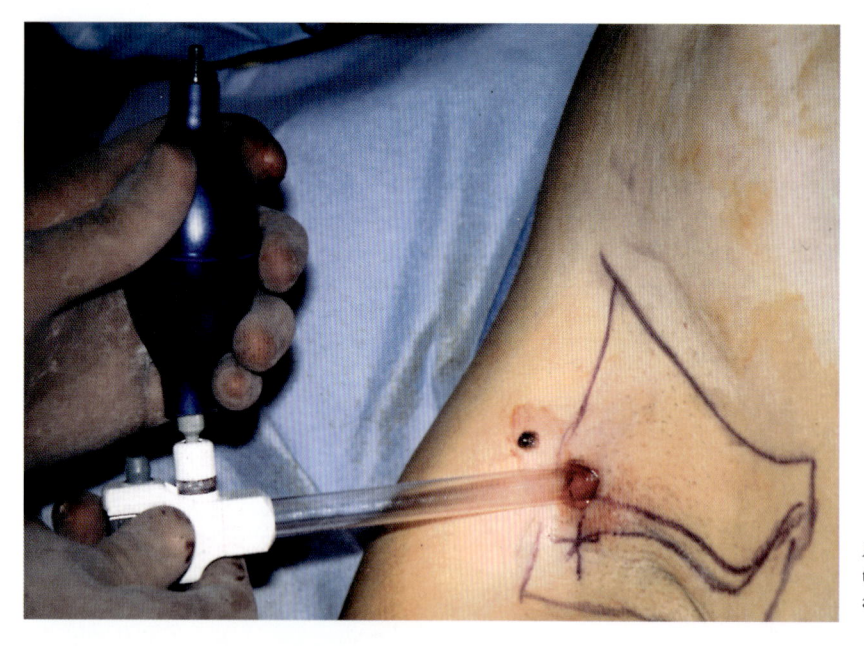

Figure 12.2 - Balloon distension of the axillary space during endoscopic axillary exploration.

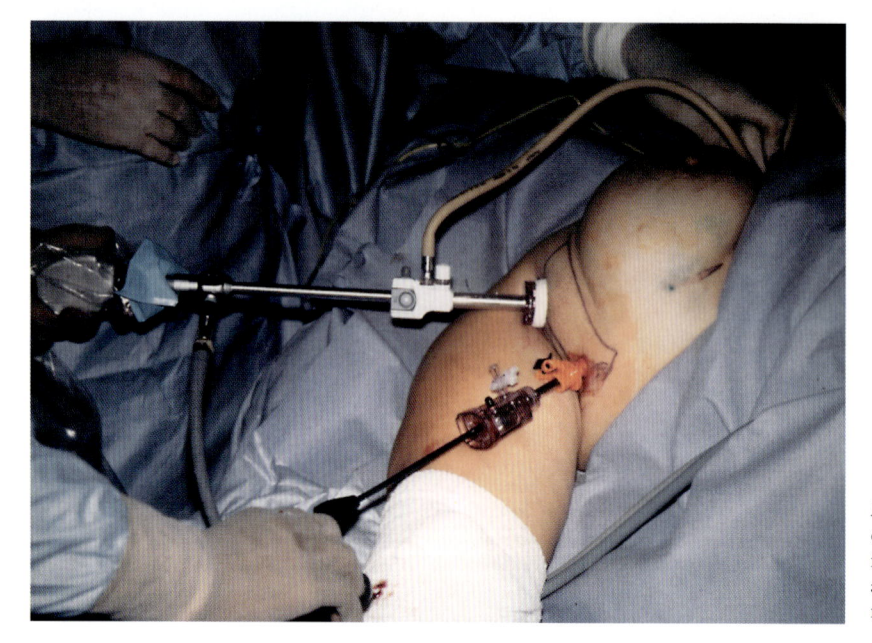

Figure 12.3 - Endoscopic axillary exploration: a 30° endoscope is inserted through a 10 mm trocar and dissecting forceps through a 5 mm trocar.

anatomic locations. In each of the 23 patients, we were able to identify all the anatomic landmarks and specifically preserve and protect the axillary vein, long thoracic and thoracodorsal nerves. The axillary contents were then inspected and manipulated in all patients.

Sentinel node identification was attempted in 19 of the 23 patients, in 16 of which the endoscopic axillary exploration correlated with what was visualized once the axilla was opened. The sentinel lymph node or blue dye was identified in 11 of the 19 patients. In 5 patients no sentinel node or dye was seen in the axilla either endoscopically or by an open procedure. In a further 3 patients, the sentinel node or dye was seen upon opening the axilla but this was missed with the endoscopic procedure.

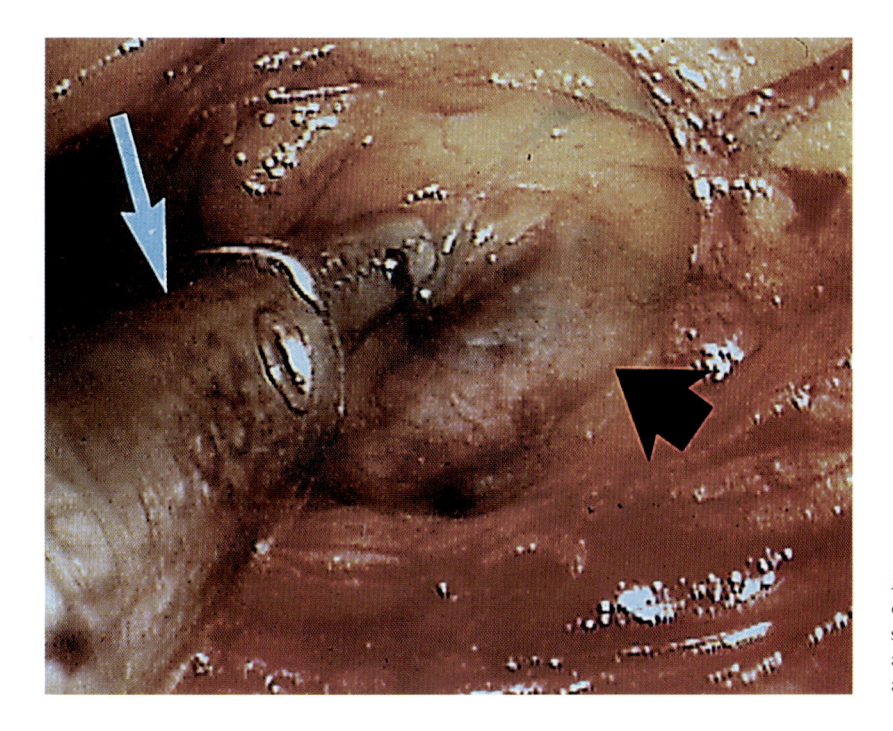

Figure 12.4 - Endoscopic axillary exploration: identification of the sentinel lymph node (black arrow) and dissecting forceps (white arrow) through a 30° endoscope.

We identified no complications in the 23 patients following endoscopic exploration as confirmed by formal open axillary dissection. Specifically, there were no injuries to the axillary vein, long thoracic nerve or thoracodorsal nerve. No patient developed subcutaneous emphysema as a result of insufflation of the axilla or showed variation from the expected postoperative course. The operative blood loss and wound complication rate were not evaluated because all patients were opened following the endoscopic exploration, but these were no more frequent or extensive than those seen for the conventional open technique.

Endoscopic axillary exploration utilizes a number of well-accepted techniques developed for laparoscopic hernia repair. Combining minimally invasive techniques with the new sentinel node technique may allow a further reduction in the morbidity caused by skin incision and excision of the entire axillary pad. If the sentinel lymph node technique proves to stage the breast cancer patient reliably, using it in combination with endoscopic exploration of the axilla may allow a truly minimal access approach to staging. The exact utility of this procedure remains to be determined. A new protocol is currently underway to determine if EAE is best suited as a substitute for open axillary dissection or is more appropriately coupled with the sentinel node technique. It remains to be seen if other approaches and new endoscopic instruments facilitate endoscopic axillary exploration.

CONCLUSION

The correct approach toward the axilla in breast cancer patients is controversial[50-58] but it appears, with the development of exciting new techniques, that the standard level I and II dissections may become the exception rather than the rule in the next few years. The approach to the axilla and use of minimally invasive techniques might be considered in the following way (Fig. 12.5): 1) eliminate axillary dissection for non-invasive breast cancers; 2) for those with invasive breast cancer where an axillary dissection will not alter or determine adjuvant therapy,

Figure 12.5 - Algorithm for the management of the axilla in breast cancer patients.

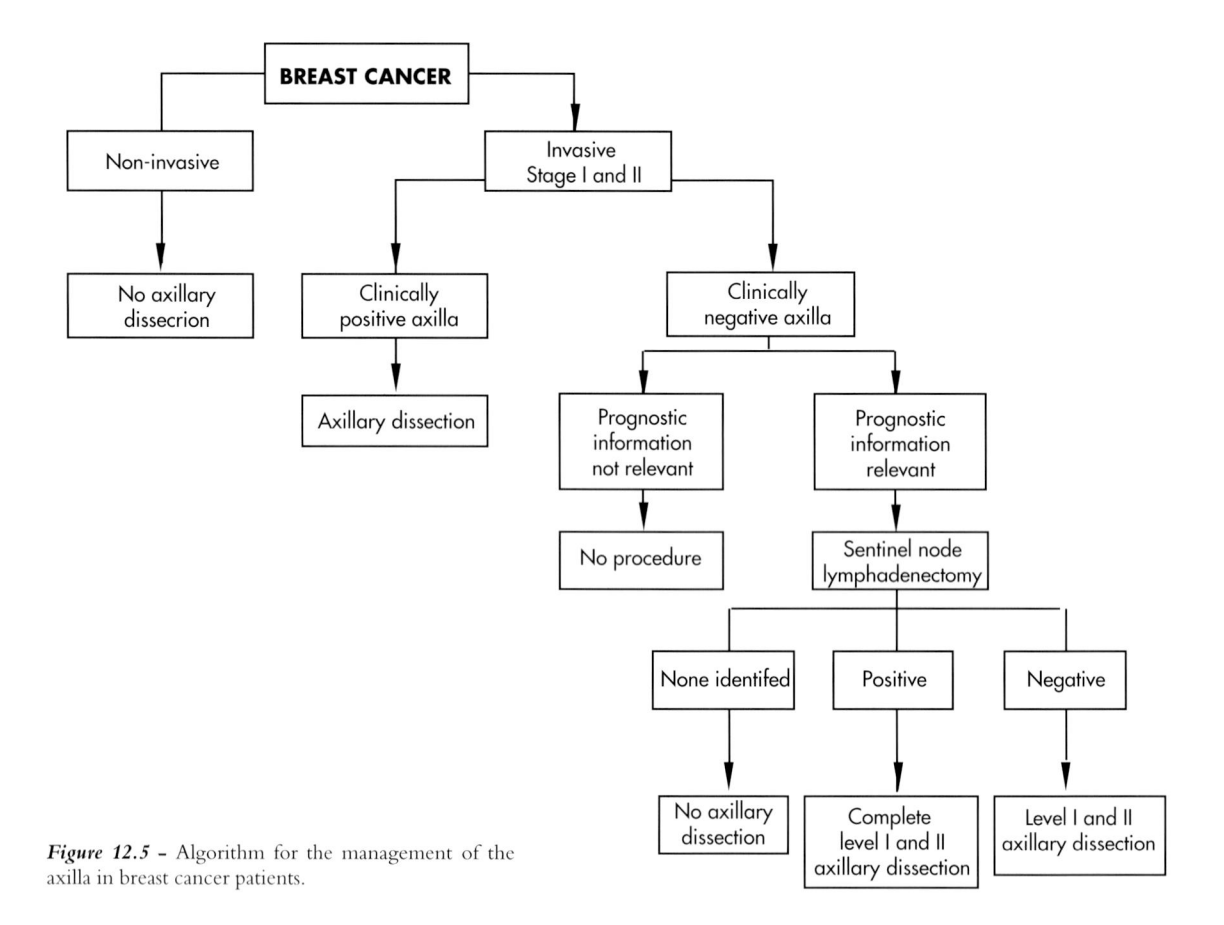

it should also be eliminated; 3) in patients with clinical stage I and II, and with clinically negative axilla, sentinel node lymphadenectomy should be considered. If positive, a complete axillary dissection could then be completed. If sentinel node is not identified then complete dissection should be performed; 4) for clinically positive axillae, standard level I and II dissections should still be considered.

Further investigation is needed to determine if other minimally invasive techniques, such as endoscopic axillary exploration, are of use in breast cancer patients. There is also little doubt that tumors of the colon, lung, testes and others will undergo similar screening in this era of minimally imnvasive surgery.

REFERENCES

1. American Cancer Society. *Cancer Facts and Figures*. American Cancer Society, 1996

2. Tabar L, Fagerberg G, Chen HH et al. Efficacy of breast cancer screening by age. New results from the Swedish two-county trial. *Cancer* 1995;**75**:2507-2117.

3. Cady B, Stone MD, Schuler JG, Thakur R, Wanner MA, Lavin PT. The new era in breast cancer invasion, size, and nodal involvement dramatically decreasing as a result of mammographic screening. *Arch Surg* 1996; **131**:301-308.

4. Smart CR, Hendrick RE, Rutledge JH, Smith RA. Benefit of mammography screening in women aged 40-49: current evidence from randomized controlled trials. *Cancer* 1995; **75**:1619-1626.

5. Shapiro S, Venet W, Strax P et al. *Periodic Screening for Breast Cancer: The Health Insurance Plan Project and its Sequelae, 1963-1986*. Baltimore: The Johns Hopkins University Press, 1993.
6. Kopans DB. Mammography screening and the controversy concerning women aged 40 to 49. *Radiol Clin North Am* 1995;**33**:1273-1290.
7. Fisher B, Costantino J, Redmond C et al. A randomized clinical trial evaluating tamoxifen in the treatment of patients with node-negative breast cancer who have estrogen-receptor-positive tumors. *N Engl J Med* 1989;**320**:479-484.
8. Early Breast Cancer Trialist' Collaborative Group. Systemic treatment of early breast cancer by hormonal, cytotoxic, or immune therapy: 133 randomized trials involving 31,000 recurrences and 24,000 deaths among 75,000 women. *Lancet* 1992;**339**:1-15, 71-85.
9. Goldhirsh A, Wood WC, Sean HJ et al. Fifth International Conference on Adjuvant Therapy of Breast Cancer, St. Gallen, March 1995: International Consensus Panel on the Treatment of Primary Breast Cancer. *Eur J Cancer* 1995;**31A**:1754-1759.
10. Bonadonna G, Valagussa P, Moliterni A, Zambetti M, Brambilla C. Adjuvant cyclophosphamide, methotrexate, and fluorouracil in node-positive breast cancer: The results of 20 years of follow-up. *N Engl J Med* 1995;**332**:901-906.
11. Neff PT, Bear HD, Pierce CV, et al. Long-term results of breast conversation therapy for breast cancer. *Ann Surg* 1996; **223**: 709-717.
12. Fisher B, Anderson S, Redmon C et al. Reanalysis and results after 12 years of follow-up in a randomized clinical trial comparing total mastectomy with lumpectomy with or without irradiation in the treatment of breast cancer. *N Engl J Med* 1995;**333**: 1456-1461.
13. Jacobson JA, Danforth DN, Cowan KH et al. Ten-year results of a comparison of conservation with mastectomy in the treatment of stage I and II breast cancer. *N Engl J Med* 1995;**332**:907-911.
14. Arriagada R, Le MG, Rochard F, Contesso G. Conservative treatment versus mastectomy in early breast cancer: Patterns of failure with 15 years of follow-up data. *J Clin Oncol* 1996;**14**:1558-1564.
15. Fisher B, Redmond C, Fisher E et al. Ten year results of a randomized clinical trial comparing radical mastectomy and total mastectomy with or without radiation. *N Engl J Med* 1985;**312**: 674-681.
16. NIH Consensus Development Conference. *NIH Consensus Statement* 1992;**8**:1-19.
17. Rosen PP, Lesser ML, Kinne DW, Beattie EJ. Discontinuous or "Skip" metastases in breast carcinoma. Analysis of 1228 axillary dissections. *Ann Surg* 1983;**197**:276-283.
18. Veronesi U, Rilke F, Luini A et al. Distribution of axillary node metastases by level of invasion. *Cancer* 1987;**59**:682-687.
19. Ivens D, Hoe AL, Podd TJ et al. Assessment of morbidity from complete axillary dissection. *Br J Cancer* 1992;**66**:136-138.
20. Hladiuk M, Huchcroft S, Temple W, Schnurr BE. Arm function after axillary dissection for breast cancer: A pilot study to provide parameter estimates. *J Surg Oncol* 1992;**50**:47-52.
21. Werner RS, McCormick B, Petrek J et al. Arm edema in conservatively managed breast cancer: Obesity is a major predictive factor. *Radiology* 1991;**180**:177-184.
22. Lin PP, Allison DC, Wainstock et al. Impact of axillary lymph node dissection on the therapy of breast cancer patients. *J Clin Oncol* 1993;**11**:1536-1544.
23. Haagensen CD. *Diseases of the Breast*, 3rd ed. Philadelphia: WB Saunders, 1986.
24. Silverstein MJ, Gierson ED, Waisman JR, Senfosky GM, Colburn WJ, Gamagami P. Axillary lymph node dissection for T1a breast carcinoma. *Cancer* 1994;**73**: 664-667.
25. Schwartz GF, Patchefsky AS, Finklestein SD et al. Non-palpable in-situ ductal carcinoma of the breast. Predictors of multicentricity and microinvasion and implications for treatment. *Arch Surg* 1989;**124**:29-32.
26. Lagios MD, Westdahl PR, Margolin FR, Rose MR. Duct carcinoma *in situ*. Relationship of extent of non-invasive disease to the frequency of occult invasion, multicentricity, lymph node metastases, and short-term treatment failures. *Cancer* 1982;**50**: 1309-1314.
27. Gump FE, Jicha DL, Ozello L. Ductal carcinoma in-situ (DCIS): A revised concept. *Surgery* 1987;**102**: 790-795.
28. Silverstein MJ, Gierson ED, Colburn WJ et al. Axillary lymphadenectomy for intraductal carcinoma of the breast. *Surg Gynecol Obstet* 1991;**172**:211-214.
29. Silverstein MJ, Gierson ED, Waisman JR, Colburn WJ, Gamagami P. Predicting axillary node positivity in patients with invasive carcinoma of the breast by using a combination of T category and palpability. *J Am Coll Surg*. 1995;**180**:700-704.
30. Walls J, Boggis CRM, Wilson M et al. Treatment of the axilla in patients with screen detected breast cancer. *Br J Surg* 1993;**80**:436-438.
31. McGhee JM, Youmans R, Clingan F, Malnar K, Bellefeville C, Berry B. The value of axillary dissection in T1a breast cancer. *Am J Surg* 1996;**172**:501-505.

32. Wazer DE, Erban JK, Robert NJ et al. Breast conservation in elderly women for clinically negative axillary lymph nodes without axillary dissection. *Cancer* 1994;**74**: 878-883.

33. Feigelson BJ, Acosta JA, Feigelson HS, Findley A, Saunders EL. T1 Breast carcinoma in women 70 years of age and older may not require axillary lymph node dissection. *Am J Surg* 1996;**172**:487-490.

34. Kuznetsova M, Graybill JC, Zusag TW, Hartsell WF, Griem KL. Omission of axillary lymph node dissection in early-stage breast cancer: Effect on treatment outcome. *Radiology* 1995;**197**:507-510.

35. Haffty BC, McKhann C, Beinfield M, Fischer D, Fischer JJ. Breast conservation therapy without axillary dissection. A rational treatment strategy in selected patients. *Arch Surg* 1993;**128**:315-1319.

36. Cabanes PA, Salmon RJ, Vilcoq JR et al. Value of axillary dissection in addition to lumpectomy and radiotherapy in early breast cancer. *Lancet* 1992;**339**: 1245-1248.

37. Christensen SB, Jansson C. Axillary biopsy compared with dissection in the staging of lymph nodes in operable breast cancer. *Eur J Surg* 1993;**159**:159-162.

38. Noguchi M, Minami M, Earashi M et al. Intraoperative histologic assessment of surgical margins and lymph node metastasis in breast conserving surgery. *J Surg Oncol* 1995;**60**: 185-190.

39. Krag DN, Meijer SJ, Weaver DL et al. Minimal access surgery for staging of malignant melanoma. *Arch Surg* 1995;**130**:654-658.

40. Alex JC, Krag DN. Gamma-probe guided localization of lymph nodes. *Surg Oncol* 1993;**2**:137-143.

41. Alex JC, Weaver DL, Fairbank JT, Rankin BS, Krag DN. Gamma-probe guided lymph node localization in malignant melanoma. *Surg Oncol* 1993;**2**:303-308.

42. Albertini JJ, Cruse CW, Rapaport D et al. Intraoperative radio lymphoscintigraphy improves sentinel lymph node identification for patients with melanoma. *Ann Surg* 1996; **223**:217-224.

43. Dale PS, Foshag LJ, Wanek LA, Morton DL. Metastasis of primary melanoma to two separate lymph node basins: Prognostic significance. *Ann Surg Oncol* 1997;**4**:13-18.

44. Giuliano AE, Kirgan DM, Guenther JM, Morton DL. Lymphatic mapping and sentinel lymphadenectomy for breast cancer. *Ann Surg* 1994;**220**:391-401.

45. Giuliano AE, Dale PS, Turner RR, Morton DL, Evans SW, Krasne DL. Improved axillary staging of breast cancer with sentinel lymphadenectomy. *Ann Surg* 1995;**222**: 394-401.

46. Giuliano AE. Sentinel lymphadenectomy: A new axillary staging procedure for primary breast carcinoma. *Breast Diseases: A Year Book Quarterly* 1996;**7**:16-17.

47. Krag DN, Weaver DL, Alex JC, Fairbank JT. Surgical resection and radiolocalization of the sentinel lymph node in breast cancer using a gamma probe. *Surg Oncol* 1993;**2**:335-340.

48. Albertini JJ, Lyman GH, Cox C H et al. Lymphatic mapping and sentinel node biopsy in the patient with breast cancer. *JAMA* 1996; **276**:1818-1822.

49. Tsangaris TN, Trad KS, Brody FJ, Jacobs LK, Sackier JM, Tsangaris NT. Endoscopic axillary exploration: Description of a novel technique. (In press)

13

Future of Minimal Access in Surgical Oncology

Amy L. Halverson and Jonathan M. Sackier

Since the earliest recorded surgical intervention for the treatment of tumors found in the Edwin Smith papyrus from the Egyptian Middle Kingdom (about 1600 BC)[1] to today's current practices, advances in surgical oncology have been tied to advances in technology. Research in medicine gives an insight into tumor biology and leads to improved medical treatment. The first elective abdominal operation in the modern era was performed in 1809 by Ephraim MacDowell. He removed a 22-pound ovarian tumor from a patient who survived for 30 years after the operation.[2] The subsequent expansion of the use of surgery to treat tumors was dependent on the development of general anesthesia by two dentists, William Morton and Crawford Long. The first major operation using general anesthesia was the resection of a submaxillary tumor at the Massachusetts General Hospital in 1846 by John Collins Warren.[2] A second important development in surgical oncology was the introduction of carbolic acid in 1867 by Lister and the application of the principles of antisepsis.[3] Further advances in microsurgical techniques allowing free grafts for reconstruction and improvements in critical care have allowed more aggressive surgery in patients with advanced disease.

The most recent advances in surgery stem from the development of minimally invasive surgery. Since the first laparoscopic cholecystectomy, credited to Mühe in 1985,[4] utilization of minimally invasive surgery has expanded to include numerous procedures in most surgical disciplines. Its increase in popularity has been accompanied by an explosion in technological advances. The telescopes used in endoscopic surgery are smaller and provide improved resolution and even a 3D stereoscopic view.[5] A new ultrasonic scalpel offers an efficient alternative to electrosurgery or hemostatic clips and facilitates the resection of liver tumors and the division of vessels during splenectomy or colon resection.[6] New instruments designed to improve efficiency and safety and to reduce the overall cost of a procedure are continually being introduced. Some of the most exciting advances are in the areas of robotics, telepresence and virtual reality.

ROBOTICS

Current use of robotics in surgery is exemplified by the AESOP (Automated Endoscopic System for Optimal Positioning) robot (Fig. 13.1). AESOP is a robotic arm with 9 degrees of freedom and is designed to manipulate the laparoscope during procedures. It replaces the surgical assistant who would otherwise operate the laparoscope. The robotic arm, which is attached to the operating table, adjusts the camera

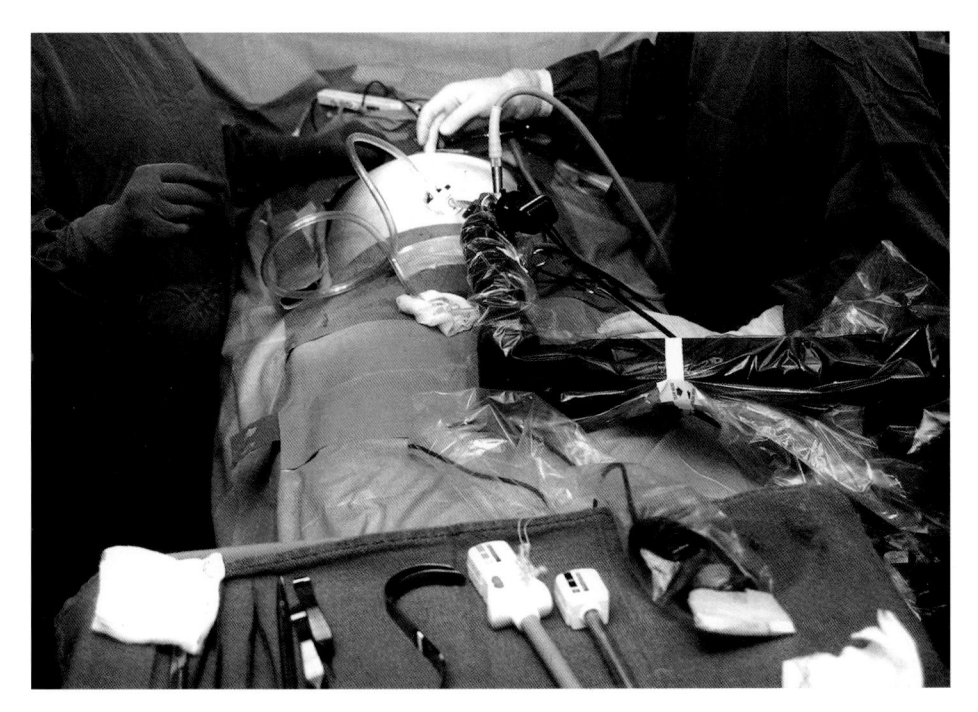

Figure 13.1 – AESOP robotic arm holding laparoscope

view under the direction of the surgeon either via a foot pedal or in response to a voice command interface. The robot has memory which allows the surgeon to 'save' certain positions so, for example, the view may be expanded and then returned to the previous position for safe exchange of instruments.[7] Advantages of the AESOP system include better surgeon control over movement of the laparoscope, a steadier picture and reduced personnel costs.

With the development of laser-etched circuits came the birth of nanotechnology or micromachines. Anita Flynn and others have developed a wide range of 'Gnat' robots with simple levels of intelligence capable of tasks such as moving from a light to a dark place and seeking sound.[8] A theoretical application for such a device would be the development of a tiny robot which could advance via remote control through the colon with an attached camera and biopsy forceps to aid in the diagnosis and treatment of colonic neoplasms.

TELEMEDICINE

Telemedicine is defined as the practice of medicine without direct physician-patient interaction via an interactive audio–video communication system employing tele–electronic devices.[9] With the goals of delivering medical care into underserved geographic areas and increasing access to specialized consultants, the practice of telemedicine is gaining popularity. Teleconsultation is being used in the fields of radiology and pathology where X-ray images or pathology slides may be transmitted over variable distances to a physician for evaluation. This system allows a single person to evaluate clinical data from different locations. At some institutions, physicians are using telemedicine to evaluate patients at remote sites. The Medical College of Virginia has implemented programs to provide care at a rural satellite clinic and at a state correctional facility. Through these telemedicine systems, education is provided to medical students, residents and practitioners. Specialty consultation is also provided in infectious disease, dermatology and cardiology.[10] Ongoing evaluation will help to determine when patients should be seen in person and when they can be followed over the telemedicine systems as well as the potential cost savings of such a system.

The main thrust for technologic advancement in telemedicine originated in the military. In an effort to manage battlefield casualties more effectively, the United States Army, under the direction of Richard Satava at Walter Reed Army Medical Center, is developing methods to evaluate and treat soldiers in the front, away from medical facilities. One product of this research is a wrist-worn device which will not only indicate the position of a soldier on the battlefield via a global positioning system (GPS), but also transmit information concerning the soldier's physiologic status. The first-generation prototype monitors heart rate, blood pressure, temperature, electrocardiogram and oxygen saturation.[11] Second-generation sensors are intended non-invasively to measure blood electrolytes and metabolites, respiration and levels of consciousness.[11] Devices like these may be useful to monitor hospital patients and patients in their homes.

VIRTUAL REALITY

True telepresence takes telemedicine one step further, whereby the physician may not only observe and communicate with a patient, but actually have control over a slave manipulator and sensory feedback.[12] The Green Telepresence Surgery System is a prototype that permits precise, accurate, remote surgery. This system brings 3D vision, enhanced dexterity and the sense of touch to the surgeon and allows surgery to be performed in one location by a surgeon at another location.[11]

Current applications of virtual reality are mostly limited to the classroom. A number of simulators are being developed to display and teach anatomy. Students may practise dissecting a 'virtual cadaver' and, just as pilots train on flight simulators, surgeons may rehearse a procedure prior to operating on a patient. Essential elements to these systems include high-resolution graphics and the model's ability to represent movement or deformation of organs and to react, i.e. show bleeding when a vessel is 'cut'. To convey a believable response, high-speed, real-time transmission of the image is required. Sensory feedback may be achieved by wearing special gloves which allow the surgeon to 'feel' what the instrument feels.[11]

Physicians at the Bowman-Gray School of Medicine have developed a model of 'virtual bronchoscopy'. They reconstructed a 3D image of the tracheobronchial tree using a helical CAT scan (Fig. 13.2). This representation of the tracheo-

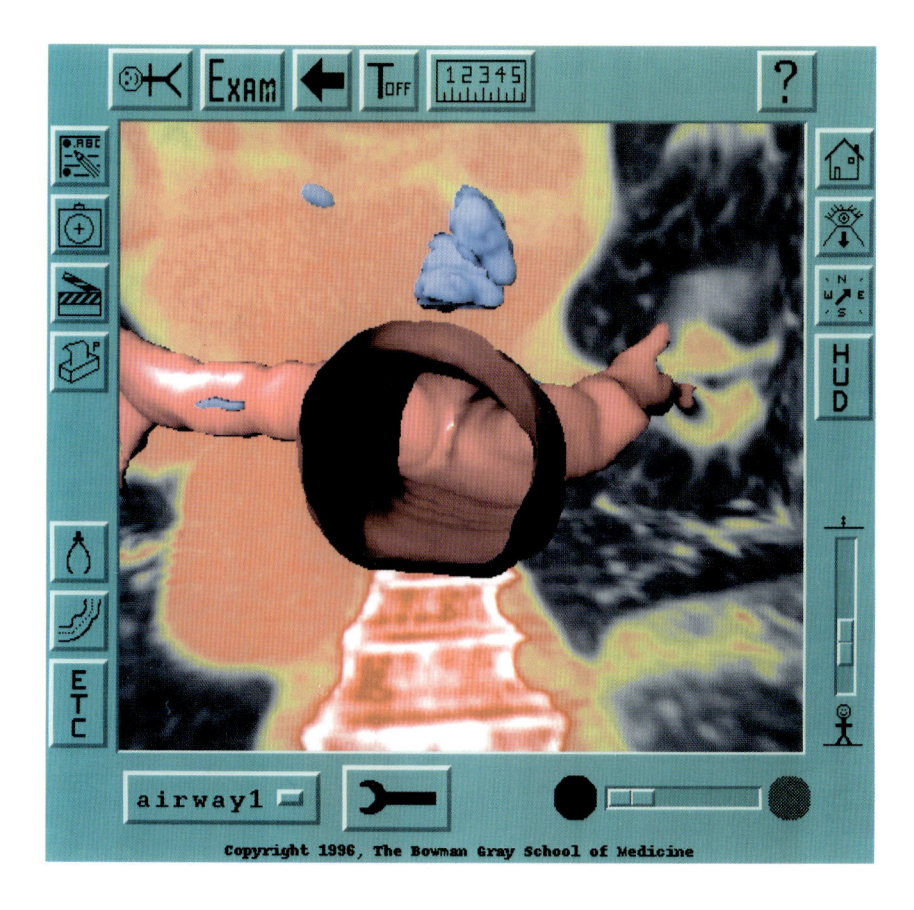

Figure 13.2 – Virtual bronchoscopy. Looking down the airway. (Surface-rendered airway (pink), lymph nodes (blue), heart and great vessels (orange) and lungs (grey).

Contributed by David J. Vining, Wake Forest University School of Medicine.

bronchial tree aids in prebronchoscopy planning, patient selection, endoscopy training and pulmonary research. One advantage of this system is the ability to render the simulated airway walls semitransparent, revealing extrabronchial structures from a perspective within the airway which may assist in transbronchial needle aspiration biopsy procedures. Another advantage is the image guidance for endobronchial treatment modalities such as laser therapy, brachytherapy and tracheobronchial stents. The virtual representation also provides the advantages of being able to 'bypass' an obstructing lesion or measure its dimensions better. Compared to traditional bronchoscopy, virtual bronchoscopy has only a limited ability to show mucosal detail and currently does not enable the practitioner to obtain biopsy specimens.[13]

LEGAL ISSUES

As telemedicine becomes more prevalent in clinical practice, several legal and ethical questions may be raised. Telemedicine may be practised within a region or across regional or international boundaries. It is important to determine the legality of consulting beyond the boundaries of one's medical licence. Several states in the US bar physicians without a state license from practising within that state. There is no definite decision on what constitutes 'practice'. It may be argued that a physician evaluating a patient via telecommunications is acting as a consultant only and is not the primary practising physician. The Joint Commission on Accreditation of Healthcare Organizations (JCAHO) recently concluded that as long as there is a referring physician primarily responsible for the patient, a consultant is not be required to be credentialed locally.[14] In the US, a possible solution to this problem might be the implementation of a federal licensing board which would allow interstate medical practice.

A second issue is malpractice. To what degree is the consulting physician responsible for the patient who has been evaluated via telemedicine? In addition, if legal action is brought, which malpractice laws apply - those of the region where the physician or where the patient is located? Many physicians and lawyers would agree that the best prophylaxis against malpractice claims is a strong physician-patient relationship. However, it would be expected that the distance between a physician and a patient communicating via an electronic interface would hinder the development of good rapport with the patient.

A third important issue to be determined is physician reimbursement. Medicare already requires documentation of 'face to face' interaction between the physician and the patient for reimbursement of services. Does a two-way, real-time, audio-video teleconferencing system satisfy this requirement? Telemedicine has the potential to reduce healthcare costs and, as the Americal Medical Association has argued, reimbursement should be designed to encourage the growth of telemedicine.[14] The Telemedicine Center at the Medical College of Georgia has been approved for Medicare and Medicaid reimbursement as long as a physician is present at both ends of the communication.[14] Louisiana is the first state to recognize telemedicine as a reimbursable service and mandate specific private health insurance coverage for it.[14]

THE FUTURE

In addition to unresolved legal issues, obstacles to the widespread application of telemedicine and virtual reality are computing and communications technology. In current systems, the fidelity of the graphics is sacrificed for faster, real-time transmission; however, these technologies are evolving rapidly. A second consideration is the high cost of this technology. A telecommunications workstation may cost more than US$100 000.[10] Network costs are equally important; satellite communication may cost up to US$3000 per hour. The Medical College of Virginia pays more than US$18 000 per month for one fiberoptic high capacity line.[10] Despite these challenges, the possibilities for the future extend to the limits of the imagination and beyond. If anyone should doubt the potential that lies ahead, they should review the following quote by the British surgeon Sir John Erichsen in 1873 during his introductory address to the medical institutions at University College London:

"There must be a final limit to the development of manipulative surgery, the knife cannot always have fresh fields for conquest and although methods of practice may be modified and varied and even improved to some extent, it must be within a certain limit. That this limit has nearly, if not quite, been reached will appear evident if we reflect on the great achievements of modern operative surgery. Very little remains for the boldest to devise or the most dexterous to perform."

REFERENCES

1. Brested JH. *The Edwin Smith Surgical Papyrus*. University of Chicago Press, Chicago, 1930.

2. Rosenberg SA. Principles of Surgical Oncology. In: DeVita VT, Hellman S, Rosenberg SA (eds). *Cancer: Principles and Practice of Oncology*, 5th edn. Lippincott-Raven, Philadelphia, PA, 1997, pp 238-247

3. Hill GJ. Historic milestones in cancer surgery. *Semin Oncol* 1979;6:409.

4. Muhe E. The first cholecystectomy through the laparoscope. *Langenbecks Arch Chir* 1986;**369**:804.

5. Southgate D. Stereoscopic imaging for laparoscopy. In: Arregui ME, Fitzgibbons RJ, Katkouda N, McKernan JB, Reich H (eds) *Principles of Laparoscopic Surgery*. Springer-Verlag, New York, 1995, pp 811-817

6. Laycock WS, Trus TL, Hunter JG. New technology for the division of short gastric vessels during laparoscopic Nissen fundoplication. A prospective randomized trial. *Surg Endosc* 1996;**10**:71-73.

7. Sackier JM, Wang Y. Robotically assisted laparoscopic surgery: From concept to development. Surg Endosc 1994; 8:63-66.

8. Flynn AM, Jones JL. *Mobile robots: Inspiration to implememtation*. AK Peters, Wellesley, MA,1993.

9. SAGES. *Guidelines for the Surgical Practice of Telemedicine*. 1996.

10. Hampton CL, Mazmanian PE, McCue MJ, Krick RS. Telemedicine in use: The Medical College of Virginia, The Powhatan Correctional Center and the Blackstone Family Practice Center. *Va Med Q* 1996; **123**:167-170.

11. Satava RM. Virtual reality and telepresence for military medicine. *Comput Biol Med* 1995; **25**:229-236.

12. Sheridan TB. *Telerobotics, Automation and Human Supervisory Control*. MIT Press, Cambridge, MA, 1992.

13. Vining DJ, Liu K, Choplin RH, Haponik EF, Virtual bronchoscopy: relationships of virtual reality endobronchial simulations to actual bronchoscopic findings. *Chest* 1996;**109**:549-553.

14. McMenamin JP. Telemedicine and the law. *Va Med Q* 1996;**123**:184-189.

Index

A

Abdominal
pain; 47, 139-140
wall hernias; 116
wall tumors; 11, 13

Abdominoperineal resection; 14, 71, 74, 79

Abscess; 112, 115, 117, 141

Absorption atelectasis; 104

Achalasia; 47, 50, 58

Acid
burns; 47
ingestion; 48

Acute cholecystitis; 63, 111, 119

Acute lung injury; 104

Adenocarcinoma; 42, 47-48, 50-53, 56-58, 63, 67, 72, 77, 79-80, 82, 101-102, 105, 131

Adenomatous polyps; 52

Adhesiolysis; 40, 127

Adhesion; 77-78, 82, 116
formation; 77-78, 82, 116

Adjuvant
radiation; 21
radiotherapy; 65
therapy; 38, 131, 138, 148-149, 153, 155

Adnexal masses; 130, 132

Adrenal
gland tumors; 141
glands; 141-142
metastases; 142

Adrenalectomy; 141-144

Advanced tumors; 20, 26

Aerodigestive tumors; 51

Aerosolization of tumor cells; 14

AESOP; – *See* Automated Endoscopic System for Optimal Positioning

Afterloading device; 54

Air
leak; 92
pneumoperitoneum; 9-10

Alcohol abuse; 50-51

Alkali ingestion; 48

Alveolar overdistension; 104

AMM; – *See* Myeloid metaplasia

Analgesics; 7, 91

Anastomosis; 5, 7-8, 55, 71-72, 80, 103-104, 109, 112-113

Anastomotic narrowing; 48

Angiography; 25, 27, 31-32, 36, 38

Angled telescopes; 86

Antibiotic prophylaxis; 111

Anus; 71, 115

Aortopulmonary window; 87, 102

Aparoscopic-assisted gastric bypass; 109

Appendectomy; 71

Arginine vasopressin (AVP); 19, 22

Arteriovenous;
malformation; 55

fistula; 140

Ascites; 25, 28, 112, 115, 118

Assessment; 9, 21, 26, 28-30, 33, 35-38, 40-42, 53, 80, 82, 101-103, 105-106, 125, 139,149, 155-156

Astler-Coller B; 75

Astler-Coller C colorectal cancer; 75

Atelectasis; 104, 140

Athymic mice; 8-9

Automated Endoscopic System for Optimal Positioning (AESOP); 159

Avary-Guillard bougies; 53

AVP; – *See* Arginine vasopressin;

Axillary
dissection; 147-151, 153-156
vein; 148, 151-153

Azygous vein; 103

B

B-cell function; 138

B-mode images; 31

Backwash ileitis; 57

Bacteremia; 112

Bacteria; 6, 112

Bags or wound protectors; 14, 75

Balloon
devices; 48
expandable endoprostheses; 110

163

Barium
  contrast studies; 55
  enema; 55

Barrett's esophagus; 50, 58

Benign
  lesions; 57, 87, 95-96
  stricture; 48
  thymomas; 95

Bile
  duct obstruction; 33, 41, 110, 112
  gastritis; 48, 113
  leakage; 110
  leaks; 111-112

Biliary
  bypass; 26, 110, 112-113
  drainage; 110-112, 119
  sepsis; 112
  stents; 36, 111

Billroth
  I reconstruction; 52
  II reconstruction; 52

Biloma; 117-118

Biopsies; 21, 33, 43, 48-52, 85, 87, 89, 91, 94, 96, 102, 128, 130-131, 137

Bleeding; 48, 52, 54-55, 57-58, 92-93, 96, 110-112, 115-118, 160
  complications; 92
  – See also Chronic -rectal bleeding

Blood-clot formation; 116

Blunt transhiatal approach; 103

Bouginage; 53

Brachytherapy; 19, 53, 58, 161

Breast
  biopsies; 89
  cancer; – See Carcinoma
  imaging; 147

Bronchogenic
  carcinoma; 37, 97
  cysts; 95

Bronchus; 104

Brush cytology; 48, 51

C

C-reactive protein; 4

Cancer; – See Carcinoma

Cannula-site metastasis; 64

Capsular liver lesions; 37

Carbon dioxide embolism; 117

Carcino-embryonic antigen; 117

Carcinoma;
  ampullary; 109
  breast; 37,19, 21, 114, 145, 147-151, 153-156
    - metastatic 114, 117
    - mouse mammary (MMC); 6-9
    - non-invasive breast; 148, 153
  colon 3, 9-10, 16, 57, 65, 77, 80, 82, 114, 117-118, 144
    - metastatic 114
    - family history of, 57
  colorectal; 57, 72, 79-80
  cervical; 81, 123-125, 131-133
  cholangiocarcinoma; 36, 114
  ductal - in situ (DCIS); 148, 155
  duodenal; 52, 109
  esophageal; 33, 42, 47, 49-55, 58, 99, 101-103, 105-106, 114
    - mucosal of the; 104, 106
  gall bladder; 36, 63-68, 81, 114
  gastroesophageal; 26
  gastroduodenal; 33-35, 42
  gastric; 29, 34-35, 42, 48-49, 52, 101, 105-106, 109, 118-119
  hepatocellular; 22, 37-38, 43, 82, 139
  in situ; 51, 63-64, 68, 148, 155
  lung; 20, 87, 89-90, 93-94, 96-97, 118
  non-small cell lung; 87, 89-93
  ovarian ; 39, 118, 123, 128, 130-133
  pancreatic; 21, 25-26, 28, 31-32, 35, 40-42, 109, 114, 118-119
  rectal; 57, 80
  squamous; 50
    - cell carcinoma; 47, 51, 101, 105

Carcinomatosis; 11, 32, 75, 144

Cardiac
  arrhythmias; 91
  obstruction; 109
  tamponade; 94

Cardinal ligaments; 124

Catheter
  migration; 116
  - related complications; 112
  - site infections; 116

Caustic
  injury; 51
  stricture; 47

Cavernous hemangioma; 139

CCD; – See Charged couple devices

CEA; – See Carcino-embryonic antigen

Cecal resection; 4-5, 7, 15

Celiac
  axis; 29
  ganglia; 109
  nodes; 29

Cell
  proliferation; 9, 65
  suspension; 11-14

Cervical
  cancer; – See Carcinoma
  dissection; 104

Charged coupled devices (CCD); 47

Chemical destruction; 109

Chemotherapy; 19, 21, 53, 65-67, 75, 87, 90, 96, 101, 103, 105, 116, 125, 128, 132, 137-139, 141, 147

Chest tube; 85, 90-91

Cholangiocarcinoma;
  – See Carcinoma

Cholangiography; 29, 33, 36, 41, 112

Cholangitis; 110-111, 113, 119

Cholecystectomy; 4, 15, 22, 36, 42, 61, 63-68, 71, 77, 81-82, 93, 112, 118, 144, 159, 162

Cholecystoduodenostomy; 114

Cholecystojejunostomy; 110-114, 119

Choledochoduodenostomy; 114

Choledochojejunostomy; 110-114

Chronic
  atrophic gastritis; 51
  lymphocytic leukemia (CLL); 139, 141

myelogenous leukemia (CML); 139, 141
rectal bleeding; 55
ulcerative colitis; 57

Chylous leak; 103

Circular stapling gun; 103-104

Cirrhosis; 25, 37-38, 118

Clinical Outcomes of Surgery Trial (COST); 3

CLL; – See Chronic lymphocytic leukemia

CML; – See Chronic myelogenous leukemia

CO_2 pneumoperitoneum; 4-5, 9-14, 16, 19, 140

Coagulation; 19

Coagulopathy; 110, 115, 117

Colectomy; 4, 10-11, 14-16, 21-22, 57, 69, 71-75, 77, 79-82, 144, 147

Colon; 3, 8-10, 14-16, 20, 22, 26, 35, 39, 52, 55-57, 59, 63-65, 68, 71-73, 75, 77-82, 114-118, 130, 139, 142, 144, 154, 159-160
cancer; – See Carcinoma
resection; 3, 20, 52, 65, 72-73, 78-80, 82, 159
tumor; 8
-26; 7

Colonoscope; 55, 57

Colonoscopy; 55, 57, 75

Colorectal; 3, 15-16, 20, 22, 25, 37-40, 43, 57, 71-73, 75, 77, 79-82
cancer; – See Carcinoma
malignancies; 3, 77

Common bile duct; 39, 41, 112-113, 119

Complications of cryosurgery; 117

Computed tomography; (CT) 21, 25-28, 31-32, 34-38, 42-43, 64-67, 85, 87-89, 92-93, 101-102, 105-106, 117, 119, 138-139
arterioportography (CTAP); 38, 43
-guided methylene blue injections; 89
-guided needle localization; 89

Contact
laser application; 53
agents; 53

Contrast radiography; 28

COST; – See Clinical Outcomes of Surgery Trial

Creatinine; 138

Crohn's disease; 57

Cryoprobes; 117

Cryosurgery; 109, 116-118, 120

CT; – See Computed tomography

CTAP; – See Computed tomography arterioportography

Cuff extrusion; 116

Cup biopsy forceps; 39

Cystectomies; 127

Cystic schwannoma; 95

Cystoscope; 25, 85, 96

Cytokine levels; 19

Cytopenia; 139

D

2 Deoxycofomycin; 139

DCIS; – See Carcinoma;

Deep
vein thrombophlebitis; 19
vein thrombosis; 19

Deep-seated
intra- hepatic lesions; 37
intrahepatic metastases; 31

Delayed type hypersensitivity (DTH); 4-5, 15

Dermatitis; 115

Desufflation; 11-12, 14

Diagnostic
imaging; 20, 66
laparoscopy; 25, 37, 40-43, 66

Dialysate leakage; 116

Diaphragm; 11, 35, 102-103, 118, 126, 131, 138

Diaphragmatic
biopsies; 128
plication; 94

Diffuse; 36-39, 51, 64-65, 88, 96, 138
peritoneal seeding; 65

Distal bile duct tumors; 36

Distant metastases; 3, 102

Diverticulosis; 55

Diverting Colostomy; 115

DNA synthesis; 9

Doppler US; 32

Double lumen
endotracheal tube; 85-86, 103

Double-stapling technique; 103-104

Drug-delivery catheters; 109, 116, 118

DTH; – See Delayed type hypersensitivity

Ductal carcinoma in situ (DCIS); – See Carcinoma

Dukes'
A lesions; 77
B lesions; 77
C lesions; 77
classification; 72

Duodenal
obstruction; 109
perforation; 111
polyps; 51-52

DVT; 19

Dysgerminoma; 131

Dysphagia; 47, 53-54
melena; 47

Dysplasia; 48, 50-52, 57

E

EAE; – See Endoscopic axillary exploration

Echogenicity; 36

Ectopic spleens; 140

Edema; 104, 111, 116, 120, 148, 155

EGD; – See Esophagogastroduodenoscopy

EMS; 111, 114

Endodissection; 104-106

Endometrial cancer; 123, 125-128, 132-133

Endoprosthesis; 41, 66, 68, 110-111

Endoscopic
  axillary exploration (EAE); 151-154, 156
  cautery; 110
  cholecystojejunostomy; 113
  dilation; 110
  lymphadenectomy; 151
  metal stent; 111, 114
  palliation; 52-53, 110, 114, 119
  plastic stent (EPS); 111, 113-114
  retrograde cholangiography; 29
  retrograde cholangiopancreatography; 33, 47, 111, 119
  screening; 48-49, 51-52, 58
  sphincterotomy; 111, 113
  stent placement; 54, 110-111, 113
  ultrasonography (EUS); 21, 28, 31, 35-36, 102, 106

Endoscopy; 40-43, 47-48, 52-53, 55, 57-58, 67, 81, 114-115, 119, 123, 161

Endotoxin; 6

Enteral feeding; 109, 114

Enterobacter; 141

Enterotomies; 127

Environmental factors; 49, 51

EPS; – See Endoscopic plastic stent

ERCP; – See Endoscopic cholangiopancreatography

Escherichia coli; 141

Esophageal
  carcinoma; – See Carcinoma
  endoscopy; 47
  resection; 55, 102, 105

Esophagectomy; 50-51, 101, 103-106

Esophagogastroduodenoscopy; 47

Esophagogastric cancer; 101, 105

EUS; – See Endoscopic ultrasonography

Evisceration; 116

Exophytic lesions; 48

Extended-field radiation therapy; 125

Extraluminal malignancy; 109

Extraluminal tumor; 110

F

Factor VIII; 19, 22

Familial polyposis; 51-52, 58

Fiberoptic
  bronchoscopy; 87, 96
  bundle; 25, 47, 104
  technology; 47

Fibrinolysis; 141

Fibromas; 139

Fibrosis; 32, 37

Fibrous tumors; 95

Flexible endoscope; 47, 53, 55, 103

Flexible gastroscopy; 48

Fluoroscopy; 54, 114-115

Focal abnormalities; 39

Follow-up; 3, 10, 14, 22, 50-51, 53, 55, 58, 66, 72, 75, 78, 90, 105, 117, 132, 138, 143, 149, 155

Frost bite; 117-118

Frozen section; 67, 89, 124, 128, 149

Fundoplication; 58, 71, 162

Fungating mass; 66

G

Gadolinium enhancement; 102

Gallbladder; 10, 20, 22, 28, 36-37, 39, 42-43, 61, 63-68, 71, 75, 77, 81, 112-113, 142, 144
  cancer; – See Carcinoma
  cytology; 66

Gallium scans; 139

Gamma
  globulin; 139
  probe guided mapping; 151

Ganglioneuroma; 95

Gardner's syndrome; 51

Gas embolism; 117

Gasless laparotomy; 12

Gastric
  bypass; 109-110, 118
  cancer; – See Carcinoma
  lymphoma; 49, 58
  polyps; 51-52, 58
  ulcers; 48

Gastroduodenal
  passage; 109-110
  cancer; – See Carcinoma

Gastroesophageal
  carcinoma; – See Carcinoma
  junction; 35, 48, 50, 58, 101-102

Gastrointestinal
  bleed; 141
  hemorrhage; 110
  malignancy; 21, 42, 49, 52, 55, 58, 119
    – early detection of; 49
    – high risk groups; 49
    – screening for; 49

Gastrojejunostomy; 109-110, 113, 118

Gastrostomy; 110, 114-115, 120

General anesthesia; 19, 39, 48, 151, 159

Genital edema; 116, 120

Gram negative bacteria; 6

Granulomas; 39

Groin hematoma; 140

H

H&E staining; 150

Hairy cell leukemia (HCL); 139, 141, 143

Hamartomas; 139

Hamartomatous lesions; 39

Hand-held gamma probe; 151

Harmonic scalpel; 71

HCL; – *See* Hairy cell leukemia

HDRB; – *See* High-dose rate brachytherapy

Head and neck cancer; 51, 120

Helical CAT scan; 160

Helicobacter pylori infection; 51, 58

Helium pneumoperitoneum; 9, 12

Hemangiosarcomas; 139

Hematoma; 20, 113, 140

Hemicolectomy; 77-78

Hemidiaphragm; 130, 132

Hemobilia; 111

Hemophylis influenzae; 141

Hemorrhage; 32, 71, 85, 90, 92-93, 103-105, 109-110, 140

Hemostasis; 20, 56, 142

Hepati-cojejunostomy; 110

Hepatic parenchyma; 112, 117

Hepaticogastrostomy; 110-113, 119

Hepatitis; 38

Hepatocellular carcinoma; – *See* Carcinoma

Hepatoma; 118

Hereditary spherocytosis; 137

Herniorrhaphy; 71

Hiatus hernia; 48

High-dose
 radiation; 48
 rate brachytherapy (HDRB); 53

High-resolution
 graphics; 160
 photography; 47

Hilar
 hemorrhage; 92
 obstruction; 112, 119

Histiocytic lymphoma; 139

Histologic examination; 21, 149

Hodgkin's disease; 137-138, 140-141, 143

Hopkins rod-lens optical system; 25

Hyaluronidase membrane; 78

Hyperamylasemia; 111

Hypercoagulability; 19, 22

Hyperechoic; 31-32, 35-36

Hyperplastic lymphadenopathy; 102

Hyperplastic polyps; 52

Hypersplenism; 139, 141

Hypoechoic masses; 35

Hysterectomy; 123-128, 131-133

I

Idiopathic thrombocytopenic pupura (ITP); 137-138, 143

Ileostomy; 78

Ileus; 72, 115, 140

Imaging studies; 21, 55

Immune
 function; 3-6, 8-10, 14-15, 19
 suppression; 19

Immunogenic tumors; 9

Immunohistochemical techniques; 150

Immunologic
 deficiencies; 141
 markers; 19

Immunosuppression; 4-6, 9, 14-15

Incidence of port-site tumors; 10, 14

Incidentalomas; 142

Incisional hernia; 116

INF-alpha; 139

Infection; 3, 20, 32, 51, 58, 110, 115-116, 140-141, 143

Inferior vena cava; 29, 117

Inflammatory bowel disease; 57

Infracolic omentectomy; 128

Infragastric bursoscopy; 28

Injury; 11-12, 50-51, 92-93, 103-104, 112, 115, 117, 126, 130, 148

Intercostal
 hemorrhages; 92
 neuralgia; 91

Interleukin (IL-6); 4

Interstitial lung disease; 86, 91, 97

Intra-abdominal
 malignancy; 23, 25-27, 29, 31, 33, 35, 37, 39-41, 43
 malignant neoplasms; 26
 metastases; 26, 32, 36, 42, 105

Intrahepatic
 biliary dilatation; 36
 lesion; 37

Intraluminal
 radiation; 53
 stents; 54
 tumor spread; 35

Intraoperative
 cholangiography; 112
 colonoscopy; 75
 ultrasound (US); 37, 89

Intraperitoneal
 chemotherapy; 116
 leakage; 115

Intrathoracic hemorrhage; 92

Intubation; 22, 48

Irrigators; 14

Isolating lymph nodes 73

Isosulfan blue; 150

ITP; – *See* Idiopathic thrombocytopenic pupura

Ivor-Lewis technique; 103

J

Jaundice; 26, 28, 33, 39, 41, 63, 111, 113-114, 119

Jejunal tube placement; 115

Jejunostomy; 103, 114-115, 119-120

K

Keyhole limpet hemocyanin (KLH); 4-5

Kidney; 11-12, 137

L

LACR; – *See* Laparoscopic-assisted colon resection 3, 10, 14

Lactate dehydrogenase; 138

Laparoscopic
- assisted abdominoperineal resections; 74
- assisted colon resection (LACR); 3
- assisted surgical staging (LASS); 126, 128, 131-132
- assisted vaginal hysterectomy (LAVH); 124, 126

cholecystcholangiography; 28
cholecystectomy; 4, 15, 22, 36, 42, 61, 63-68, 71, 77, 81-82. 93, 112, 144, 159
cholecystojejunostomy (LCCJ); 111-113, 119
choledochojejunostomy (LCDJ); 111-114
colectomy; 11, 14, 16, 21-22, 69, 71-73, 75, 77, 79-82, 147
colorectal surgery; 16, 71-73, 79-82
colostomy; 116
fecal diversion; 115-116
gastrojejunostomy; 109, 113
gastrostomy; 115
- guided biopsy; 28, 39
hepaticogastrostomy; 111
hepaticojejunostomy; 111, 114
jejunostomy; 115, 119
lymphadenectomy; 123-124, 126, 131-133
para-aortic lymphadenectomy; 123, 125
pelvic lymphadenectomy; 68, 123
peritoneal cytology; 29-30, 42
proctosigmoidectomy; 74
staging; 21, 29, 32, 35, 38, 40, 42, 101-103, 106, 126, 128, 130-131, 133
3-port technique; 102
4-port technique; 102
transperitoneal pelvic lymphadenectomies; 123
ultrasonography (LapUS); 22, 25-27, 29, 31-39, 41-43, 101, 117
- 180° sector scanning probe; 38
- 360° sector scanning probe; 3, 37

Laparoscopy; 4, 6, 8-9, 12, 15-16, 20-22, 25-43, 64-68, 72, 75, 77-82, 85, 101-102, 105, 107, 109, 111-113, 115-117, 119, 121, 123-133, 140, 162

Laparotomy; 4-10, 12, 14-16, 20, 25-27, 29-30, 32, 34-39, 43, 57, 64-66, 68, 72, 74-75, 77-78, 101-103, 109, 115-116, 124-128, 130-133, 137-139, 141, 143

LapUS; – *See* Laparoscopic ultrasonography (LapUS)

Laryngeal
 nerve palsies; 96, 104

Laser
 ablation; 48, 55, 106
 probes; 111

LASS; – *See* Laparoscopic-assisted surgical staging

Lateral decubitus position; 86, 94

LAVH; – *See* Laparoscopic-assisted vaginal hysterectomy

LCCJ; – *See* Laparoscopic cholecystojejunostomy

LCDJ; – *See* Laparoscopic choledochojejunostomy

Left hepatic lobe; 39

Legal issues; 161-162

Leiomyosarcoma; 118

Leukemia; 137, 139, 141, 143

Ligament of Treitz; 29

Linear array probe; 38

Lipomas; 95, 139

Liquid nitrogen; 116-117

Liver
 abscess; 112
 biopsy; 38, 43, 139
 capsule tear; 117
 cirrhosis 25
 insufficiency; 110
 malignancies; 26, 117
 metastases; 25-28, 32, 34, 37-38, 40, 42-43, 102
 metastasis; 28, 105, 109, 113
 tumors; 36-38, 40, 43, 117, 120, 159

Lobectomy; 86, 89-90, 92-93, 96-97, 118

Locoregional staging; 29, 35-36

Long-term; 3, 14, 54, 63, 66, 71-73, 75, 77-79, 90, 93, 104, 110, 112-114, 117, 132, 149, 155

Lugols' solution; 51

Lumpectomy; 149, 155-156

Lung cancer; – *See* Carcinoma

Lye; 47, 51

Lymph node; 3, 19, 21, 29, 31-32, 36, 39, 42, 63-64, 66, 73-75, 79, 90, 94-96, 101-104, 106, 110, 123-126, 128-133, 137-139,145, 147-153, 155-156 161
 basins; 149-150, 156
 harvest; 3, 73-75, 79
 staging; 101-102

Lymphadenectomy; 15, 68, 81, 104, 123-128, 131-133, 147, 149-151, 154-156

Lymphangiogram; 138

Lymphangiography; 137

Lymphocyte; 4, 6

Lymphoedema; 147

Lymphoma; 37, 49, 58, 95, 106, 123, 132, 137-139, 141, 143

M

Magnetic resonance imaging (MRI); 21, 25, 95, 101-102, 105

Malabsorbtion; 110

Malignancy; 3, 9, 16, 21, 23, 25-29, 31-33, 35-43, 49-50, 52, 55, 58, 63, 66, 71, 79-80, 93, 102, 109-110, 112-114, 119, 128, 141-142

Malignant
  lymphadenopathy; 32, 36
  melanoma; 37, 156
  nodules; 93
  ovarian tumors; 43, 130
  peritoneal seedlings; 27

Malpractice; 161-162

Mammography; 147, 154-155

Marginal ulcer; 48

Margins; 3, 19, 21, 32, 73-75, 79, 117, 156

Mass screening; 49

Mediastinal; 21, 47, 90-91, 94-96, 98, 102-104
  lymphatic seeding; 47
  masses; 94, 96, 98
  – *See also* Video-assisted thoracic surgery (VATS)

Mediastinoscope; 85, 103-104

Mediastinoscopy; 85, 87, 94, 96, 102

Melanoma; 7, 15, 37, 149-151, 156

Melanoma B-16; 7

Melena; 47, 57

Mesenteric
  root; 29, 39
  venous thrombosis; 19

Metastases; 3, 13, 16, 20-22, 25-28, 31-40, 42-43, 67-68, 75, 79-82, 92, 94-95, 97, 101-102, 104-105, 118, 124-125, 131, 133, 138, 142, 155

Metastatic
  breast cancer; – *See* Carcinoma
  colon cancer; – *See* Carcinoma
  esophageal cancer; 114
  implants; 21
  lymphadenopathy; 102
  osteosarcoma; 92, 98
  workup; 67

Microinvasion; 148, 155

Micrometastasis; 150

Microperforations of the bowel; 77

Microscopic omental metastases; 131

Microsurgical tools; 104

Mini-laparotomy; 5, 102

MMC; – *See* Carcinoma

Monoclonal-tagged yttrium; 128

Monocyte; 5

Mouse mammary carcinoma (MMC); – *See* Carcinoma

MRI; – *See* Magnetic resonance imaging

Mucosa; 21, 35, 48-49, 63-64, 66

Mucosal
  cancer of the esophagus; – *See* carcinoma 104, 106
  resections; 105
  thickening; 66

Muscle-sparing thoracotomy; 90, 97

Myasthenia gravis; 95

Myeloid metaplasia; 137, 139, 143
  agnogenic (AMM); 139, 141
  Postpolycythemic(PPMM); 139
  – *See also* Postpolycythemia vera

N

Nanotechnology; 160

Nasobiliary catheter; 110-111

Nasogastric feeding tubes; 114

Nasojejunal feeding tubes; 114

Needle biopsy; 20, 37-39, 43, 87, 96

Neodymium-YAG laser; 53, 119

Neoplasia; 47, 49-50, 58, 133

Neurogenic tumors; 95

Neutrophil
  chemotaxis; 4
  function; 19

Nitrogen embolus; 117, 120

Nodal
  dissection; 19
  metastases; 34, 124

Nodular lymphoma; 139

Non-Hodgkin's lymphoma; 123, 132, 137-139, 141, 143

Non-invasive breast cancers;
  – *See* Carcinoma

Non-small cell lung cancer;
  – *See* Carcinoma

O

Obstructive jaundice; 26, 28, 33, 39, 41, 111, 113-114, 119

Occluded stent; 111

Occlusion; 110-112, 114

Occult hepatic metastases; 38

Odynophagia; 47

Omental; 26, 116, 125, 131
  carpet; 125

Omentum; 25, 28, 39, 64, 101, 116, 126, 128, 130-131

Open
  cholecystectomy; 4, 66
  lobectomy; 90
  resections; 93
  thoracotomy; 90, 92, 103

Ovarian
  cancer; – *See* Carcinoma
  tumors; 20, 22, 37, 43, 81, 130

Ovary; 43, 115, 126, 128, 132

P

Palliation; 6, 35, 40-41, 52-54, 58, 68, 109-110, 112-114, 118-119, 137, 141

Palliative
  bypass surgery; 109
  laparoscopic bypass; 25
  surgery; 37

Pancreatic; 20-22, 25-33, 35-37, 39-42, 50, 75, 82, 109, 111, 113-114, 118-119, 140
  cancer; – *See* Carcinoma
  necrosis; 140

Pancreaticobiliary sepsis; 111
Pancreaticoduodenectomy; 21, 110
Pancreatitis; 112, 140
Para-aortic
　lymph nodes; 125, 128, 131
　lymph; 130-132
　lymphadenopathy; 35
Parabronchial lymph node; 104
Paracolic gutters; 39, 130
Paraesophageal lymph nodes; 102
Parenchymal tears; 117
Parenteral feeding; 114
Parietal pleura; 88, 103
Partial thromboplastin time (PTT); 137
PCNA; – See Proliferating cell nuclear antigen
PEG; – See Percutaneous endoscopic gastrostomy
PEJ; – See Percutaneous endoscopic jejunostomy
Pelvic
　lymph; 123, 128, 130
　node dissection; 125, 132
　washings; 128
Pelvis; 39, 47, 67, 75, 126, 140
Percutaneous endoscopic gastrostomy (PEG); 114-115, 120
Percutaneous endoscopic jejunostomy (PEJ); 114-115, 120
Percutaneous
　non-endoscopic gastrostomy; 114-115
　stent placement; 110
　transhepatic; 29, 33, 111-114, 119
　transhepatic cholangiography (PTC); 33
　transhepatic stent (PTS); 111-114
　transhepatic stent placement; 113
Periampullary
　cancers; 52
　carcinoma; 30
　malignancies; 114
Pericardial windows; 94

Perigastric; 29
Perineal phlegmon; 58
Perineum; 71
Perioperative
　pulmonary aspiration; 104
　tumor growth; 9, 14
Peripheral lesions; 93
Periportal lymph node biopsy; 29
Peritoneal
　cavity; 5-6, 11, 15, 20-21, 25, 29-30, 38-40, 115, 141
　cytology; 29-30, 41-42, 128
　dialysis; 116, 120
　seeding; 20, 65, 81, 101
　washings; 29, 42, 128
Peritonitis; 25, 115-116
Peritube leakage; 115
Pernicious anemia; 51
Phytohemagglutinin (PHA); 4-5
Placement of feeding tubes; 114-115
Plain films; 85
Pleural
　adhesions; 85, 90, 103
　effusion; 94, 117, 138
Pleuropericardial cysts; 95
Plugging; 115
Pneumobilia; 36
Pneumonectomy; 91, 93, 97
Pneumoperitoneum; 4-5, 7-14, 16, 19-20, 25, 77, 82, 115, 140
Pneumothorax; 86-87, 112
Polycythemia vera; 139
　– See also Myeloid metaplasia
Polypectomy; 52, 72, 75
Polypoid
　disease; 49
　lesions; 48
Polyps; 51-52, 57-58, 64
Polyvalent pneumococcal vaccine; 140
Porcelain gallbladder; 64-65
Port-site
　hemorrhage; 32

　metastases; 20, 42, 75
　metastasis; 65, 67
　seeding; 32, 36
　tumor; 3, 10, 12-14
Portal; 28-29, 31-32, 36, 38-39, 64, 117, 139
　hypertension; 28, 139
　vein resection; 32
Positron emission tomography; 21
Posterior laminectomy; 95
Postoperative
　pain; 19, 57, 72, 85, 90-91, 104, 112, 141-142
　sepsis; 3
Postsplenectomy sepsis; 138, 141
PPMM; – See Myeloid metaplasia
Pre-operative endoscopic cholangiopancreatography (ERCP); 32-33, 47, 111, 119
Prebronchoscopy planning; 161
Premalignant lesions; 49-50
Preoperative
　evaluation; 21, 26, 55, 66, 139-140
　laparoscopy; 32
　staging; 19, 26, 28, 37-38, 41-42, 105
Preventive radiation; 65
Proctocolectomies; 40
Proctoscope; 25
Prolapse; 115
Proliferating cell nuclear antigen (PCNA); 9
Proliferation index; 9
Prostate; 115
Prothrombin (PT); 137, 154-155
Proximal bile duct carcinomas; 36
Pruritus; 110, 112
Pseudomonas sp; 141
PTC; – See Percutaneous transhepatic cholangiography
PTS; – See Percutaneous transhepatic stent

Pulmonary
    artery injury; 92
    complications; 103-105, 116
    edema; 104
    infection; 141
    resection; 89, 97

Pyloric obstruction; 109

Q

Quality of life; 21, 54

R

Radial scanning; 38

Radical
    cholecystectomy; 64
    hysterectomy; 123-125, 131-133
    mastectomy; 147, 155
    surgery; 101, 147
    vaginal hysterectomy; 124-125, 131, 133

Radiolymphoscintigraphy; 151

Raised mucosa; 66

Recanalization; 110-111

Rectal
    adenomas; 57
    carcinoma; – See Carcinoma

Rectoscope; 57

Rectovaginal fistula; 58

Recurrent malignancy; 39

Reduction pneumoplasty; 86

Reflex diaphragmatic dysfunction; 104

Reflux
    bile gastritis; 48
    esophagitis; 47, 50, 58

Regional lymphadenopathy; 31, 35-36

Remote manipulation; 20

Renal
    capsule; 8
    failure; 110
    insufficiency; 138

Resection; 3-8, 10-11, 13-15, 20-22, 26, 29-30, 32, 35, 37-38, 47-48, 51-53, 55-57, 64-67, 71-75, 77-80, 82, 86-87, 89, 92-98, 101-106, 109-110, 116-118, 147, 150, 156, 159
    margins; 32
    - open laparoscopic; 3

Respiratory failure; 91, 104

Retrogastric mass; 28

Robotics; 159

S

S-phase; 9, 148

Sampling errors; 50-51

Schauta procedure; 124

Screening; 47-52, 58, 148, 154-155

Sealed specimen bag; 93

Second-look
    laparoscopies; 39-40, 43 128, 130
    laparotomies; 39, 130

Secondary
    biliary radicles; 36
    tumor sites; 20

Sector scanning probe
    (180°, 360°); – See Laparoscopic ultrasonography (Lap US)

Seeding; 10-11, 20, 22, 32, 36, 38, 42-43, 47, 65-68, 77, 81-82, 92-94, 101, 120

Segmental colectomies; 71

Segmentectomy; 93

Self-breast examinations; 147

Self-expandable endoprostheses; 110, 119

Sentinel node
    biopsy; 150, 156
    lymphadenectomy; 150-151, 154

Seroma; 147-148

Serosal; 26, 33

Sertoli-Leydig cell tumor; 131

Serum amylase; 112

Sham
    laparotomy; 4-6, 9, 12
    procedure studies; 7

Simulators; 160

Single lung ventilation; 85-86

Sister Mary Joseph's nodules; 65

Skin reactivity; 19

Small-bowel enterotomy; 130

Snare wire; 57

Solid
    stents; 54
    tumors; 19-20, 141

Solitary pulmonary nodule; 87-89

Specimen bags; 14, 86

Spine surgery; 94

Spiral CT scanning; 28

Spleen; 13, 137-141, 143

Splenectomy; 13, 137-143, 159

Splenic
    artery embolism; 140
    infarction; 139
    tumors; 13, 139

Splenomegaly; 28, 139-141, 143

Spontaneous pneumothorax; 86

Squamous
    carcinoma; – See Carcinoma
    cell carcinoma; – See Carcinoma

Staging; 19-22, 23, 25-43, 63, 67, 73, 82, 87, 94, 96-97, 101-106, 112, 123, 125-128, 130-133, 137-141, 143, 148-149, 153, 156

Staphylococcus aureus; 141

Stapled anastomosis; 104

Stapling; 78, 90, 92, 97, 103-104, 106, 109, 127

Steatosis; 37-38

Stenotic lesions; 48

Stent; 21, 26, 54, 110-114, 119
    fracture; 111
    migration; 111-112, 119

3D Stereoscopic view; 159

Stoma formation; 116

Stomach; 20, 26, 35, 39, 42, 47-48, 52, 58, 63-64, 101, 103-104, 109, 114-115

Streptococcus pneumoniae; 141

Stress; 4, 15-16, 66, 140-141

Stress ulcer; 141

Stricture; 47-48, 51-55, 58, 104

Subcapsular hematoma; 113

Subclavian artery injury; 92

Submucosal spread; 47

Subphrenic
   abscess; 117, 141
   spaces; 39

Superficial; 37, 48, 117

Superoxide anion;, 5

Supragastric
   bursoscopy; 28
   pancreoscopy; 28

Surgical trauma; 4

Sympathetic denervation; 94

Symptomatic reflux; 113

T

T-cell; 4

T-fasteners; 115, 119

T1-weighted spin-echo images; 102

T2-weighted spin-echo images; 102

Table tilt mechanism; 39

Tactile
   sensation; 75
   sensor; 89, 97

Tamoxifen; 149, 155

Tapered bougies; 53

Technetium-labeled sulfur colloid; 151

Teleconsultation; 160

Telemedicine; 160-162

Telepresence; 159-160, 162

TEM; 57-58

Tenckhoff catheters; 116

Testes; 154

Therapeutic
   laparoscopy; 66
   protocols; 101

Thermal probes; 111

Third-look laparoscopies; 39, 128

Thoracic duct injury; 103

Thoracic outlet syndrome; 94

Thoracodorsal nerve; 153

Thoracoscopy; 20-21, 85-86, 90, 96-98, 102, 104, 106
   staging; 102, 106

Thoracotomy; 21, 85-87, 89-94, 96-97, 101, 103-104

Three-stage esophagectomy; 103

Thrombocytopenia; 117, 139, 141

Thymic cysts; 95

Thymomas;,94-95

Thymus gland;, 95

TNF; – See Tumor necrosis factor

TNM staging; 21, 32, 35

Tobacco abuse; 50-51

Toothed forceps; 39

Total abdominal colectomy; 57

Tracheoesophageal fistulae; 47, 54

Transabdominal US; 31, 33, 36

Transanal endoscopic microsurgery; 57, 59

Transbronchial biopsy; 87

Transhiatal esophagectomy; 103-106

Transient phrenic nerve; 96

Transthoracic
   core biopsy; 87
   fine needle aspirates; 93
   needle biopsy; 87, 96

Trocar
   injury;130
   metastases; 20
   site incision;10

Truncal vagotomies;109

Tube migration;115

Tuberculous peritonitis;25

Tumor ; 3, 6-14, 19-22, 25-26, 28, 30-31, 35-38, 40-41, 43, 48, 51-52, 57-59, 66, 81, 83, 85-87, 89-91, 93-95, 97, 101, 103, 105, 109-111, 113-115, 117, 119-120, 130, 137, 139, 141-142, 148, 151, 154-155, 159
   behavior; 8
   cell lines; 7, 10
   cell proliferation; 9
   destruction; 9
   growth; 3, 6-12, 14-16, 64, 67-68, 77, 82
   ingrowth; 32, 3, 110-111
   manipulation; 20
   margins; 19, 21
   markers; 21, 40
   necrosis factor (TNF); 5
   prognostic factors; 149
   recurrence; 16, 22, 64-65, 67, 72, 80, 92, 94
   recurrence at VATS ports; 92
   staging; 22, 25, 33, 38, 41

Two-stage ileoanal J-pouch; 78

Type A gastritis; 51

Type B atrophic gastritis; 51

U

Ulcerative colitis; 57

Ultrasonography (US); 22, 25-28, 31-39, 41-43, 49, 63-64, 66-67, 78, 91, 101-102, 106, 117 147, 161-162
   -guided fine-needle aspiration cytology; 39

Ureteral stents; 75

Uric acid; 138

US; – See Ultrasonography

Uterine vessels; 124

Utility incision; 86, 90, 92-94

V

3D Vision; 160

Vaginal cuff;124

Vaginal margin;124

Vascular
  invasion; 29, 31-32, 104, 148
  ligation; 71, 73
  staplers; 71
  trauma; 19

Vasopressin; 19, 22

VATS; – *See* Video-assisted thoracic surgery

Venous stasis; 19

Video
  recording; 47
  -assisted thoracic surgery (VATS); 82, 83, 85-87, 89-98
    - pneumonectomy; 91
    - thymectomie; 95
    - *in* diagnosis and treatment of masses in the mediastinum; 94

Videoendoscopy; 47, 55

Videolaparoscopy; 25

Virchow's triad; 19

Virtual
  bronchoscopy; 160-162
  reality; 159-160, 162

Vital dyes; 51

Von Meyenburg's complexes; 39

Von Willebrand's Factor; 19

W

Washing,
  ports; 14

instruments; 14

Wedge
  excision; 20
  resection; 64, 86-87, 89, 93, 97

Wound
  dehiscence; 117, 141
  healing; 65
  infection; 32, 91, 116, 140-141
  protection; 20, 93
  protectors; 14, 75
  seeding; 11

Z

Z-line; 48